PHYSICIANS AND SOCIETY

A Social History of the Royal College of Physicians of Edinburgh

MORRICE M^CCRAE

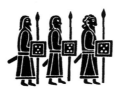

First published in Great Britain in 2007 by
John Donald, an imprint of Birlinn Ltd

West Newington House
10 Newington Road
Edinburgh
EH9 1QS

www.birlinn.co.uk

ISBN 10: 0 85976 698 5
ISBN 13: 978 0 85976 698 2

British Library Cataloguing-in-Publication Data
A catalogue record for this book is available on request from the British Library

Typeset by Creative Link, North Berwick
Printed and bound in Britain by Bell and Bain Ltd, Glasgow

CONTENTS

LIST OF ILLUSTRATIONS

PREFACE AND ACKNOWLEDGEMENTS

At the first meeting the of Royal College of Physicians of Edinburgh after its foundation on St Andrew's Day 1681, it was agreed that the College should take the lead in providing the free medical care that the many poor in Edinburgh at that time so obviously needed. Following this very early decision, the College continued to accept service to society as one of their chief commitments. During the following two centuries of rapid and profound social change in Scotland, and in the absence of any appropriately responsible central government body in all those difficult years, the College emerged as the chief agency in promoting measures to secure and maintain the health of the people of Scotland.

In this history the emphasis is not on the scholarly activities of the College or on their contribution to the advance of medical science but on the efforts made by the College to meet some of the most pressing problems of British society in the eighteenth and nineteenth centuries. The story of *Physicians and Society* does not continue beyond the end of the nineteenth century. The humiliation suffered at that time by British forces in the wars in South Africa, and the emergence of Germany as a threat to Britain's industrial supremacy, stimulated central government in London to take new powers and introduce new measures to improve the health and fitness of the nation. Thereafter, the College found themselves required to relate, not directly to society, but to central government. For these later years an appropriate history would be of *Physicians and the State*.

In writing this history, I have enjoyed the unfailing, cheerful and highly skilled co-operation of Iain Milne, John Dallas, Estela Dukan and Emily Simpson of the library of the Royal College of Physicians of Edinburgh. Malcolm Nicolson of the Centre for the History of Medicine at the University of Glasgow has been generous in providing his invariably positive criticism and helpful guidance. I am indebted to Laurence McCullough of Bayor College of Medicine, Houston, Texas, for the material that has informed Chapter 6 on John Gregory and the invention of medical ethics and to Anne Cameron of the University of Glasgow who has allowed me to base Chapter 12 on her researches on the Registration Act. Christine Short, Anne Crowther, James Williamson and Jennifer McCrae have read all or part of the text and have been kind and constructive in their comments. The illustrations have been assembled and edited by Iain Milne with the technical assistance of Malcolm Merrick. Images not in the collection of the College have been provided by Marianne Smith of the Royal College of Surgeons of Edinburgh, Tricia Boyd of Edinburgh University Library, Michael Barfoot of the Lothian Health Services Archive and Charles Ritchie of the New Club, Edinburgh. To all those who have helped me in writing this short social history of the College, I offer my very sincere thanks.

PROLOGUE

A Brief Seventeenth-century Scottish Enlightenment

The Royal College of Physicians of Edinburgh was founded towards the end of a century in which Scotland suffered civil war, depredation by invading armies, epidemic disease[1] and bloody religious persecution. When the king granted the College its Royal Charter in 1681, Scotland was impoverished and bitterly divided. And religion was still at the heart of Scotland's troubles.

In 1625, when Charles I succeeded to the throne of Scotland, England and Ireland, he was determined to follow his English predecessors, Henry VIII, Edward VI, Mary Tudor and Elizabeth I, in imposing his religious beliefs and his church on all his subjects in all three of his kingdoms. This principle of *cuius regio, eius religio* had been reluctantly abandoned by his father, James VI and I,[2] but Charles believed that it should be revived and enforced. His subjects in all his kingdoms were to be commanded to adopt his Arminian form of Protestantism and to acknowledge him as head of one national Episcopal church. When the king's intentions were signalled in Scotland by the introduction of Archbishop Laud's prayer book at a service in St Giles Cathedral, there were riots in Edinburgh followed by a rising tide of protest across the country.

In Scotland, the Reformation had been more sudden and more radical than in England; early in the sixteenth century the Roman Catholic church had been abandoned for a Presbyterian Church governed by a General Assembly of representatives of all the nation's congregations. Within months of the demonstration in St Giles, the Scottish people in their thousands had taken an oath to preserve this national church that had been growing in strength for almost a century. In 1638, in a National Covent, they pledged their loyalty to the king but at the same time denied the king's right to intervene between God and his people. They demanded that the national church should remain independent of the crown. In 1639 and again in 1640, armies of supporters of the Covenant fought to protect the Presbyterian church in Scotland from suppression by the forces of the king.

In England, in these same years, Charles I was being challenged by Parliament. The overwhelming majority in Parliament disapproved of his Arminianism but their chief objection was to his predilection for arbitrary rule. From the beginning of his reign, Charles had pursued his own policies, even taking England to war with Spain without the agreement of Parliament. When Parliament refused to vote for adequate funding for his projects, Charles

---

1. Typhus spread by the marching and counter-marching of armies may have killed a third or more of the population: T.C. Smout, *A History of the Scottish People* (London, 1969), p. 164.
2. K.M. Brown, Reformation to Union in R.A. Houston and W.W. Knox (eds.) *History of Scotland* (London, 2001), p. 185.

raised loans and levied taxes without its authority. The quarrel between King and Parliament continued over several years with varying degree of intensity and bitterness; on a number of occasions, Charles inflamed a tense situation by threatening the use of force. Then, in March 1642, tired of the indignities and frustrations he had suffered, Charles finally decided to fight. He moved his court to York and began to raise an army. The civil war that followed brought the English Parliamentary army and the Scottish Covenanter armies together. It ended with the execution of Charles I by the English Parliamentary army in January 1649. The monarchy was replaced by a Commonwealth, ostensibly a parliamentary republic but one in which the real power came to rest in the hands of an Army Council dominated by Oliver Cromwell.

Cromwell imposed a harsh settlement on Scotland. The Scottish Covenanter armies had fought the king to defend their church but not to put an end to the monarchy. When news of the king's execution reached Edinburgh in 1649, his son was immediately proclaimed Charles II, 'King of Great Britain, France and Ireland;' an act of the Scottish Parliament added the condition that he must first sign the National Covenant, a condition that he accepted.

Cromwell's troops, under the command of General George Monck, were sent north to crush Scottish support for the monarchy. The quick defeat of all the scattered Covenanter forces north of the border was followed by the murderous sacking of Dundee; all other towns in Scotland escaped the same fate but only by paying huge and crippling ransoms. Everything and anything that could be looted was carried off to England.[3] English garrisons were established everywhere except the Highlands; the construction of new fortresses was begun at Inverness and at other key military sites. Taxes were increased tenfold. The government in London asserted the 'right of England to Scotland' and the Scottish monarchy and the Scottish parliament were declared redundant.[4] In 1651, the Commonwealth of England became the Commonwealth of Great Britain and Ireland.

THE RESTORATION

In 1658 Cromwell died and the Commonwealth began to crumble. In January 1660, General Monck, still the commander of the forces in Scotland, marched south to London and persuaded the government to vote for its own dissolution. In the absence of a realistic alternative, it was agreed that the monarchy should be restored. In the spring of 1660, Charles I's son and heir was invited to return to Britain from his exile in the Netherlands. But in the next twenty years Charles II failed to heal the divisions that had led to the execution of his father. Political tensions revived and by the 1670s the monarchy was again in crisis. In each of Charles II's kingdoms the crisis had its own particular origins and now took its own particular form.

In England, Charles had promised to 'heal the wounds that had kept bleeding for so long'[5] and within weeks of his coronation he had granted a general pardon for all 'crimes' committed against the monarchy in the previous two decades. But the fall of the Republic that had brought the restoration of the monarchy had also brought the restoration of Parliament. The

3. N. Davies, The Isles: A History (London, 2000), p.501.
4. Ibid.

'Cavalier' Parliament that was elected after the Restoration was broadly royalist in its sympathies, but it contained a body of members (the 'Whigs') who were still intent on restricting the powers and privileges of the crown as a guarantee against arbitrary and absolute government. The Parliament elected in 1661 was not dissolved until 1679 and, as members died and were replaced, the number of Whigs increased until they came to completely dominate the House. The Whigs were intent, not only on preventing arbitrary government but also on banishing popery from England, and it was Whigs who had their way. A narrow and intolerant Episcopal church was re-established, backed by a severe penal code (the Clarendon Code). The six acts of the Code were designed to exclude all but members of the Church of England from public office. All non-conformist religious meetings were outlawed and participants fined, imprisoned or transported.[6] This repressive legislation was aimed principally at Catholics and its purpose was political. It was feared that a Catholic administration, backed by a strong Catholic church, would inevitably lead to alliance with Catholic France and perhaps even to absorption into the expansionist empire and the arbitrary and absolute government of Louis XIV. Religious organisations and associations outside the Church of England were therefore seen by Parliament as potentially seditious.

The King did not risk outright conflict with Parliament but he evaded its legislation. He welcomed Catholics at Court and, from 1667, his chief ministers[7] included two Catholics, Clifford and Arlington.[8] In 1670, a fake treaty with France provided cover for a secret treaty with Louis XIV in which Charles II promised, in return for French subsidies, to join France in declaring war on the Dutch and, at the same time, to announce his conversion to Roman Catholicism. The existence of the secret treaty was known only to Clifford, Arlington and the king's brother and heir,[9] James, Duke of York, but it was widely suspected. Throughout the 1670s Charles' Catholic sympathies became ever more readily apparent as he used his suspending powers to protect individual Catholics from prosecution under the Clarendon Code and more and more Catholics appeared at his Court.

Then, in 1671, it was noticed that his brother, James, Duke of York, no longer received Communion according to Anglican rights. Persuaded by the king, James made no announcement of his conversion to Roman Catholicism for over two years but, in 1673, Parliament passed a new Test Act that required all office-holders under the Crown to take the Anglican sacrament. James declined to take the oath. Later that year, he married his second wife, fifteen-year-old Mary d'Este, the daughter of the Dowager Duchess of Medina. Since Mary was a devout Catholic the marriage raised the prospect of a neverending succession of Catholic monarchs. In Parliament, a move to have James excluded from succession to the throne had begun when it first became known that he had converted to Rome. That movement now gathered such momentum that Charles felt it necessary to protect James by proroguing Parliament. But the growing discontent was not confined to Parliament. In the

5. Harris, *Restoration: Charles II and His Kingdoms* (London, 2006), p. 44
6. Ibid., p. 53.
7. The 'Cabal': Clifford, Arlington, Buckingham, Ashley Cooper and Lauderdale.
8. J. Callow, *The Making of King James II* (Stroud, 2000), p. 153.
9. Charles had numerous illegitimate children but no legitimate son.

country more generally, the early enthusiastic support for the restored monarchy had all but melted away.

In 1688, James' young wife gave birth to a healthy son, exacerbating fears of a forced restoration of Roman Catholicism in England, and diminished still further public trust in a future under the Stuart dynasty. All remaining trust was almost destroyed in the summer of 1678. Titus Oates, an ex-Anglican priest, ex-Jesuit and accomplished liar with a bogus degree from the University of Salamanca, claimed to have discovered a Popish Plot. He reported to the Privy Council that the Jesuits planned to send priests disguised as Presbyterian ministers to assassinate the king and burn London to the ground; the objective was to provoke the nation's Catholics to rise up and massacre Protestants in their thousands and re-impose the Roman Catholic faith in England. Edward Coleman, a former secretary to James, Duke of York, was said to be one of the conspirators. A search party sent to Coleman's lodgings found a large number of letters that had been exchanged between James and the French court; that many were in code was particularly damning. For a time it seemed that James would weather the storm but more incriminating letters were later discovered in the English Embassy in Paris. The political storm that erupted threatened the crown and the whole Stuart dynasty but it centred on James, Duke of York. In January 1679 Charles II dissolved Parliament, and James was sent into exile in Brussels. Rashly, he returned to London in September but was immediately sent away again, this time to Scotland.

JAMES IN SCOTLAND

When Charles II was able to return to the throne of Scotland in the spring of 1660. In 1660, the overwhelming majority of the people of Scotland expected a peaceful Presbyterian settlement. However, Charles II was firmly opposed to Presbyterianism and he deeply resented having been forced to sign the National Covenant in 1651. His hostility towards the Covenanters was matched by that of Scotland's nobility who had suffered deep humiliation and even deeper financial and material loss in the Covenanters' wars of the previous decades. When the Scottish Parliament was restored in 1661, the nobility took charge. All members were required to take an oath of allegiance to Charles II as the 'only Supreme Governor of this Kingdom over all persons and all causes'. All the legislation passed by the Covenanting Parliaments between 1639 and 1651 was repealed. The privileges and prerogatives that the king had enjoyed in 1633 were all restored. Finally it was made an offence 'to endeavour any change or alteration of the government of the church or state as it is now established by laws of the kingdom'. Within months of the Restoration, the Scottish parliament had made Charles II's power in Scotland more absolute than any of his forefathers' had ever been and more absolute than it now was in his kingdom of England.

In March 1661, Charles informed the Privy Council in Scotland that he wished 'to interpose our royal authority for the restoring of the church to its right government by bishops' in order to establish 'its greater harmony with the government of the churches of England and Wales.' The Scottish Parliament accordingly re-established the government of the church by archbishops and bishops and restored lay patronage in the parishes. All ministers appointed since 1649 were dismissed from their parishes unless they could provide evidence that they had been 'presented' by the patron of the parish and their appointments to their charges had the sanction of the local bishop. Private religious meetings and public conventicles were forbidden; to join any new league or covenant was made an act of treason. All holders of public office were required to formally renounce the National Covenant

In Aberdeenshire and the north east of Scotland, the return to an Episcopal Church was welcomed. Elsewhere, many ministers simply accepted the new conditions in order to continue with their pastoral vocation. But, in Lanarkshire, Ayrshire, Dumfries, Galloway, and later in Fife and the Lothians, some 300 ministers were forced out of their churches to preach to their flocks in private houses or at conventicles in the open. They were replaced, often by young, untrained and poorly educated Episcopalian ministers whose entry to their new churches and parishes was resisted, sometimes violently, by the local congregation. In the years that followed, many hundreds of lay people were cited before the Privy Council for supporting their ousted ministers. In 1663 troops under the command of Sir James Turner were sent to collect fines from those who refused to attend church; the fines extorted were often excessive, many people were physically abused and many, forced to provide free quartering for the troops, were reduced to poverty. Those who resisted Turner's demands risked imprisonment.

Turner's forays were repeated a number of times but to little effect and for a time the government took a more conciliatory line but, in 1666, in a period of deepening economic depression, demonstrations of opposition to government policies became more violent. In November, Turner was captured at Dumfries and the insurgents gathered a force of almost 2,000 to march to Edinburgh to demand concessions. When they reached Rullion Green in the Pentlands their numbers had fallen to only some 900. The Covenanters were easily defeated by government troops. In the battle 50 were killed; 120 were captured and taken as prisoners to Edinburgh Castle where they were brutally treated. Those who refused to tell everything they knew of the rebellion, its organisation and its leaders, were tortured by the 'boot'.[10] General Sir Tam Dalzel was sent to the south west with 3,000 of foot and 8 troops of cavalry to restore order and to hunt down everyone in any way associated with the rising. Thumb screws and other tortures were used to extract confessions and information about the whereabouts of possible conspirators and sympathisers. Only 36 rebels were captured and executed; 56 others who escaped were indicted for treason in their absence and made outlaws. Nevertheless, the resistance of the Covenanters continued and there were more heavy fines, imprisonments and executions. And the cost of the army's depredations was enormous and devastated the local economy. On 3 May 1679, James Sharp, Archbishop of St Andrews, was murdered by a small party of militant Presbyterians, sparking off further escalation of conflict between government forces and determined Covenanters culminating in the crushing defeat of the Covenanters at Bothwell Bridge. All realistic hopes that the Covenanters might have had of forcing Charles II and his ministers in Scotland to re-establish a strictly Presbyterian national church had come to an end. However, before he was killed, the Covenanters'

---

10. A metal device strapped round the lower leg and gradually tightened until the bones were crushed.

charismatic leader, Robert Cameron, had issued a declaration urging his followers never to abandon the struggle. The Privy Council and the king's ministers in Edinburgh now faced, not a war but a drawn-out guerrilla campaign.

It was now that Charles II sent James, Duke of York, to Edinburgh. In London in 1679 he was an embarrassment but in Scotland his talents could be put to some use. In the 1650s he had served with distinction with the French Army and had been noted for being 'unstinting in his predilection for the use of physical force'.[11] James was given no clear brief or any formal office but he was allowed to sit on the Scottish Privy Council. There he encouraged and helped direct a reign of terror. Covenanters were hunted by Claverhouse's dragoons. Anyone who refused to acknowledge Charles II as head of the church was shot, hanged or tortured by the 'boot' or by thumbscrews. A few were tied to stakes and left to be drowned by the incoming tide.

By March 1682, Charles II had resolved the 'Exclusion' crisis in London. He had remodelled his Privy Council. He called Parliament away from London to the more royalist ambience of Oxford and when, even there, it had proved to be less amenable than he had hoped, he dissolved it and, supported by French subsidies, he did not call another in his lifetime. Without Parliament, 'Exclusion' became impossible except by mass public insurrection. He removed Whigs and dissenters from local government and the court system. The alarm and agitation caused by the Popish Plot faded. By the summer of 1682 the monarchy was as secure as it had been at any time since the Restoration.

James, Duke of York, was allowed to return from Scotland, now the unchallenged heir to the throne. He had spent the early months of the Exclusion crisis in exile in Scotland but, in October 1680, James had been sent once again to Edinburgh, now in the office of High Commissioner but effectively as Viceroy. As Viceroy and Heir to the crown of Scotland, England and Ireland he had used his time in Scotland to demonstrate his capacity for constructive government. Between October 1680 and March 1682 he set out to show that he could improve the condition of Scotland, not only by enhancing its commercial life to relieve its abiding poverty but also by promoting its intellectual and cultural life. Even against a background of continuing sporadic violence in the Covenanting counties of Scotland, his few years in Edinburgh proved to be a brief period of enlightened government. The institutions founded at this time were at the heart of a Scottish revival that led later to the Scottish Enlightenment of the eighteenth century. The Royal College of Physicians of Edinburgh was one of those institutions.

11. Callow, *The Making of King James II*, p. 176.

1

THRESHOLD OF THE MODERN WORLD
The Foundation of the College

The Royal College of Physicians of Edinburgh was founded on St Andrew's Day, 1681. It was the creation of Robert Sibbald. For Scotland, a whole century had been wasted by internal strife, wars and foreign invasion.[1] As a young man of twenty-one, Sibbald had become determined to marshal the talents and resources of Scotland and carry his county forward into the modern world; the creation of a College of Physicians was to be the beginning.

Robert Sibbald was born in 1641 into an ancient and prosperous landed family in Fife. His father was David Sibbald of Rankeillor,[2] a descendant Sir Thomas Sibbald of Rankeillor, a fourteenth-century Lord High Treasurer of Scotland and the brother of Sir James Sibbald, Bt. Keeper of the Great Seal of Scotland. His mother was the daughter of Robert Boyd of Kipps in West Lothian. Robert's family lived first at Kipps but in 1645, to escape an outbreak of the plague, they moved to the Sibbalds' country house in Fife; while in Fife, Robert was a pupil at the high school in Cupar. When, in 1650, Cromwell ordered the invasion of Scotland, the family, like most of Fife's landed gentry, left their isolated country house for the supposed security of the city of Dundee; but it was a false hope. In 1651, General Monck's troops plundered Dundee and the family lost everything they had carried with them and, for a time they, were left almost destitute.

When the crisis had passed and the family had moved back to the Lothians, Robert was enrolled first at Royal High School in Edinburgh and, in 1653, at the Town's College.[3] In 1659, he graduated MA and began to prepare for a career in the church. His theological studies lasted for only six months. In his memoirs, he recalls that 'there were then great divisions amongst the Presbyterians [that] occasioned factions in state and private families. I saw none could enter the ministry without engaging in these factions and espousing their interests. I was disposed to affect charity to all good men of any persuasion and I preferred a quiet life wherein I might not be engaged in factions of Church or State. Under this consideration I fixed upon the study of medicine.'[4]

In March 1660, he set off to study at Leiden. There he was taught anatomy and surgery by Franciscus Sylvius (Francois de Boe) and Johannes van Horne, botany by Adolph Vorstius, chemistry by Christian Marcgraf and natural philosophy by Miels Stenson. Soon after he arrived in Leiden, his father died and, although he received some financial support from his

1. Prelude, pp. 1–17.
2. He was also the nephew of George Sibbald, an Edinburgh physician.
3. The Town's College was not raised to the status of a university until 1685.
4. F.G. Hett (ed.), *The Memoirs of Sir Robert Sibbald (1641–1722)* (London, 1932), p. 55.

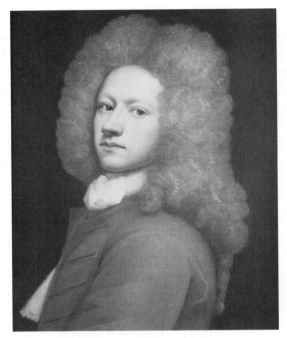

Robert Sibbald as a young man

maternal uncle, he was obliged to cut short his medical education. After only eighteen months at Leiden, he moved to study in Paris for nine months. Then, as was the common practice for Scottish students who had studied in Holland, he presented himself to be examined for 'his patent as Doctor' at Angers where the fees were lower than that at Leiden.[5] After graduating, he spent three months in London where his cousin, Andrew Balfour, introduced him to Sir Robert Moray, the president, and to a number of Fellows of the Royal Society; throughout his subsequent career he continued to correspond with the *virtuosi* he met in London in the summer of 1662.

When he returned to Scotland in October 1662[6] he had already conceived a compelling ambition to re-create in Scotland the learned institutions he had come to admire in the Netherlands, in France and in London; without such institutions, he believed, Scotland would never be fit to take its places among the modern nations of Europe. He was now a physician and he first turned his attention to founding the institutions necessary for the advancement of medicine. But he was also a landowner and from his father he had inherited an estate that, at the end of the seventeenth century, was inevitably burdened with debt. Throughout his life he concerned himself not only with medicine but also with the improvement of agriculture, mining, industry and commerce.[7]

5. E.A. Underwood, *Boerhaave's Men at Leyden and After* (Edinburgh, 1977), p. 89.
6. In his memoirs Sibbald claimed that on his return to Scotland he intended 'to pass quietly through the world'. Given his achievements this comment seems disingenuous.
7. R.G. Emerson, Sir Robert Sibbald, Kt, the Royal Society of Scotland and the origins of the Scottish Enlightenments, *Annals of Science*, 1988, Vol. 45, p. 44.

THE PHYSIC GARDEN

Sibbald's first project for the improvement of Scotland was the creation of a physic garden to rival the King's Garden in Paris where he had studied botany in 1661. He enlisted the help of his cousin, Andrew Balfour, and a neighbour, Patrick Moray. Balfour had spent fourteen years studying medicine in France, Italy and finally in London where he had been a pupil of William Harvey. On returning to Scotland in 1666, he had practised first in St Andrews and then in Edinburgh where he had established his own physic garden. When he studied botany at the King's Garden in Paris, Balfour had been a pupil of Robert Morison. Morison had since become Professor of Botany at Oxford and from Oxford he continued to send Balfour a supply of interesting medicinal plants. Patrick Moray was a prosperous landowner and well-known plant collector whose property at Livingstone was within a few miles of Kipps;[8] in his collection he had more than a thousand plants, many of them from overseas.

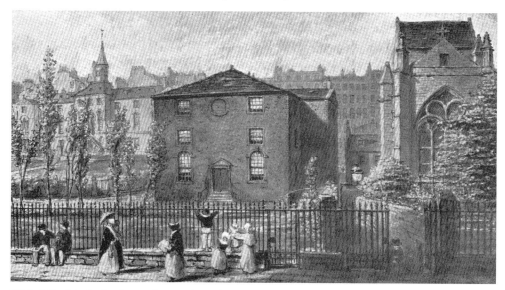

Sibbald's third physic garden and (right) Trinity College Church, now the site of Waverley Station

On his return to Scotland, Sibbald had established a small physic garden of his own. In 1667 he joined forces with Balfour to create a larger garden ('40 foot of measure every way'[9]) at St Anne's Yards near Holyrood Abbey; Partick Moray donated rare and interesting specimens from his garden at Livingstone; and there were contributions from a number of other gardens in the Lothians. Within a very short time Sibbald and Balfour had created a garden of over 800 medicinal plants[10] and James Sutherland, a young man who 'by his own industry had attained a great knowledge of plants', had been employed as gardener. Balfour, at

8. Sibbald had inherited his mother's estate of Kipps, near Torphichen.
9. This garden measured only 1,600 square feet. It was later moved to a larger site at the east end of the Nor' Loch, then to the west of Leith walk in 1770 and, in 1824, to its final site as the Royal Botanic Garden at Inverleith.
10. V.F. Barker and I.A.D. Bouchier, Robert Sibbald, *Journal of the Royal College of Physicians of Edinburgh*, 1976, Vol. 10, p. 414.

that time a much more influential figure in Edinburgh society than Sibbald, brought in new financial support from various friends, from the Town Council, from the Town's College and from the Faculty of Advocates. He even succeeded in persuading the Incorporation of Surgeons, which had a garden of its own, to contribute to this new and much more ambitious physic garden.[11] The garden was fully established in 1670; in 1699 it received its royal warrant and James Sutherland was appointed King's Botanist. After various moves to more convenient sites and years of expansion and development it opened on its present site in 1820. Since then it has continued to be the world-renowned scientific garden that Sibbald would have wished but could only have dreamt of.

GEOGRAPHER ROYAL FOR SCOTLAND

With the Physic Garden well established, in the 1670s Sibbald found the patronage that was to make it possible for him to launch the second of his ambitious schemes for the advancement of Scotland. His cousin, Patrick Drummond had given him letters of introduction to the head of the Drummond family, the Earl of Perth, then an ambitious and rising royalist politician. Lord Perth began to consult Sibbald from time to time and when Perth's personal physician died in 1678 Sibbald was appointed in his place. This was to be a relationship of the greatest importance in Sibbald's life; in his memoirs he records how it began:

> The Earl was of great parts and of serious temper, read much and was very observant of the rites of the Church of England and had the service always in his family. He was temperate and was of excellent conversation and very desirous to learn. I, by his order, acquainted him with curious books, especially pieces of divinity, history, memoirs of ministers of state and discoveries in philosophy. There was a great friendship betwixt us and few weeks passed without letters either when he was in England or here. I gave him the best advice I could for ordering his life, wrote many letters to him and had many discourses with him to dissuade him from meddling with the Court and public employments and to follow the directions left him by his grandfather who did advise his descendents to keep at home and manage their private affairs aright. But the low condition of his estate, having sustained great loss and paid many fines in the late troubles, and the persuasions of his friends who expected great advantages by his [being at] Court, prevailed with him to embrace public employments and go frequently to Court.

Lord Perth became an important figure in Scottish political affairs. In 1678 he became a Privy Councillor, then Justice General and, later still, Chancellor of Scotland. Sibbald meanwhile became one of the king's physicians with Perth as his increasingly powerful patron.

For some time Sibbald had been making his own modest investigations into the natural resources of Scotland. Now with the encouragement and support of his patron, Lord Perth,

---

11. The surgeons had initially 'opposed the garden, seeing that the inception of a powerful College of Physicians could follow from such a venture'. Barker and Bouchier, Robert Sibbald.

he expanded his researches to include a study of the geography of the country. Perth, now one of the king's most influential advisors in Scotland, persuaded the king that Sibbald's studies could be of the greatest importance in the management of the country and its economy. Sibbald was awarded a patent as Geographer Royal and embarked on what was intended to be a comprehensive survey of all the natural and cultural resources of Scotland. The results were to be published in two volumes. The first volume *Scotia Antiqua* would cover the historical development of the nation, its customs and its antiquities. The second, *Scotia Moderna* would give an account of the geography, natural history, demography and political economy of Scotland. Although the project had been encouraged by the king and approved by the Privy Council, Sibbald received no financial support 'except a hundred pounds sterling', his salary for one year as one of the King's physicians. Without the necessary resources, the comprehensive survey Sibbald had planned was never completed and his *Scotia Antiqua* and *Scotia Moderna* were never written. But, in 1683, he managed to publish two more modest volumes, *Scotia Illustrata, sive Prodromus Historiae Naturalis* and *Nuncius Scoto-Britannicus, sive admonoto deatlante Scotico seu descriptione Scotiae antique et modernae*. The first was a general account of the geography of Scotland with sections on the flora, the fauna and the human inhabitants. The *Nuncius* was based on questionnaires in which some seventy contributors from across Scotland provided detailed accounts of their own burghs or districts.

These researches fell far short of what Sibbald had hoped to achieve. By 1698, it had become clear that he would never be able to carry out the work that he had begun as Geographer Royal under King Charles II. The Revolution of 1688 had brought William III to the throne; Sibbald's patron, the Earl of Perth, was a prisoner in Stirling Castle and Sibbald himself had suffered public humiliation.[12] However, he had not lost his vision for Scotland. He remained confident that by uncovering and exploiting all of Scotland's natural resources Scotland could be rescued from its besetting problem of poverty. In 1698, he wrote *A Discourse anent the improvements that may be made in Scotland for advancing the wealth of the kingdom*.[13]

The nationwide survey of Scotland that Sibbald had in mind was not completed in his lifetime but a century later his concept was taken up and completed by Sir John Sinclair in his *Statistical Account of Scotland* in 1790–99.

A ROYAL SOCIETY OF SCOTLAND

Undaunted by his lack of success in making a complete inventory of the material resources of Scotland, Sibbald embarked on a scheme to bring together the nation's intellectual resources. When he wrote his *Discourse anent the improvements that may be made in Scotland for advancing the wealth of the kingdom* he also wrote *Improving of Learning as means to enrich the country and therefore regard to be had for it*. He had in mind the academies in 'every city' in Italy and France 'where men of learning and polite breeding of all conditions meet and have exercises, lectures, harangues and they read their poems and give censures and several pieces of wit'.[14] In 1698

12. Chapter 2.
13. National Library of Scotland, Advocates, MS 33.5.16, ff. 29-30.
14. Emerson, Sir Robert Sibbald, p. 48.

(and again in 1701) he tried to found a Royal Society of Scotland on the model of the Royal Society of London.[15] Again he achieved only partial success. His efforts did not immediately lead to the founding of the great prestigious body he had in mind. However, a number of those who had been involved in the movement to form a Royal Society came together in 1703 as a forerunner of the Society of Antiquaries that received its charter in 1783. Sibbald's concept of learned society of all-embracing intellectual interests was not lost. In 1731 a Philosophical Society was formed in Edinburgh and in 1783 it became the Royal Society of Edinburgh.

A COLLEGE OF PHYSICIANS FOR SCOTLAND

Of the several concepts that made up Sibbald's grand design for the advancement of Scotland the one that was fully achieved in his lifetime was the foundation of a College of Physicians. As a student, he had come to admire the medical colleges in the Netherlands and in France where they had been in place for many years. At their foundation Europe's medieval universities had been given the authority to license their graduates to practise medicine in all its branches. It had later become the practice for major towns, where there was no university, to establish colleges of medical graduates (usually graduates of specified universities) to license medical men with no university degree who wished to practise in the town.

In England, until the sixteenth century, only the universities of Oxford and Cambridge had powers to license physicians.[16] Since the number of medical graduates from England's two

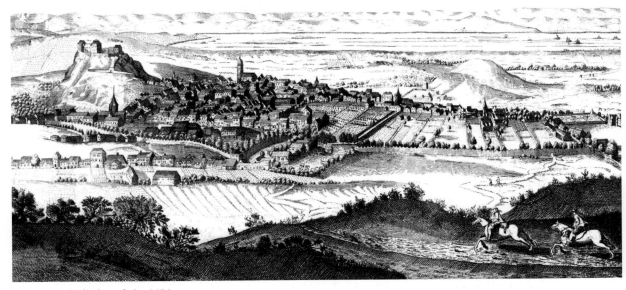

Edinburgh in 1681

15. Ibid., p. 46.
16. A surgeon in England could be licensed by the bishop of the diocese in which he intended to practise. Medical graduates of Oxford and Cambridge were licensed to practise both medicine and surgery anywhere in England.

universities was very small, the great majority of those practising medicine in England were not only unlicensed but of very uncertain training. In the early years of his reign, Henry VIII had cause to complain that medicine was being practised 'by a great multitude of ignorant persons of whom the greater part have no manner of insight in the same nor in any kind of Learning'.[17] It was within Henry VIII's power to limit these abuses. He had inherited a kingdom in which the authority of the crown was unchallenged.[18] He had 'more ready money than any Prince in Christendom'[19] and could afford to finance his own very effective administration without resort to Parliament. And, in England, the church, even before Henry made himself head of the Church of England, provided the king's administration with a bureaucratic network that extended into every part of the kingdom.

In 1512 Henry VIII made it illegal for anyone other than medical graduates of Oxford or Cambridge to practise as physicians in London or within seven miles of London until examined and licensed by the Bishop of London or the Dean of St Paul's; the equivalent church authorities in England's other sixteen dioceses were given the same powers. This was an extension to physicians of a system already in place for the licensing of surgeons, and for surgeons that system continued to be accepted as satisfactory. However, experience during an outbreak of plague indicated that stricter regulation was needed for physicians. New legislation was drawn up for London, creating a college loosely modelled on the colleges in place in those major towns in Europe which, like London, did not have a university. However, unlike the European colleges, this new college was given no powers to regulate the activities of surgeons or apothecaries. Henry's Act of 1518 founded a College of Physicians (all graduates of Oxford or Cambridge) to license and supervise physicians in London and within seven miles of London.

EARLY ATTEMPTS TO CREATE A COLLEGE IN SCOTLAND

What was achieved by Henry VIII in England was impossible in Scotland. It was not that Scotland was without learned physicians. Like Oxford and Cambridge, the universities of St Andrews, Glasgow and King's College, Aberdeen had the power to grant degrees in medicine but they had made almost no provision for the teaching of the subjects most relevant to the study of medicine. It had long been the practice for Scottish medical students to go abroad to study wherever the most eminent teachers of the day were to be found.[20] When the post-Reformation universities were founded at Edinburgh and Marischal College, Aberdeen, that practice had continued. In the sixteenth and seventeenth centuries there were therefore numbers of graduates of Lieden, Padua, Paris, Montpellier and the other leading medical schools of Europe who might have formed one or more colleges of physicians in Scotland. But, unlike Tudor England, Scotland did not have a monarchy able to make the necessary

17. G. Clarke, *A History of the Royal College of Physicians* (Oxford, 1964), Vol. 1, p. 54.
18. R. Bucholz and N. Key, *Early Modern England, 1485-1714* (Oxford, 2004), p. 50.
19. W. S. Churchill, *History of the English Speaking People* (London, 1956), p. 24.
20. In Gaeldom, the office of physician to the clan chief was usually hereditary and traditionally the physicians were educated either at Padua, Paris or Montpellier or at small local medical schools where they were taught by those who had been trained abroad. For these small schools, the whole Galenic collection of texts had been available, translated into Gaelic, since the fourteenth century.

intervention in the social administration of the country. In the fifteenth and sixteenth centuries Scotland had a succession of child monarchs. James I succeeded at the age of 10, James II was 6, James III was 8, James IV was 15, James V was 1, Mary Queen of Scots was 1 week and James VI was 1 year old. In this long period of minority rule and unstable regencies, competing groups of nobles fought for power and used that power, not for the commonweal, but to advance the interests of their own families and factions. Across almost the whole of Scotland government and the administration of the law was not exercised directly by the crown but was franchised to hereditary jurisdictions held by the great territorial magnates and to the ruling bodies of the burghs; what power remained to the crown was in the hands of the nobles who acted as the king's regents during his minority. And while in Tudor England the church continued as a nationwide bureaucratic arm of central monarchical government, in Scotland the old Roman Catholic Church continued to decay almost to the point of collapse while a new reformed church grew up disputing the authority of the king.

It was not until the last years of the sixteenth century that a Scottish king was able to begin to gather power into his own hands. In 1592, James VI reached the age of twenty-five, the age of majority for young kings when their regents could be discarded. In his few years of unfettered power in Scotland before he succeeded to the English crown and departed to London, he was able to impose a degree of peace and political stability. In that brief period he also took a first small step in the regulation of medical practice in Scotland. Like Henry VIII almost a century before, James had good reason to complain …

> of the great abuse done and practised by a number of ignorant and unskilful persons, who without knowledge of the science and faculty of medicine being neither learned nor graduate therein, presume at their own hand to profess and practise physic and medicine to the great and evident hazard and danger of the lives and health of many of our subjects.[21]

The king's first response to this problem was prompted by an appeal from the medical practitioners in Glasgow. The leading petitioner was Peter Lowe, who had trained in Paris and had been surgeon to the King of France before returning to Scotland as surgeon to James VI. Glasgow University had never made it a practice to license physicians to practise;[22] Peter Lowe's proposal was therefore for a college on a similar model to those he had seen established in major cities in France that did not produce and license their own graduate physicians. His proposal was for a body that included surgeons and apothecaries as well as physicians. In November 1599, the King granted a charter to a body with powers to examine and license all practitioners in Glasgow[23] and in the area of the old Roman Catholic diocese of Glasgow. As Scotland was now forty years into the Reformation, the rights and privileges of the new body

---

21. R. Sibbald, Memoirs of the College of Physicians, *Analecta Scotia* (Edinburgh, 1837), p. 113.
22. From its foundation King's College, Aberdeen made provision for the teaching of medicine and a small number of physicians graduated in the sixteenth century. At the Reformation the *First Book of Discipline* proposed the creation of a medical school at St Andrews but the plan was not implemented for almost two hundred years. Glasgow University established a Chair of Medicine in 1637 but it was abolished five years later.
23. The total number of physicians, surgeons and apothecaries at that time was seven.

were to be enforced by the secular authorities of Glasgow and the counties of Dumbarton, Renfrew, Lanark and Ayr. The new body assumed the title of the Faculty of Physicians and Surgeons of Glasgow in imitation of the Faculte de Medicine in Paris, the corporate body of medical men with which Lowe was most familiar.[24]

Four years later, in 1603, James VI of Scotland became also James I of England. King and court moved to London and Scotland was once again a 'kingless kingdom'. The creation of further medical colleges or faculties for Scotland again became difficult. Petitioners for the necessary royal warrants needed access to the King and for almost a century there were few opportunities. James VI & I returned only once to Scotland and then only for two weeks in 1617. Charles I came to Scotland only to be crowned in 1633 and, again briefly, in 1641 when he was already powerless. Charles II came to Scotland only to be crowned and in the hope of military support in 1651. During these many years, Parliament could have taken some action to improve the regulation of the practice of medicine but the Scottish Parliament met seldom, always briefly and only to grant new taxes and settle disputes among its members;[25] in the whole of the seventeenth century it met only seventeen times and never for more than two or three days.[26]

In spite of the difficulties of those years, a number of attempts were made to found a medical college in Scotland. In 1621, James VI & I issued a royal warrant for the establishment of a College of Physicians in Edinburgh. There had been no petition from Scotland. The initiative came from King James himself as part of his earnest but ultimately unsuccessful endeavour to rule his two kingdoms as one United Kingdom of Great Britain. In the warrant, King James stated explicitly that his aim was to 'establish convenient and comely order as it is observed in this our Kingdom of England'.

James VI & I clearly intended that, like the Royal College of Physicians in London, this new College should include only physicians and have supervision only of physicians in Edinburgh. However, George Sibbald, on behalf of the physicians of Edinburgh, submitted an amendment to the king's proposal that would have given the proposed college jurisdiction over surgeons and apothecaries as well as physicians and not only in Edinburgh but in every part of Scotland. Since George Sibbald's amendment called for the privileges of Scotland's ancient universities, the Incorporation of Surgeons of Edinburgh and the Faculty of Physicians and Surgeons of Glasgow all to be set aside, it met widespread and vigorous opposition. No agreement had been reached when King James died in 1625.

In 1630, Dr John McClure, a young but already prominent physician in Edinburgh, took advantage of the appointment of his friend Sir William Alexander to the post of Master of Requests for Scotland to submit a petition to Charles I for the creation of a college.[27] The Privy Council, on behalf of the king, asked Edinburgh's physicians to submit 'heads and articles' for

24. J.Geyer-Kordesch and F. Macdonald, *The History of the Royal College of Physicians and Surgeons of Glasgow 1599–1858* (London, 1999), p. 12.
25. K. Brown, *Kingdom or Province* (London, 1993), p.13.
26. In the years of the Commonwealth and Cromwell's occupation of Scotland there was no Scottish Parliament.
27. J.F. McHarg, Dr John Makluire and the 1630 Attempt to Establish the College, *Proceedings of the Royal Colllege of Physicians of Edinburgh Tercentenary Congress 1981*, p. 49

further consideration. The physicians abandoned their earlier demand to have authority across Scotland but again proposed that, in Edinburgh, the new college should have jurisdiction over surgeons and apothecaries as well as physicians. Again there was opposition from the universities and especially from the Incorporation of Surgeons; their resistance continued until 1633 when the physicians, who had now been campaigning for a college in Edinburgh for over twelve years, 'being become many of them aged but all of them wearied out with toil did of necessity desist'.

Twenty-three years later, during the years of the Commonwealth and Cromwell's occupation of Scotland, a group of Edinburgh physicians, led by George Purves, tried again. They submitted to Cromwell a list of 'public abuses in matters of medicine' in Scotland. Cromwell appointed a Commission to decide what action should be taken. It quickly drew up a draft Charter for a College in Edinburgh that would have jurisdiction over all physicians, surgeons and apothecaries in Scotland with the exception of surgeons in Glasgow and Edinburgh. The opposition of the universities, the Incorporation of Surgeons in Edinburgh and the Faculty of Physicians and Surgeons of Glasgow was renewed and continued until Cromwell was dead and the recommendations of his Commission had died with him.

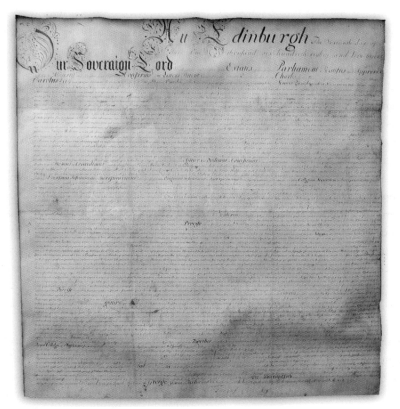

College Charter

MEDICAL PRACTICE IN SEVENTEENTH-CENTURY SCOTLAND

In Scotland in the late seventeenth century the provision of medical aid went virtually unnoticed and unregulated by the state. Scotland was then one of the poorest nations in Europe. The population, which had been massively reduced by war, famine and disease (probably typhus) in the 1640s, numbered less than a million. The great majority of the people of Scotland depended for their subsistence on the land and the land suitable for cultivation or for the raising of stock was widely scattered over a countryside divided by mountains, bogs and large expanses of water. For this widely scattered population, central government, in the form of the Privy Council and the great officers of state, was far off and irrelevant to every day life. In each rural community the people still lived within a social structure headed by the local magnate – in the Highlands, a clan chief; in the Lowlands, the head of some great ducal family. The great house of the local magnate, whether Highland or Lowland, would have its own physic garden[28] and the great man would have a physician as a member of his household. The extent to which the physician's services were available to the great man's many dependants was at best uncertain. For medical aid the great majority of the rural population relied on folk medicine. They looked to their own traditional cures, the support of their families, the advice of the local wise woman, the services of a bonesetter (traditionally the blacksmith) or perhaps a visit to one of Scotland's many healing wells.

In the 1680s, Scotland's urban population was still very small. Edinburgh, with some 20,000 people, was by far the largest city. Glasgow, Aberdeen and Dundee may each have housed as many as 10,000 but other regional centres at Perth, Inverness, Stirling, Dumfries and Jedburgh were little more than villages. However, in these urban centres the provision of medical aid had taken a new form. Scotland's burghs had been established specifically as markets and for trade; in the burghs the craft of surgery and the preparation and provision of medicines were practised on a commercial basis and had come under a degree of local regulation. In the middle ages all forms of trading in the towns had been regulated by a single guild but, by the sixteenth century, those crafts that had become particularly important and well represented in the town, were given independent status as craft guilds, with a monopoly in their own trade and with powers to regulate the training and standard of performance of their members. Often the chief attraction of the guild for its members was that it acted as a mutual aid society providing relief in times of distress. Independent guilds were therefore never set up without a sufficient number of members to support a mutual aid scheme. In the seventeenth century even in Dundee, Perth, Aberdeen or Stirling there were not enough surgeons or apothecaries to form independent guilds; there surgeons joined with the apothecaries and were admitted as members of one of the large guilds, usually the Grocers' Guild.

The arrangement in Edinburgh was unique. In the first years of the sixteenth century Edinburgh already had a sufficient number of surgeons to support a guild and the Incorporation of Surgeons and Barbers was founded in 1505. In 1645, Edinburgh's

---

28. H.G. Graham, *The Social Life of Scotland in the Eighteenth Century* (London, 1928), p. 5.

Incorporation of Surgeons and Barbers began to admit a number of apothecaries and thereafter those who had served the dual apprenticeships in surgery and pharmacy formed, within the Incorporation, a Fraternity of Apothecaries and Surgeons whose members were able to undertake all forms of medical activity. These surgeon-apothecaries, the general practitioners of the time, became the largest body of incorporated medical men in Edinburgh.

In Edinburgh, and indeed in Scotland, physicians were relatively few. The classical medicine of Hippocrates and Galen had been practised in Scotland for over three hundred years by physicians trained at the leading medical schools of Europe. However, in seventeenth-century Scotland, physicians had few profitable opportunities to exercise their professional skills. In rural Scotland, success as a physician was dependent on patronage, preferably the patronage of one of the great territorial magnates. But as Scotland's towns grew in size in the seventeenth century,[29] numbers of graduate physicians came to practise in the medical market place of the towns. There, unlike the surgeons and the apothecaries, they did not enjoy a locally protected monopoly. It was not open to physicians to incorporate themselves as a guild; they were not trained by apprenticeship and their education and standards of performance were not subject to the sanction of the Council of the town in which they set up practice. Educated at universities in Europe, they saw themselves as members of an elite cosmopolitan learned society. However, without the protection of a guild, they were open to the competition of the surgeon-apothecaries and the activities of anyone who falsely 'presumed to profess and practise physic'.

These last came in different guises. There were the itinerant troupes of mountebanks who regularly descended on all the major towns in Scotland but especially on Edinburgh. Almost automatically they were granted permission by the Town Council to erect their stages at popular parts of the town, usually on the High Street. There they would perform comic plays, juggling acts, acrobatics; a tightrope walk high up across the High Street was a particular favourite. Having collected a crowd they would then deliver pseudo-scientific lectures on the ills they claimed to be able to treat, extol the wondrous properties of their powders and potions and then sell their 'cures' at vast profit to the gullible. There were also unscrupulous apothecaries who bought in the mountebanks' fake medicines to sell in their shops and plausible impostors who passed themselves off as qualified physicians.[30]

RENEWED EFFORTS TO FOUND A COLLEGE

In this unseemly free-for-all that still persisted in Scotland, physicians as well as patients stood in need of protection. Robert Sibbald wrote:

> It is certain that no man can be secure in his particular interest in the service of
> any faculty, without such constitution be made as may both encourage each one
> in their interests and be a bulwark against the invasion of others.[31]

29. T. M. Devine, *The Scottish Nation* (London, 1999), p. 152.
30. R. Thin, Medical Quacks in Edinburgh in the Seventeenth and Eighteenth Centuries, *Book of the Edinburgh Club*, 1938, pp. 132–59.
31. Ibid.

The 'constitutions' that Sibbald had in mind were of course the medical colleges he had admired on his travels abroad. As Sibbald observed, these colleges had been founded 'in all well constituted kingdoms and commonwealths so soon as the arts of peace began to flourish amongst them'.[32] For much of the seventeenth century in Scotland, the arts of peace had not flourished. Scotland had suffered armed rebellion, bloody civil war and years of military occupation and the restoration of the monarchy in 1660 had failed to bring peace to Scotland. The years that followed the accession of Charles II were intolerant and violent. The bitter campaigns to suppress Presbyterianism (Prologue) had led to an exodus of many of those who refused to renounce the National Covenant. Large numbers of the lower orders were shipped off to the plantations of South Carolina.[33] But for those who could afford the cost of transporting their families abroad, the obvious place of refuge was the Netherlands where the state had a long tradition of harbouring exiles.

Of the 419 Scots in enforced exile to the Netherlands some twenty were doctors or medical students.[34] In 1672, Charles II issued an Indulgence that allowed these exiles to return to Scotland. Returning to Scotland at the same time there was also the usual (and larger) number who had gone quite freely to study medicine at Leiden and the other great medical schools of northern Europe. In the 1670s therefore, there were many young physicians in Scotland who had been trained at the most progressive schools in Europe at a time when the principles on which European medicine was practised were changing.[35] Galen's ancient unquestioned authority was being challenged by the notion promoted by Francis Bacon that the reverence for the authorities of the past had been over done and that learning must be advanced by observation and reasoning. University students were also being introduced to the mechanical world of Isaac Newton.

It had long been believed that every event of every day was at all times subject to the immediate intervention of God; man could only submit. In Newton's mechanical world, events were subject to unchanging natural laws set by God at Creation; once God's laws were set, natural events continued like the mechanical workings of a clock. The work of Isaac Newton was introducing university students to a new concept of the day-to-day responsibility of man and his gift of reason. In Europe, from the middle years of the seventeenth century young Scottish physicians were being introduced to a new, more critical and more responsible approach to the practice of medicine. With their new learning and new responsibility came a new consciousness of their status.

As a student Robert Sibbald had been greatly influence by the teachings of Francis Bacon but unlike some other more mathematically minded physicians in Scotland, he still rejected Newton and the iatromechanism that was becoming fashionable in his time. He remained true to Galen. Nevertheless he was very conscious of the enhanced status that the new learning had given to the physician; he cited the authority of the Bible:[36]

32. Ibid.
33. T. M. Devine, *Scotland's Empire* (London, 2003), p. 38.
34. G. Gardner, *The Scottish Exile Community in the Netherlands, 1660-1690* (East Lothian, 2004), pp. 17-20.
35. By the last quarter of the seventeenth century there were over 150 Scottish medical students who had studied at Leiden and the leading medical schools of Europe.
36. Hett, *The Memoirs*, p. 114.

Honour a physician with the honour due unto him for the uses you may have of him for the Lord hath created him.

For of the most High cometh healing and he shall receive honour of the king.

The skill of the physician shall lift up his head and in the sight of great men he shall be in admiration.

(Ecclesiasticus 38)

Sibbald believed that a college was needed not only to regulate the practice of medicine but also to secure the status of physicians and to advance the learning on which that new status was based. All earlier attempts to secure a royal charter for a college of physicians in Scotland had failed but Sibbald had put himself in a position to take full advantage of any opportunity that might occur.

For the story of events that finally led to the foundation of the College of Physicians in 1681, we must depend on Sibbald's own account in his *Memoirs of My Life*.[37] Sibbald tells us that when he returned to Edinburgh as a newly graduated physician he had made it his business to win the confidence of the leading physicians in Edinburgh by showing 'a great deal of deference and respect to them'. In 1680, he felt that he was in a position to invite them to meet regularly at his lodgings off the High Street. Most, but by no means all, of the sixteen or so who attended were of Scotland's landed gentry. The group included David Hay, from the family of the Earl of Errol. Andrew Balfour, the son of Sir Michael Balfour of Denmylne, a former Lord Lyon King of Arms, and a welcome figure at the Court of Charles II. Thomas Burnet was the son of Lord Crimond of Keys and the brother of the historian and politician, Gilbert Burnet, the Bishop of Salisbury. But the group also included John McGill and William Stevenson, both of more humble origin, and John Hutton who had been a herd-boy in a country parish until the parish minister paid for his education at Edinburgh and at Padua. It was also notable that at a time in Scotland when passionately held confessional and political differences were the cause of persecution, rebellion and bloodshed, the group meeting peacefully at Sibbald's lodgings included both Covenanting Presbyterians and Royalist Episcopalians. The meetings convened by Sibbald provided a space where political and religious differences could be forgotten at least for a time.[38]

The common interest that brought this very disparate group together was their commitment to science and medicine. They met to discuss 'rare cases [that] had happened in our practice'[39] and 'books that tended to the improvement of medicine'. But they were also more generally interested in philosophy and natural history. They had 'discourse upon letters from abroad giving account of what was most remarkable a doing by the learned'. They had all studied at leading universities in Europe and they all maintained their association with the physicians and scientists they had come to admire during their student years. They also kept

37. The manuscript has been lost. A transcript is held by the Advocates Library in Edinburgh (MS Adv.33.5.1). There are two published editions: *Memoirs of my Lyfe*, J. Maidment (ed.) (Edinburgh, 1833); *The Memoirs of Sir Robert Sibbald (1641-1722)*, F.G. Hett (ed.) (London, 1932).
38. Emerson, *Sir Robert Sibbald*, p. 42.
39. Hett, *The Memoirs*, p. 76.

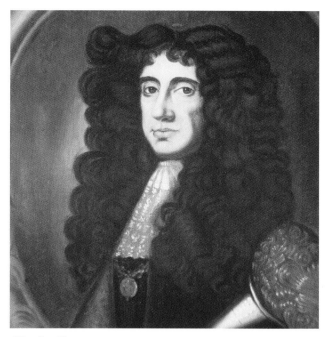

Charles II

themselves informed of the activities of the Royal Society in London. Robert Sibbald was in regular communication with Sir Robert Moray, the first President of the Royal Society and his 'letters, excellent and full of good advice and discoveries' kept Sibbald 'acquainted with the curious experiments made by him'. An accomplished mathematician, Archibald Pitcairn was already corresponding with Isaac Newton.

At these meetings, Sibbald did not declare an intention to renew the struggle to establish a college of physicians in Edinburgh. However, the group that he had brought together had helped promote the new physic garden at Holyrood and a number of its members had begun to draw up a pharmacopoeia for general use in Edinburgh. Certainly Edinburgh's Incorporation of Surgeons saw the emergence of this group as ominous, 'dreading that it might usher in a College of Physicians [that] would mightily encroach upon their privileges and tend to other prejudices'. It seems probable that Sibbald did indeed have the foundation of a college in mind long before 1681 but it was not until that year that an opportunity presented itself.

An apothecary, Patrick Cunningham, was charged by the Faculty of Surgeon-Apothecaries with performing a surgical operation. When the case was heard by the Lords of Session, the Court sought the guidance of four of Edinburgh's leading physicians:

> about the surgeon-apothecaries, whether there was any such conjunction of these employments in other countries, and whether or not it was expedient for the lieges, they should be joined in one person here.

Those consulted were Drs Hay, Burnet, Stevenson and Balfour, all of whom had travelled extensively abroad and were familiar with the regulation of the practice of medicine in a number of different countries in Europe. It was a question of great relevance and importance for Edinburgh's physicians since surgeon-apothecaries, offering as they did the full range of medical services, were their most potent rivals and a growing threat to their prosperity. On a matter of such general concern, Hay and his colleagues thought it appropriate to convene a meeting of all the physicians in Edinburgh. The meeting had little hesitation in agreeing to recommend that the licensing of surgeon-apothecaries should be abolished; but before the meeting could disperse, Sibbald seized his opportunity. As he recorded in his memoirs:

> I took the occasion to represent to them, that this being the first time we had all
> met, I thought it in our interest to improve the meeting to some further use,
> and I downright proposed we might take into consideration the establishment
> of a College to secure the privileges belonging to us as doctors.

Sibbald had good reason to believe that, this time, a move to establish a College would be successful. For the first time for almost a hundred years there was a royal court in Edinburgh. James, Duke of York, was in residence at Holyrood, in effect, as the Viceroy of Scotland. While in Edinburgh, it had become clear that James meant to win the goodwill of the intellectual and professional classes and, in this, his closest advisors were Sibbald's friend and patron the Earl of Perth and his brother, the Earl of Melford. Sibbald was confident that, if approached, the Duke of York would prove willing to extend his favour to Edinburgh's physicians. He was also confident that he and Andrew Balfour would be given an appropriate introduction to the Duke to present their case. James had brought with him to Edinburgh the king's Physician, Sir Charles Scarborough. Scarborough and Andrew Balfour had both been pupils of William Harvey and had been friends for many years. Sibbald records in his memoirs that 'we consulted with Sir Charles and found him our great friend and very ready to give us his best assistance with the King and the Duke'. Sibbald and Balfour were granted an audience with the Duke of York and presented their petition for the creation of a College of Physicians in Edinburgh. At the audience, Sibbald dramatically produced the warrant that James VI & I had issued in response to the petition presented by his uncle, George Sibbald in 1618 (above). In that warrant the king had entrusted the foundation of a College of Physicians to the Scottish Parliament but nothing had been achieved. Sibbald records that, on looking at the warrant, the Duke of York 'said he knew his grandfather's hand and would see our business done'.

A small committee of the Privy Council was set up to draw up a code of its privileges and responsibilities. One of the four members of that committee was Sibbald's friend and patron, the Earl of Perth. Perth and his brother Lord Melfort (who were soon to become respectively Chancellor of Scotland and Secretary of State) were two of the Duke's closest advisors. Together they were able to command the support of the Court party in Parliament for the proposed College and, as the most influential member of the Privy Council Committee, Lord Perth made it clear that he would do everything necessary to promote the scheme.

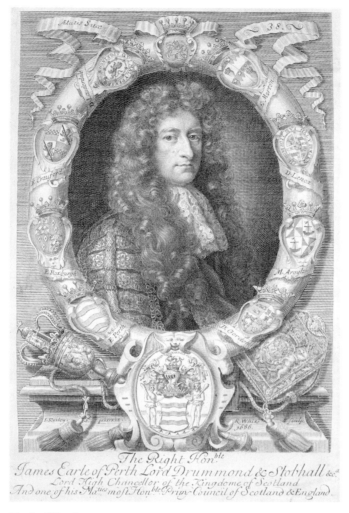

Earl of Perth

As they stood, the proposals for a charter submitted by George Sibbald to King James VI & I in 1621 and now submitted once more in 1681 by Robert Sibbald to the Duke of York would have given the new college in Edinburgh jurisdiction over all physicians, surgeons and apothecaries in Scotland. Such a creation would have been as vigorously resisted as before by the Scottish universities, the Incorporation of Surgeons of Edinburgh and the Faculty of Physicians and Surgeons of Glasgow. Andrew Balfour forestalled their foreseeable objections. To prevent opposition from the Faculty in Glasgow, he insisted that the new College of Physicians must be 'metropolitan and not national'. To reassure the surgeons in Edinburgh, he promised that the new College of Physicians would 'not rival them in trying to obtain the body of even one malefactor for dissection'. He also persuaded Sibbald and the other physicians that:

the Universities will be reconciliated by our relinquishing the idea of giving degrees whilst their opposition will be further countered by agreeing to admit Scotch University graduates in medicine to the College license to practise and ultimately to the Fellowship of our Society without examination. Better have the College established though more restricted than we desire than to have no College at all.

Balfour's diplomatic concessions were agreed. A Charter was drawn up by the Scottish Privy Council and dispatched to London. It was signed and the Great Seal was appended on St Andrew's Day, 1681.

While James, Duke of York was in Scotland as the king's representative, he continued the brutal suppression of the Covenanters. But, in Edinburgh, he presided over a period of national revival. Under the direction of the Duke of York, the Privy Council introduced measure to improve the economy. He revived the moribund Council of Trade, new industries were introduced, new skills were recruited from abroad and taxes on raw materials were reduced;[40] Edinburgh University was given a new charter and projects in mathematics, cartography, engineering and surgery were awarded royal patronage; the Advocates Library was founded; there was royal support for what later became the Royal Botanic Garden. There had now begun the movement that led to the foundation of the Philosophical Society, the Royal Society of Edinburgh and the Society of Antiquaries. The Royal College of Physicians of Edinburgh was founded at the height of what, in retrospect, has been recognised as a brief but ground-breaking royalist seventeenth-century Scottish Enlightenment.[41]

40. R. Mitchison, *Lordship to Patronage* (Edinburgh, 1983), p. 86.
41. Emerson, *Sir Robert Sibbald*, p. 42.

2

SURVIVAL

Royalists and Covenanters, Newtonians and Traditionalists

At the inaugural meeting of the College on 18 January 1682, Archibald Stevenson was elected president. The son of a distinguished Professor of Philology and Philosophy at the Town's College and one of Edinburgh's most successful physicians, Stevenson had been one of the earliest supporters of Sibbald's scheme to form a college and had paid a large share of the legal costs of drawing up and securing the College Charter.

A council of six members was chosen and they, 'having retired to another room', elected the other officers of the College. James Livingstone, the most senior in age of the physicians practising in Edinburgh, and Andrew Balfour, who had played such an important part in founding the College, were appointed as censors with 'the power, authority and jurisdiction to call before them all persons practising and exercising within the jurisdiction of the City, its liberties and its suburbs the said profession of Medicine without a licence and to impose on them the fines specified'.[1]

Robert Sibbald was appointed Secretary. John Hutton became the College's first Treasurer. Archibald Pitcairn was appointed as Procurator Fiscal, a legal office not mentioned in the College charter. Pitcairn had studied law at Edinburgh for four years before going to Paris to study medicine; he was the youngest of the founding members of the College but the only one with legal expertise.

With the ominous exception of John Hutton – a staunch Presbyterian and one of the few members of the College who had not been born into Scotland's landed gentry – the newly elected officers of the College were made welcome at Court at the royal palace of Holyroodhouse.[2] Within a few weeks of the foundation of the College, Archibald Stevenson, Robert Sibbald and Andrew Balfour were knighted.

MEDICAL AID FOR THE POOR

As its first act at its inaugural meeting, the College drew up a scheme to provide free medical aid for the poor of 'the City and its suburbs'. It was not an obligation set down in the College charter but it was a service that was urgently needed. Scotland was then one of the poorest nations in Europe and although Edinburgh was by far its richest town, many of its people lived in poverty. Some 200 licensed beggars, in their blue coats and pewter badges, were to be seen

---

1. The College Charter as translated from the Latin in W.S. Craig, *History of the Royal College of Physicians of Edinburgh* (Edinburgh, 1976), p. 1045.
2. M. Clough, Lady Rabat and the Physicians, *Proceedings of the Royal College of Physicians of Edinburgh*, 1991, Vol. 21, p. 474.

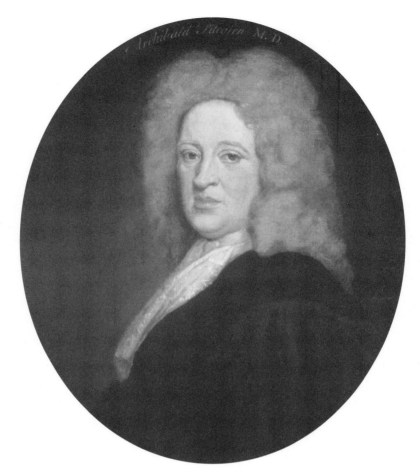

Archibald Pitcairn

everywhere in the streets. An equal number of paupers were maintained on a permanent basis by their kirk sessions and ten times that number of Edinburgh's citizens became dependent on parish aid at some time during the year.[3] In 1681, Edinburgh's perennial problem of poverty became even more pressing as failed harvests and unemployment brought destitute refugees from the countryside flooding into Edinburgh to search for work or simply in the hope of finding sustenance. The College agreed that each year two designated Fellows would make themselves available to give medical aid to the poor. The Town Council was asked to establish a fund to meet the cost of the necessary medicines and 'to nominate some person to be apothecary'. The ministers of all ten kirk sessions in the town and suburbs of Edinburgh were 'desired to give certificates to the poor that are sick and in their bounds'. Those certified as in need of medical attention were then visited at home by one of the designated Fellows of the College.

3. R.A. Houston, *Social Change in the Age of the Enlightenment* (Oxford, 1994), p. 258.

QUACKS, MOUNTEBANKS AND DRUGS

At its foundation the College immediately assumed the responsibilities set down in its charter. Required to ensure that 'no person not examined and admitted by the Fraternity of Apothecaries' was permitted to sell medicines, in its first months the College investigated a number of reports of unlicensed trading by 'stationers and merchants' and successfully prosecuted seven quacks and mountebanks. The College had also been charged with a duty to 'examine and inspect the drugs and medicines sold within the jurisdiction, suburbs and liberties of Edinburgh' and, if found to be worthless quack remedies, to 'throw them into the public street or destroy them'. To make clear which drugs and medicines would be acceptable a committee was appointed to revise and publish the pharmacopoeia that Sibbald and some others had begun to draw up at their meetings at Sibbald's lodgings in 1680. As an unexpected extension of the College's duties in the supervision of the preparation and use of drugs, in April 1682 the Privy Council delegated to the College the investigation of a charge of homcide: it was alleged that an apothecary, by 'composing and vending poisonous tablets had caused the death of one, Mrs Elizabeth Edmonston'.

A LIBRARY AND THE COLLEGE DISSERTATIONS

In these first months, the College also began to develop its scholarly and intellectual resources. A librarian was appointed and a library built up from the 'presse with three shelves of books' donated by Sir Robert Sibbald. His donation included 'Galen's works, 5 voll Greek and five Latin, Hippocrates in Greek, of Aldus's edition, Gesner his history of animals 3 voll, Paris bind, and some other valuable books'. This first donation was quickly followed by a gift by John Hope of Hopetoun of the ten volumes of the collected works of Jerome Cardan, who had been Professor of Medicine at Padua before Padua was overtaken by Leiden as the leading medical centre in Europe.

Before the College was founded, dissertations had been presented at the informal meetings of physicians held at Sibbald's lodgings. In 1683, this practice was revived and formalised by the College; it was agreed that, each month, a Fellow of the College would present, in Latin, a dissertation on an aphorism of Hippocrates or on a medical subject of his own choice. Dissertations that won the approval of the College were to be 'given to the Secretary to be inserted in the Register'. Those presented in the first year were all received 'with great satisfaction' (Table 2.1).

TABLE 2.1 First dissertations to the college

Sir Archibald Stevenson	De Polypus cadis
Sir Andrew Balfour	Aphorism 22, Section 1 (Use drugs only when the disease for which you employ them has come to a head)
Sir Robert Sibbald	De Concha Anatifera
Robert Crawford	De Natura et usu succi pancreatici
Robert Trotter	De Essentia ffebris
Matthew Sinclair	De Dysenteria
Alexander Cranston	De Alienatione Mentis
John Learmonth	De Longa media

In its first year the College made some notable progress. But it had not survived unscathed from the religious and dynastic conflicts of the time. King Charles II and James, Duke of York, his 'Viceroy' in Scotland were not content only to destroy all those who might take up arms against the monarchy. They meant to establish that although a Catholic, James, Duke of York had an undisputable right to succeed to the throne. They also meant to root out every man of influence in the country who might use that influence against the interests of the monarchy and particularly to root out those Presbyterians who refused to abjure the National Covenant. In July 1681, the Scottish Parliament was convoked for the first time since 1673 with James, Duke of York, as the king's High Commissioner. On 13 August it passed an act that asserted that the kings of Scotland derived 'their Royal power from God almighty alone' and that 'no difference in religion nor act of parliament could alter or divert the right of accession and lineal decent of the crown'.[4] On 31 March it passed an act requiring all holders of public office to swear and sign a Test Oath. Those required to take the Test included not only all Members of Parliament, all officers in the armed forces, all judicial officers, but also all clergymen and all school and university teachers. They had to swear, firstly, their loyalty to the crown and, secondly, their commitment to the protestant religion.

The Bill had been carelessly drawn up and when it was first presented to Parliament it was unclear how the protestant religion was to be defined; James Dalrymple of Stair, Lord President of the Court of Session, moved that definition should be conformity to the Confession of Faith of 1560. Since the Confession of Faith explicitly excluded the king from authority over the church, the two parts of the oath became mutually contradictory. In Parliament, Stair's aim had been to sabotage the Bill and prevent it being passed.[5] But virtually no one other than the lawyer Stair was familiar with the wording of the Confession of Faith and his definition was accepted without the protest and debate that he had intended to provoke. The result was a confused Act open to manipulation. Yet to refuse to take the Test Oath was deemed an act of treason and punishable by death.

4. T. Harris, *Restoration: Charles II and His Kingdoms* (London, 2005), p. 345.
5. Ibid.

To avoid taking the oath, some men of conscience went into voluntary exile. Many more gave up public office; several members of the nobility resigned their hereditary jurisdictions and large numbers of ministers vacated their pulpits. The Privy Council soon came to recognise that many useful men who presented no possible threat to the crown or the succession were being lost to the public service because they found it impossible, with a clear conscience, to take the Test Oath as it stood. It became acceptable for useful holders of public office to take the Test Oath with evasive modifications of their own devising. Administered in this way, the Test came to be applied selectively and used as an instrument to weed out all those most likely to threaten the monarchy or the succession.[6] The Earl of Argyll was a Presbyterian with an extensive power base in the Highlands; the government feared that he would emerge as the leader of a Protestant in opposition to the Catholic court party in Edinburgh. As a Privy Councillor he took the oath but with the reservation that he did so only 'as far as it was consistent with the Protestant religion' and 'not repugnant to it or his loyalty'.[7] His reservation was not accepted; he was found guilty of treason and condemned to death. Dalrymple of Stair, who had opposed the imposition of the Test, made no attempt to even offer a politic modification of the Oath and was convicted of treason; but, like Argyll, he escaped to the Netherlands before sentence could be carried out.

Apart from such prominent men who were driven into exile, there were many others who found they could not, in conscience, take the Test even in modified form and were simply deprived of their offices. In January 1682 the Privy Council in Scotland wrote to King Charles that the Test was proving 'a most happy expedient for filling offices with persons from whom your Majesty and your people may expect the unanimous and firm prosecution of your laws against all manner of irregularities'.

In 1682, the imposition of the Test began to cause the College the damaging loss of members. On 1 May, it was recorded in the College minutes that John Hutton, the College's first Treasurer, had 'necessarily gone forth from the Kingdome'. A Presbyterian and a moderate but committed Covenanter, he had fled to the Netherlands. (There he became physician to William of Orange and Princess Mary. He returned to Britain in 1688 and was their physician when they became respectively King William III and Queen Mary of England, Scotland and Ireland.) A year later, William Stevenson, who had succeeded Hutton as Treasurer, asked 'that some fit person might be named in his place'.[8] As he had never disguised his sympathy with the Covenanters it seems highly probable that he too had gone into exile; after his sudden resignation he is not mentioned again in the College records. A few months later a third upholder of the Covenant, John McGill, also disappeared from the records of the College.

The College also lost a royalist. When the Duke of York left Edinburgh for London in March 1682 he was accompanied by an entourage that included James Livingstone, the College's first Censor. When the Duke of York sailed north again in May to wind up his affairs in Scotland and bring home his household from Edinburgh, Livingstone was again one of the

6. J. Callow, *The Making of King James II* (Stroud, 2000), p. 293.
7. W. Churchill, *Marlborough: His Life and Times* (London, 1966), Vol. I, p. 154.
8. College Minute, August 1683.

Duke's party on board the frigate *Gloucester*. On 6 May 1682, the *Gloucester* was wrecked on a sandbank near the Wash. The Duke of York, John Churchill (later the Duke of Marlborough), Sir Charles Scarborough and several priests were among the forty survivors but James Livingstone was one of the three hundred who were drowned.

There was some delay in appointing Livingstone's successor as Censor. At the end of May, Sir Robert Sibbald was proposed but, he 'desired a little time to consider of it if he should accept'. Before being Censor he was obliged to take the Test Oath. It was only in June, after an amended form of the oath had been agreed with his political patron, the Earl of Perth, that 'he did take the oath of allegiance and did swear and sign the Test'.

The College had never been able to muster the twenty-one physicians who had signed the patent for the creation of the College. James Stewart had died before the College was founded. Six of the signatories (Sir David Hay, Mathew Brisbane, Mathew Sinclair, William Wright, William Halliburton and William Lauder) took no part in College activities once it was established. The loss of Hutton, Stevenson, McGill and Livingstone meant that, within a year of its foundation the College was already having difficulty in gathering a quorum for its meetings.

THE SHORT-LIVED PRESIDENCY OF SIR ROBERT SIBBALD

In March 1682, the Duke of York's period as the king's Commissioner in Scotland came to an end. He and his closest English advisors and courtiers, including John Churchill and Charles Scarborough, were made burgesses and guild brothers of the City of Edinburgh. His departure from Leith was marked by all the customary professions of affection and devotion. But, he left behind the resentment he had caused by his open and deliberate display of his commitment to the Roman Catholic faith. He had removed the Protestant congregation which had worshipped in the Royal Chapel at Holyroodhouse to a new church to be built in the Canongate;[9] the Royal Chapel had been re-equipped as a place of Roman Catholic, consecrated with holy water and reopened for the celebration of the mass. Edinburgh's students had rioted in protest but had been ignored. When James, Duke of York returned to England his closest supportes were left in charge. The Earl of Aberdeen became Chancellor, the Marquis of Queensbury the Lord Treasurer, the Earl of Perth the Justice General, Lord John Drummond, Perth's brother the Deputy Treasurer and the Marquis of Atholl the President of Parliament. In 1683 the king agreed that policy in Scotland should be managed by a 'Secret Committee' of Aberdeen, Queensbury, Atholl, Perth and Lord John Drummond reporting to the Duke of York in Whitehall. In little over a year, in 1684 the Earl of Perth and his brother, Lord John Drummond,[10] had engineered the downfall of both the Protestant Earl of Aberdeen and the Protestant Marquis of Queensberry.[11] The brothers, as the agents and acolytes of the Duke of York, had now achieved complete control of the government in Scotland, the Earl of Perth as Chancellor and Lord John Drummond as Secretary of State. Sir Robert Sibbald was quick to take advantage of his patron Lord Perth's rise to power.

9. The Canongate Kirk completed in 1688.
10. Harris, *Restoration.*, p. 342.
11. Aberdeen and Queensberry were Episcopalians. Aberdeen's father had been captured and executed by the Covenanters.

In December 1684 Sibbald had succeeded Sir Archibald Stevenson as President of the College. He immediately revived one of his original ambitions for the College that had been thwarted during the negotiations that settled the terms of the College Charter. To Sibbald's great disappointment the College had agreed not to compete with the universities in the teaching of medical undergraduates. To circumvent the restriction accepted in 1681, Sibbald now planned to have the College create a school of medicine within Edinburgh's university.

At the first meeting after his election as president, Sibbald moved to secure the necessary political patronage for his scheme: he had a patent drawn up for the creation of Honorary Fellows. Among those immediately made Honorary Fellows were the Lord Chancellor, the Earl of Perth, and the Secretary of State, Lord John Drummond. With that accomplished, he wrote to Lord Perth asking him to prevail upon the Town Council to appoint three Fellows of the College as professors of medicine at Edinburgh University, then still the 'Town's College'. The Town Council found it impossible to disoblige Lord Perth and Sir Robert Sibbald, Archibald Pitcairn and James Halket were duly appointed. Although the Town Council could not refuse to make the appointments, it could and did refuse to finance them or make the professorships more than empty titles. The Fellows of the College appointed as Edinburgh's first university professors of medicine never succeeded in teaching undergraduates; Sibbald's hopes had once again been thwarted. And almost immediately thereafter there followed a threat to the College's very survival.

Quite unexpectedly in February 1685, the king died and the Duke of York succeeded to the throne as James II and was now an openly professed Catholic. The Earl of Perth, and his brother, now the Earl of Melfort, quickly converted to Roman Catholicism and were confirmed in office, now even more powerful than before. More politic conversions followed; in September, Sir Robert Sibbald was persuaded by the Earl of Perth that he too should embrace the Roman Catholic faith.[12] Only nine months before, on becoming President of the College, Sibbald had signed the Test and had sworn to reject 'the Pope's authority and jurisdiction' and 'the Pope's erroneous doctrine'. As a Catholic his position at the College was now untenable and he was obliged to resign.

Out of office, Sibbald was nevertheless a member of the powerful Catholic community that the Earl of Perth had gathered round him in Edinburgh. In his memoirs Sibbald records that, 'notwithstanding the great opposition I met with from all my relations and acquaintances I continued more and more resolute. I frequented their services and became seriously enamoured with their way'. However, within a few months, he found that the Catholic priests

---

12. We must depend heavily on Sibbald's own Memoirs for an account of events. The records of the College for the period from 21 December 1684 until 22 March 1693 have not survived. In December 1684 it was agreed that the Clerk, Hugh Stevenson, W.S., would attend meetings of the College only 'when there is any use for him in any acts of Jurisdiction'. The responsibility for keeping College minutes was to be assumed by the newly elected College Secretary, Archibald Pitcairn. If the minutes were indeed kept, they have not survived; there is now no record of the proceedings of the College during the years from 21 December 1684 until 22 March 1693. The records may have been lost; there are similar gaps in the records of other Edinburgh institutions during this period. However, it seems more probable that the absence of any formal written account of College affairs should be attributed to the disruptions within the College that resulted from the religious, political and dynastic conflicts that engulfed Scotland at that time. The gap in the records of the College coincides with the years leading up to the Gloriou Revolution in England, the hesitant acceptance of William and Mary as joint monarch in Scotland and the years of disillusionment that descended on Scotland in the first years of their reign.

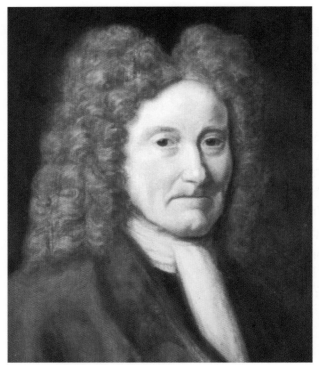

Robert Sibbald in old age

in Edinburgh had 'become too forward in their methods, having their services in the streets. They did it more like bigots than wise men and provoked the rabble against them and me'. In February 1686, when the mob, angry at the number of Catholic placemen being put in positions of power, did eventually break out in riot against Perth and his acolytes, Sibbald was one of its chosen targets. Forewarned, Sibbald managed to escape to the safety of Holyroodhouse. Next day, escorted by James Graham of Claverhouse and a detachment of the Life Guards, he was taken to Berwick. From there he travelled post to London.

In London, Sibbald was received briefly by the king. He renewed his acquaintance with Sir Charles Scarborough and was made an honorary Fellow of the London College of Physicians. For nine weeks he lived quietly, giving himself 'entirely to devotion'. However, he disliked the food ('few good fish could be had'), he found the air of the river and the city disagreeable and he became unwell. He had also discovered that 'the Jesuites, who had the greatest influence at court [were] pressing the King to illegal and unaccountable undertakings'. In his memoirs he records that he 'perceived also the whole people of England was under a violent restraint and foresaw they would overturn the Government. I began to think that I had been precipitant in declaring to the Romish Church, though I joined in the simplicity of heart. I repented of my rashness and resolved to come home and return to the church I was born in'. After a voyage of eight days he arrived at Leith and in September 1686 he was received again into the protestant church in Scotland by the Bishop of Edinburgh.

However, the damage had been done. Sibbald had lost the trust of the Fellows of the College. He was lampooned in verse by the College Secretary, Archibald Pitcairn. Pitcairn, the most brilliant of the original Fellows, was a considerable mathematician, a poet and a wit whose genius was seldom tempered by discretion. He was also a passionate Jacobite. His satire on Sibbald was vitriolic.

There is lost, there is lost
On the Catholic coast
A quack of the College's quorum
Tho' his name be not shown
Yet the man may be known
By his *opus viginti annorum*

With each wind he steer'd
And hath often so veered
That at last he split on ambition
While the Whigs were in vogue
He was the arrantest rogue
Of that damnable tribe of sedition

Day and Night did he work
In erecting a kirk
And gathering gold to a preacher
But he turned as soon
As the Whigs were undone
And left the poor destitute teacher

By the kirk he erected
By the gold he collected
By all that fanatical rabble
He ne'er could expect
Such wealth and respect
As he doth from the whore of Babel

For his taking the Test
Which he foreswore at last
A pardon he'll get from the Pope
But though he so do
I confess it to be true
He very well merits a rope

> 'Tis not the way to appear
> A true Cavalier
> To quit the protestant road
> To the King I avow
> He can never be true
> That so oft had played booby with God.

The College was now split into factions and their internal differences continued as religious bigotry and escalating political rivalry brought the nation to Revolution and years of recrimination.

THE 'GLORIOUS' REVOLUTION

In 1685, James came to the throne unopposed but within three years he had lost the support of Parliament. He had begun to dismantle the legal restrictions on the Roman Catholic population of England, not through Parliament but by using his Dispensary Powers (of very doubtfully legality[13]) to issue Indulgencies allowing freedom of worship. The hostility of the English Parliament was rekindled and, as Sibbald had observed while exiled in London, 'revolution was in the air.'[14]

In Scotland at this time, resistance to James VII and II's regime amounted to little more than a deliberate failure of co-operation. In England however, tension mounted and when the birth of a male heir to James II in June 1688 seemed to promise a Catholic monarchy continuing indefinitely into subsequent generations, a small aristocratic group of Protestant parliamentarians mounted a military coup. William of Orange, with an army of Dutch and mercenary troops, was encouraged to invade England. James, abandoned by all those he had looked to for support, deserted his throne and was replaced as joint monarchs by his daughter Mary and her husband, William of Orange.

Although Scotland had played no part in England's 'Glorious Revolution' the Scottish Parliament was now forced to choose. It could vote to continue in allegiance to a Catholic monarch who had fled for support to a Catholic country and could not be fully restored to his three kingdoms without war. Alternatively, it could bow to events in England and offer the throne to William and Mary. In February 1689, the Scottish Parliament voted for William and Mary and a Protestant succession. The decision was not unanimous and for a quarter of a century in Scotland the restoration of the Stuart dynasty remained a realistic and, in bad times, even an attractive proposition.

However, from the moment of James II's flight from Whitehall the position of the Catholic faction in the Scottish Privy Council had become untenable. Sibbald's former patron, the Catholic Earl of Perth was arrested and imprisoned; his brother, the Earl of Melfort had escaped with the deposed king to exile in France. There followed eighteen months of uncertain government in Scotland by a Convention Parliament. A royalist rising in

13. R. Mitchison, *Lordship to Patronage* (Edinburgh, 1983), p. 115.
14. F.P. Hett (ed), *The Memoirs of Sir Robert Sibbald (1641–1722)* (London, 1932), p. 93

the Highlands was defeated but Parliament was unable to control the 'rabblings' of armed Covenanters which ejected over two hundred Episcopalian ministers from their parishes.[15] When William of Orange finally settled with Parliament[16] the terms on which he would accept the crown in Scotland, it was agreed that no Catholic could be monarch or hold office. In what was seen by many as a necessary concession to the extreme Covenanters whose armed troops were then standing guard over the meeting of Parliament it was also agreed that episcopacy was to be condemned as an 'insupportable grievance and trouble to this nation'. What followed was a militant purge, not only of the small number of Catholics but the very much larger number of Episcopalians who had held public office. In the years that followed, two-thirds of Scotland's parish ministers were driven from their churches, a loss that was not made good for more than a generation.

Archibald Pitcairn and James Halket were dismissed from their positions as Professors of Medicine. It seems probable that this active prejudice against Episcopalians, especially those with declared Jacobite sympathies, influenced Archibald Pitcairn's decision to resign as Secretary of the College and accept an invitation to become Professor of Medicine at Leiden.

DISSENT AND DECLINE

Pitcairn's time at Leiden lasted only from April 1692 until the early autumn of 1693. Pitcairn and his friend David Gregory, both notable mathematicians, had been sent a copy of Isaac Newton's *Principa* soon after its publication in 1687. Pitcairn who had already been interested in early concepts of iatromechanics now became inspired by Newton's ideas. On his way to Leiden he visited Newton at Cambridge and was given a copy of Newton's (not yet published) *De Natura Acidorum* which set out his new theory of matter. Newton and Pitcairn had become friends and when Newton, in the autumn of 1693, suffered a period of apparent insanity, Pitcairn resigned his chair at Leiden to help care for him at Cambridge.[17]

On his return to Edinburgh at the end of 1693, Pitcairn became an enthusiastic exponent of a new Newtonian version of iatromechanics (the theory that all physiological phenomena could be explained in terms of physics and mathematics). Pitcairn's new ideas were unacceptable to the more conventional Fellows of the College and, along with personal and political differences, became yet another cause of the conflicts that divided the College.

These were also troubled times in Scotland. The massacre at Glencoe in February 1692 had damaged the reputation of the government. The new king's continental wars had closed down Scotland's trade with Europe and the deficit could not be made up in the English markets because of the tariffs and restrictions imposed by the English at the border.[18] Poor harvests at home led Scotland further into a long period of intense poverty and widespread famine. Sibbald wrote at this time that 'everyone may see death in the faces of the poor'. In the 1690s, Scotland experienced a level of collective misery and misfortune that was never approached

15. M. Lynch, *Scotland: A New History* (London, 1999), p. 302.
16. Properly a Convention rather than a Parliament since it had not been called by a reigning monarch.
17. L. Shirlaw, Dr. Archibald Pitcairn and Sir Isaac Newton's Black Years, *RCPE Chron*, 1975, Vol. 5, pp. 23-6.
18. T.C. Smout, *A History of the Scottish People* (London, 1969), p. 242.

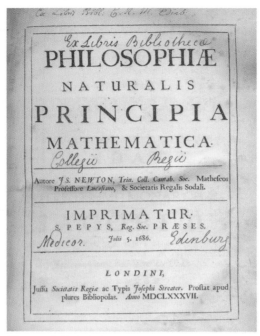

Newton's *Principia*

again. At this time of the deepest distress, almost two in three of parishes across the country were deprived of their accustomed leadership as 'all inefficient, negligent, scandalous and erroneous [i.e. Episcopalian] ministers'[19] were purged by a fiercely Presbyterian General Assembly. By 1693, it had become uncertain whether the hopes and faith of the majority of the people of Scotland were with Covenanters or with Episcopalians or with the Whigs rather than the Jacobites.

This was also true of the College. When Sir Archibald Stevenson was again elected President on St Andrew's Day 1693, his Council was equally divided between Whigs and Jacobites. And, in the years since 1684, the College had not prospered. The total number of Fellows had been sadly reduced and not every Fellow continued to take an active part in College business.

Sir Archibald Stevenson now introduced a series of reforms to restore the life of the College. From its first years the College had met at the lodgings of the Presidents. A reference in the minutes to bills paid to 'masons and wrights' for work 'approved by the landlord, Patrick Inglis' suggests that in February 1694 the College moved into rooms of its own. To take account of the decline in numbers, the quorum for business meetings was reduced to three; and in the following year seven new Fellows were elected. The monthly presentation of dissertations was revived, the day and time of the meetings was changed to the afternoon of the first Thursday of each month. A committee was appointed 'to inspect the former laws [of

19. Lynch, *Scotland*, p. 304.

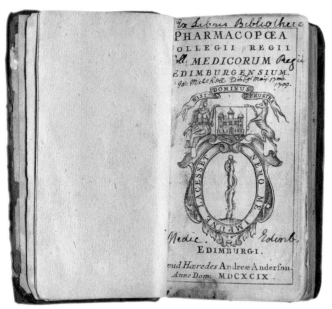

College *Pharmacopoea*

the College] and report to the President'. A second committee was appointed to review the finances of the College and a third committee was appointed to review the conditions on which a non-graduate could be given a licence to practise. And yet another committee was directed to prepare a new draft of the College's pharmacopoeia.

These attempts at reform did nothing to revive the fortunes of the College. They introduced a decade of discord in which the College was almost destroyed. Personal antipathies and antagonism between Whig and Jacobite intensified the rancour engendered by factional disputes over the adoption of the 'new science'. Sibbald, his medicine firmly based on the works of Galen, was resistant to all modern hypotheses, including the theories of the iatromechanists.[20] Sibbald could count on the support of Sir Thomas Burnet, author of the standard medical text of the time, *Thesaurus Medicinae Practica*[21] and the conservative Whig faction within the College. The Jacobite, Archibald Pitcairn, was the leading exponent in Scotland of iatromechanism and Newton's new science. Pitcairn, Sir Archibald Stevenson (his father-in-law) and the younger Fellows of the College regarded the Sibbald faction as reactionaries.

The most long-lasting of the College disputes was over the new pharmacopoeia. Sibbald and Andrew Balfour had begun to prepare a pharmacopoeia for Scotland in 1680. A committee of the College had taken on the work in March 1682 but an agreed draft had not been produced by 1693. In 1694, overall responsibility for the pharmacopoeia passed to Sir Archibald Stevenson and for the next five years, under his chairmanship, a succession of

20. A. Cunningham, Sir Robert Sibbald and Medical Education, Edinburgh, 1706, *Clio Medica* , 1978, Vol. 13, pp. 136-7
21. Twelve editions of *Thesaurus Medicinae Practica*, were published in London and Geneva between 1673 and 1698.

committees struggled to draw up an agreed version that could go forward for publication. In his *Memoirs* Sibbald attributes this further long delay to 'malice' and 'faction'.[22] Malice there may well have been but it is probable that the opposing attitudes to the 'new science' were at the heart of the matter. Some of the classical galenicals favoured by Sibbald and the herbal remedies that made up the 'simple method of Physic' he had learned in Paris[23] were discounted by Stevenson and Pitcairn as outdated while any Newtonian spagyric remedies suggested by Pitcairn were rejected by Sibbald. At last, in 1699, a text was produced that met with the approval of the College and, nineteen years after the work had begun, the *Pharmacopoeia Collegii Regii Medicorum Edinburgensis* was published.

Agreement on the contents of the *Pharmacopoeia* had been made possible by a division within the College that saw Pitcairn, Stevenson and the 'moderns' of their party suspended from their Fellowships. In 1691 Dr Andrew Brown, a graduate of Aberdeen and at one time a pupil of Sydenham, published a small book, *A Valedictory Schedule Concerning the New Cure of Fevers*. In it, he followed Syndenham in advocating the generous use of blood letting, emetics, and purgatives. Although Brown did not practise in Edinburgh he was well known there since it had become fashionable for patients from Edinburgh to travel to Dolphinton in Lanarkshire to consult him. The appearance of a pamphlet advertising his methods was deplored by a majority of the Edinburgh College and sparked off a controversy that continued for years.[24]

In November 1694, soon after his return to Edinburgh, Archibald Pitcairn presented a dissertation to the College in which he set out to justify Brown's practices in terms of his new Newtonian mechanicotistic theories. His presentation caused uproar and in the following year he went on to stir up more trouble by publishing his arguments in a pamphlet *Dissertatio De Curatione Februm Quae Per Evacuations Instituitur*.

An anonymous author replied, mocking Pitcairn's theories in a pamphlet, *Apollo Mathematicus or the Art of Curing Diseases by Mathematics According to the Principles of Dr. Pitcairn*. Pitcairn at first assumed that the pamphlet had been written by Sibbald but it was soon revealed that the author was Dr Edward Eizat. Eizat's satirical condemnation of Pitcairn's 'new science' was applauded by the Sibbald faction and he was quickly presented for admission as a Fellow of the College; as a graduate of a Scottish university, he could be elected by the College without examination. The meeting to elect Eizat was held on 14 September 1695, not at the College rooms[25] but at the lodgings of the president, Dr Trotter[26] and in the absence of both Pitcairn and Stevenson.

Eizat was duly elected but only by a narrow majority. The President, Dr Trotter, and the other members of the Sibbald faction immediately contrived to strengthen their support

---

22. Hett, *The Memoirs*, pp. 85 and 96.
23. Ibid., p. 64.
24. In the College library there are fourteen pamphlets published between 1691 and 1700 either supporting or condemning Brown's views.
25. The rooms of the College were in the same building as Sir Archibald Stevenson's lodgings and Stevenson had acted as curator of the rooms and their contents. In his Memoirs, Sibbald reports that Stevenson refused to make the keys of the College rooms available for the meeting on 14 September 1695.
26. 'Stevenson seems to have seen Trotter as something approaching the devil incarnate', W.S. Craig, *History of the Royal College of Physicians of Edinburgh* (Edinburgh, 1976), p. 413.

within the College. For some years it had been the practice for candidates for admission to the College to be examined by three Fellows drawn from a panel of five appointed to serve for a full year. Of the panel of five examiners who had been appointed for 1695, four were of the Stevenson party and supporters of Pitcairn.[27] Following the contested election of Dr Eizat on 14 September, and again by a majority, the panel of examiners was abolished and an earlier arrangement had been reintroduced; thereafter the examination of candidates for admission to the College was again to be carried out on an ad hoc basis by three examiners appointed specifically for each candidate. From 14 September, no examiner was chosen from among the Fellows sympathetic to Pitcairn. Over the following seven weeks, five new Fellows were admitted, all adding to the strength of the Sibbald party and giving it a secure overall majority in the College.[28]

Those who continued to support the 'new science' and the principles of Dr Pitcairn were not overawed. George Hepburn published a pamphlet entitled *Tarrago Unmasked*. A parody of a popular comic opera, *Turrago's Wiles*, the pamphlet aimed to 'expose the cunning address of Edward Eizat in studying to attain his objects as a medical practitioner'. A meeting of the College on 14 November found that Hepburn had acted improperly in publishing his pamphlet without the permission of the College and that the pamphlet itself was censurable. Hepburn was summoned to appear before the College on 20 November.

On 18 November Pitcairn, attending a College meeting for the first time since the break-away meeting of 14 September, submitted a paper attacking the conduct of the President, Dr Trotter and his party over the preceding months. The paper was referred to a special committee for consideration. The committee, consisting of the President, Sibbald and four others of their party, found the paper 'calumnious, scandalous, false and arrogant'.[29] On 22 November, Pitcairn was suspended. Two weeks later Hepburn was suspended for the publication of *Tarrago Unmasked*. Olyphant, the Treasurer, followed a few days later; he was suddenly ordered give in his accounts and when he had not done so by the next day, he too was suspended.

When the College met in December 1695 for its annual St Andrew's Day elections, Pitcairn and the others who had been suspended tried to join in the proceedings. Their appearance had been expected; one of Edinburgh's bailies[30] and a number of Town Officers were present and on the orders of the President, Pitcairn and his party were forcibly removed from the meeting.[31]

The College at once complained to the Privy Council, accusing Pitcairn and his supporters of causing a riot. When the Privy Council later found them guilty, Stevenson, Eccles, Smellholme, Robertson and Melville were all suspended from their Fellowships. In 1696, both parties took their grievances to the Court of Session. Stevenson, Pitcairn and their party

27. Stevenson, Pitcairn, Eccles and Olyphant. Only Halket belonged to the Sibbald faction.
28. W.B. Howie, Sir Archibald Stevenson, His Ancestry and the Riot in the College of Physicians at Edinburgh, *Medical History* 1667, II, p. 272.
29. Ibid., p. 273.
30. Bailies were magistrates and next in precedence to the Lord Provost.
31. The ejected group held a meeting of their own and elected Sir Archibald Stevenson as their President. However, this was no more than a futile gesture.

claimed for the restitution of the rights of which they had been deprived by their suspension. The College sought confirmation of its rights and authority. Three years later, the Court found in favour of the College in both actions.

These prolonged legal actions were expensive but achieved little. The suspension of so many of its most active Fellows inevitably proved damaging to the College. The provision of medical aid for the poor continued. Work continued on revising the pharmacopoeia and books were added to the library. But meetings of the College became irregular. Only two dissertations were presented in a period of over five years. Attendance at meeting declined and on a number of occasions a quorum could not be achieved.

SURVIVAL

In January 1700, the College, in a tentative attempt to effect a reconciliation, made a conditional offer to lift all the suspensions imposed over the previous four years. The conditions were unacceptable and the offer was refused. It was not until 7 January 1703 that the College finally decided to 'show to the world … that nothing may be wanting on their part to restore the peace of the society'.[32] It was agreed that the suspensions should be lifted unconditionally. For reasons unknown, the College did not meet again for eleven months but in December 'an act of oblivion' was drawn up 'to the end that no memory may remain of what is past and all Acts whereby censures were inflicted are not only annulled but likewise razed and deleted out of the records'. The Act was given the unanimous approval of the College. The first meeting of the reunited College took place on St Andrew's Day 1704 and, as final evidence of conciliation, Sir Archibald Stevenson, William Eccles, Andrew Melville and John Smellholme were elected to the Council.

RECOVERY

In the decade that followed, the College enjoyed a remarkable period of recovery. A few weeks after the reconciliation, the College bought the house in Fountain Close that was to serve as the College Hall for almost seventy years. The College yards extended southward from Fountain Close on the High Street to open on the Cowgate. The College later bought the buildings that adjoined the Cowgate entrance to the yards and replaced them with a Cold Bath House where members of the public could bathe and drink the waters of St Michael's Well.

In January 1705, the monthly dissertations were resumed. It was also arranged that 'any members that please may meet at the College every Monday betwixt three and four in the afternoon to confer about medicine and other parts of learning'. The library was extended and the number and generosity of the donations of books increased; as the library grew it was agreed that 'where there where several copies of the same edition they be auctioned off'.

By October 1705 the services for the poor were improved. In addition to visiting the sick poor in their homes it was agreed that 'two Fellows would attend at the College every Monday, Wednesday and Friday for giving advice to the sick poor'.

32. Craig, *History*, p. 417.

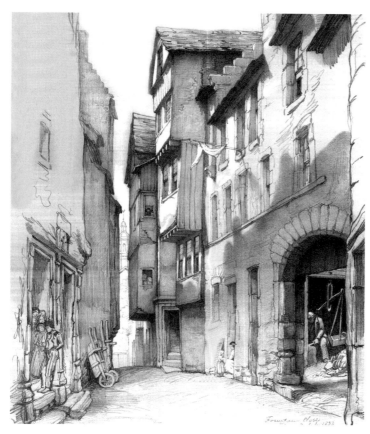

**Fountain Close,
Edinburgh**

In October 1706 the College found that it 'stood in need of money'. Large sums had been spent on the College buildings and in extending the College physic garden. Even before these investments had been made, the College had been far from rich. The many legal suits in which the College had become involved the late 1690s and early 1700s had been costly. In 1698 the College had also bought shares in the Scottish Company Trading with Africa and the Indies; when that company's great Darien Venture ended in disaster the College had lost its investment. In 1706 the President and Censors had to ask for authority to borrow money. However, a year later the financial crisis was resolved. In September 1707 the Commission for the Disposing of the Equivalent granted to the College 60 per cent of the amount that the College had lost by the failure of the Darien Venture.[33] The finances of the College were further improved by the election of new Fellows; between 1704 and 1708 the number of Fellows almost doubled to a total of thirty-two. By February 1711 the College was not only solvent but the Treasurer was able to invest a surplus.

33. The failure of the venture of the Scottish Company Trading with Africa and the Indies at Darien had been in large part due to the hostility of the English Government. As part of the agreement reached at the Union of Scotland and England in 1707, the English government undertook to make some compensation for the losses incurred. The sum set aside for that purpose was known as the 'The Equivalent'.

The College had now recovered from what had been the most regrettable years in the history of the College. The ostensible cause of the division within the College had been the difference in views of the theories of iatromechanism and 'the new science'. That bitter conflict had taken the place of rational debate was a reflection of the troubles that beset Scotland in these same years.

Scotland had been divided by conflict between Presbyterian and Episcopalian, and between Catholic and both; by conflict between Whig and Jacobite; and by conflict between monarchist and theocrat Covenanter. In the 1690s the country had suffered famine in which thousands perished; in Midlothian, the rural community nearest to the nation's capital, one in five of the population starved to death. Recurring seasons of unusually severe weather had caused years of poor harvests and King William's continental wars had cut Scotland off from its long standing trading partners in Europe. Attempts to find new outlets on the other side of the Atlantic trade had come to a disastrous end with the failure of the Darien Venture and the loss of a third of Scotland's working capital. Efforts, in 1702 and 1703, to establish a form of union with England that would allow open access to markets south of the border had come to nothing.

In 1707, in its own interest, the English Parliament manoeuvred the Scottish Parliament into accepting a union of both Parliaments into a single British Parliament. It was expected in Scotland that the economic advantages of the Union would compensate for the loss of independence. These expectations were soon disappointed. In the first years of the union the people of Scotland became more conscious of the burden of new taxes than of any boost to the Scottish economy. When, in 1715, the Earl of Mar raised a rebellion against the Hanoverian King and his government in London, recruits flocked to his banner from every part of Scotland. Most were motivated by resentment over the 'lean years' that had followed the accession of King William in 1688 and the disappointing outcome of the Union in 1707 rather that any deep commitment to the Jacobite cause.

The failure of the rebellion brought an end to any realistic prospect of a return to an independent Scotland or a restoration of a Stuart monarchy. In the peace that followed, the bitter conflicts between Tory and Whig, Covenanter and Episcopalian, Protestant and Catholic that had divided Scotland and divided the College of Physicians faded from centre stage. As these wounding differences healed both Scotland and the College were able to move on to find their places in the modern world.

3

A RIVAL TO LEIDEN
An Edinburgh Faculty of Medicine

In 1469, Andrew Garleis was admitted *Doctor in Medicinus* at the University of Glasgow. He was the first medical graduate of a Scottish university and until the eighteenth century there were very few others. At their foundation, Scotland's medieval universities of St Andrews (1411), Glasgow (1451) and King's College, Aberdeen (1494) had all been granted the privilege of awarding degrees in medicine. But, for over three centuries, Scots intent on studying medicine had continued to go abroad to Padua, Montpellier, Paris, Leiden or whichever of the other great university medical schools of Europe had the leading teachers of the time.

In 1560, in *The First Book of Discipline*, John Knox had set out his plan for the reform of Scotland's universities. In it he proposed that St Andrews should be a 'complete' university with faculties of Philosophy, Medicine, Law and Divinity.[1] However, Knox's scheme came to nothing. In the seventeenth century, St Andrews still had no medical faculty and no professor of medicine. Nevertheless the university continued to exercise its ancient privilege of granting medical degrees. Some were awarded *honoris causa*; some were awarded to medical graduates of reputable universities; but many others were granted a degree *in absentia* simply on payment of a fee.[2]

When Andrew Garleis graduated at Glasgow University it is probable that his degree was granted *honoris causa* since at that time the university did not have a medical faculty or a professor of medicine. A professor of medicine, Robert Mayne, was appointed in 1637 but three years later a Commission of the General Assembly of the Church of Scotland judged that a chair of medicine at Glasgow was 'unnecessary' and after Mayne's death the chair was allowed to lapse. When two medical degrees were awarded early in the eighteenth century, one 1703 and the other in 1711, the candidates were examined by the professor of mathematics and two local physicians, both graduates of foreign universities. The chair of medicine at Glasgow was not revived until 1713.

King's College, Aberdeen, has some claim to be the first university in Britain to make provision for the teaching of medicine. King's College was founded by James I, who was an amateur physician and a skilful surgeon; in 1494, he made a grant of royal lands to endow the appointment of a Mediciner (professor of medicine). However a number, perhaps a majority, of those appointed as Mediciner regarded the post as purely titular. Those who did teach did so as part of the three or four years of general studies (*stadium generale*) then thought appropriate for the education of a gentleman; on the rare occasions when a student was

---

1. In John Knox's plan St Andrews was to be the only 'complete university' in Scotland.
2. J.D. Comrie, *History of Scottish Medicine to 1860* (London, 1927), p. 178.

awarded the degree of MD it was on the evidence of his scholarship and not as an endorsement of any skills he might have as a physician.[3] At Aberdeen the great majority of the medical degrees were conferred not on students who had completed a course of study at the university but were awarded as a mark of distinction to medical men already established in practice and they were granted simply on the recommendation of two or more of their colleagues.[4]

Scotland's two post-Reformation universities, Edinburgh founded in 1556 and Marischal College, Aberdeen founded in 1593, did not have faculties of medicine and did not award medical degrees. As a result, even in the last years of the seventeenth century, St Andrews and King's College, Aberdeen were the only universities in Scotland awarding medical degrees in significant numbers and many of their degrees were being granted, without examination, to candidates who had not studied medicine at a reputable university. Although Scotland's ancient universities had shown little interest in the study of medicine or in promoting high standards in its practice, they were nevertheless jealous of their monopoly in the conferring of medical degrees. For that reason they had successfully opposed the creation of a College of Physicians in 1621, in 1630 and again in 1655. In order to forestall their opposition yet again in 1681, the College had agreed, first, to relinquishing the right 'to the erection of schools to teach medicine or any part of the same or to the conferring or granting of degrees in the same' and, second, to license any medical graduate of a Scottish university to have 'the liberty and power to practise within the jurisdiction of the Magistrates of the City of Edinburgh' without examination. These two concessions effectively excluded the College from the pursuit of its chief aim, the promotion and maintenance of the highest possible standard of medical practice. For over half a century, the College struggled to obviate the first of these unfortunate concessions by establishing a faculty of medicine, made up of Fellows of the College but within the university. The struggle to overcome the second concession was to take even longer.

EDINBURGH'S FIRST FACULTY OF MEDICINE

In the first years of the College of Physicians, the Scottish universities were caught up in the Duke of York's remorseless campaign to exclude from the church, the schools, the universities or any other office of influence and anyone who might challenge the absolute authority of the crown. University students were not allowed to graduate until they had sworn an oath of allegiance to the monarch. At Edinburgh, the great majority of the students refused to take the oath;[5] those few who were determined to graduate, took the oath in private since to take the oath in a public ceremony was to invite violent 'retaliation'[6] from militant supporters of the National Covenant. While James, Duke of York was in Scotland, the number of students graduating at Edinburgh became so few that the public graduation ceremony was abandoned.

---

3. Ibid., p. 140.
4. In 1690 Archibald Pitcairn, a graduate of Rheims, became MD *ad eundem dignitatais gradum ab Universitate Aberdonensis evectus.*
5. R.H. Campbell and A.S. Skinner, *The Origins and Nature of the Scottish Enlightenment* (Edinburgh, 1982), p. 53.
6. A. Bower, *A History of the University of Edinburgh: Chiefly Compiled from Original Papers and Record Never Before Published* (Edinburgh, 1817), Vol. I, p. 308.

The Duke of York also curbed the independence of Edinburgh University's governing body, the Town Council.[7] He ordered that elections to the Town Council should not be called until his pleasure was known and, even then, that the elections should not proceed until all the nominations for election had been approved by his Privy Council.[8] On his departure for London in 1682, the tight control he had established over the Town Council and its university passed into the hands of his representative in Scotland, the Chancellor, the Earl of Perth. When James succeeded as James VII and II on 6 February 1685, Lord Perth was confirmed as Chancellor and became the *de facto* governor of the university.

Sir Robert Sibbald, the President of the College of Physicians immediately seized the occasion to write to Lord Perth. He reminded his friend and patron, that 'the chief end' of the College was 'the debarring of illiterate and unqualified persons from the practice of medicine' and that 'the College of Physicians humbly conceive our universities cannot regularly confer degrees in medicine until they be provided with a sufficient number of professors to constitute a faculty of medicine'. Lord Perth at once made his wishes known to the Town Council of Edinburgh as the patrons of the university, and on 27 February 1685, Sir Robert Sibbald was appointed as Professor of Medicine; on 16th September James Halket and Archibald Pitcairn were also made Professors of Medicine 'that they might unite their endeavors with Sir Robert Sibbald in teaching that science in this University'.[9]

Edinburgh, alone among Scotland's universities, now had the number of professors that Sibbald had set as the minimum required to constitute a faculty of medicine. Sibbald pressed home his advantage. On 6 July 1686 he wrote again to Lord Perth to ask that:

> His Majesty would be graciously pleased to ordain that all persons, in any time coming wherever they be graduate either at home or abroad shall be first tried and examined by the said College to the effect that they may be admitted if they shall be found sufficiently qualified or otherwise that they may reject them, notwithstanding of any clause or provision contained in the patent of erection of the College.

Lord Perth and his brother the Earl of Melfort, the Secretary of State, both wrote at once to King James II in support of Sibbald's case, their letters following almost word for word Sibbald's memorandum.[10] The response was equally prompt; from the Court at Whitehall on 19th November 1686 King James issued a 'Warrant for a Grant in favour of the College of Physicians in Edinburgh authorising them to try and examine Graduates in medicine before their being allowed to practise there'.

It must have seemed that all that the College hoped to achieve in its relationship with the universities had been accomplished. Then, two years later, there was a further unexpected but welcome royal intervention in the affairs of the university. Early in 1688, a new royal charter

7. Unlike Scotland's mediaeval universities which had been founded by Papal Bull, that at Edinburgh had been founded after the Reformation in 1583 by Edinburgh's Town Council and the Town Council had continued as its governing body.
8. R.D. Anderson, M. Lynch and N. Phillipson, *An Illustrated History of the University of Edinburgh* (Edinburgh, 2003), p. 47.
9. Bower, *A History*, p. 308.
10. College Archive, MS 13/97.

recreated what had always been known as 'the Town's College' as King James' University with rights to teach and grant degrees in 'philologie as well in the Hebrew, Greek, Latin, Oriental French and other languages as in all its other parts the professions of History, Mathematics, Philosophy, Medicine, Law and Theologie in all their parts and all other faculties and professions of arts and sciences what somever'.[11]

But, almost immediately, everything that the College seemed to have achieved was lost in the Revolution of 1688. The Warrant that King James had issued authorising the College 'to try and examine' all graduate physicians before they were allowed to practise in Edinburgh was set aside by the new Parliament as 'an act of arbitrary power'. Then, in 1690, the fiercely Presbyterian Parliament passed an act for the 'visitation of universities, colleges and schools'. The Visitors were authorised to 'inquire into and take exact trial of the masters, professors, principals regents &c if any of them be erroneous in doctrine'. Robert Sibbald, the first professor of medicine at Edinburgh had already been forced to resign in 1685 after his sudden conversion to the Catholic faith in 1685; now in 1690 the second and third professors of medicine, Archibald Pitcairn and James Halkett, as Episcopalians were found to be 'erroneous in doctrine' and were ousted without ever having taught or examined students. Edinburgh University's first faculty of medicine, if it had ever really existed, was no more.

THE YEARS BETWEEN

These were now difficult years for Edinburgh's university. The purge that followed the 'visitation' of 1690 deprived the University of its Principal, Alexander Monro.[12] Monro's successor was Gilbert Rule, a hard line Presbyterian and militant Covenanter who had been imprisoned, tortured and forced into exile in the Netherlands during the regime of Charles II and James II. Now, after the Revolution, his aim was to turn Edinburgh University into a seminary for a new generation of orthodox Presbyterian clergy in his own image.[13] Although he was a graduate of Leiden and had practised as a physician for several years in Scotland[14] he made no attempt to advance the study and teaching of medicine or even to replace the professors of medicine who had been dismissed in 1690.

Rule died in 1701. In May 1703, he was succeeded as Principal by William Carstares. Like Rule, Carstares was a committed Presbyterian who had suffered torture by the 'boot' and by thumbscrews and had then been exiled in the Netherlands. While at university there he had been recruited as one of William of Orange's secret agents in England and when William of Orange became King William III of England and Scotland, Carstares became one of his closest advisors. Although, like Rule, Carstares was a Presbyterian who had suffered persecution for his faith, he did not share Rule's fanaticism. His aim was to train a moderate minded clergy to replace the radical and uncompromising Presbyterians who had come to dominate the church in the immediate aftermath of the Revolution. Even before becoming Principal at Edinburgh,

11. Draft Charter of King James quoted by Sir A. Grant, *The Story of the University of Edinburgh* (London, 1884) Vol. I , p. 256.
12. Those ousted from their Chairs included the Professor of Divinity, the Professor of Hebrew and the Professor of Mathematics, David Gregory, who became Professor of Mathematics at Oxford.
13. Anderson et al., *An Illustrated History*, p. 55.
14. His son was a Fellow of Edinburgh's College of Physicians.

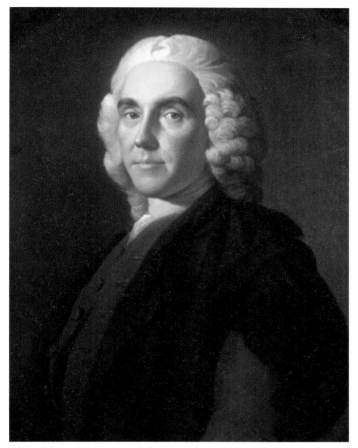

Alexander Monro (Royal College of Surgeons)

Carstares had used his influence with King William to divert funds that had formerly been used to support Scotland's bishops to the Scottish universities. At Edinburgh, Carstares meant to reform the university on the model of Leiden and the Dutch universities he had come to admire during his years of exile.

It may have been Carstares' appointment as Principal at Edinburgh that, in July 1704, encouraged the President of the College of Physicians, Alexander Dundas, to put forward his 'proposals for an agreement betwixt the Universities of St Andrews, Aberdeen, Glasgow and Edinburgh of the one part and the Royal College of Physicians in Edinburgh on the other part'. These were:

> That until they had professors of medicine and medical faculties of their own, the universities should grant medical degrees only to those with a recommendation and declaration that they had been examined and found qualified by the College.

1. That the College should undertake to admit as licentiates or Fellows of the College only medical graduates of one of the Scottish Universities; medical graduates of foreign universities should first be referred to a Scottish university with an appropriate recommendation and declaration from the College.

2. That when medical faculties became established within any of the Scottish universities, the medical graduates of those universities should be licensed to practise in Edinburgh without further examination.

3. That, together, the College and the universities should seek to obtain an Act of Parliament that would ensure that only medical graduates of Scottish universities would be allowed to practise medicine in Scotland.

There is no record of any response from the universities of Aberdeen or Glasgow; in a very few casual lines the Principal of St Andrews agreed to Dundas's proposals but indicated that the establishment of a faculty of medicine at St Andrews would be, 'for what I know, *ad callendas graecas*' [i.e. never].

On 28 July 1704, a much more positive response was received from Principal Carstares of Edinburgh:

I no sooner had a proposal made by you to this university in the name of the College of Physicians when I took the first opportunity of calling the professors together, who after deliberating upon what was proposed to them about conferring degrees of Doctor of Medicine, did desire me to signify in their name to the College of Physicians ... that they are ready to agree with the proposals as made until medicine be taught in the College of Edinburgh, providing always the candidates apply to the university first who are to remit them to the College of Physicians for examination ... This is, Sir, what I am desired to give in reply to your letter and doubt not but it will show how willing this university is to keep up a friendly correspondence with the College of Physicians.

This rapprochement with the university was followed a few months later by an offer of friendly co-operation with the Incorporation of Surgeons. For well over a decade the new College of Physicians and the Incorporation had continued in cautious rivalry, each one carefully guarding its privileges against any possibility of infringement by the other. Then, on 27 September 1704 it was reported to a meeting of the College of Physicians that the 'Deacon of the Surgeons had proposed to several members of the College his earnest desire for an accommodation betwixt the College and their Calling'. The Incorporation was at that time in the midst of negotiations with the Town Council to restore the association of Incorporation of Surgeons with the apothecaries that had been dissolved in 1681. Since the association had been dissolved on the advice of Edinburgh's physicians (Chapter 1) the Incorporation now expected to meet renewed opposition from the College of Physicians. However, in words that recalled the bloody disputes that had raged for many years on Scotland's border with England, the

President of the College acknowledged that 'we have ridden the marches with the Surgeons of Edinburgh' but proposed that the College should now 'settle with the surgeons'. The College made no objection to the Incorporation's plan to restore the profession of Surgeon-Apothecary in Edinburgh. In return, the Incorporation of Surgeons withdrew its opposition to the moves then being made by College of Physicians to promote the establishment of a faculty of medicine at Edinburgh University.

MEDICAL GRADUATES AND EXTRAMURAL PROFESSORS OF MEDICINE

The first candidate for the degree of Doctor of Medicine was put forward by Edinburgh University on 5 April 1705. In a letter to the College, Principal Carstares wrote: 'Mr David Cockburn, student in physic having addressed for the degree of doctor of medicine, the professors of that university desire that the College of Physicians give themselves the trouble to examine him.' On 17 April 1705, Cockburn was examined by Dr Smellholme and Dr McKenzie on the Institutes of Medicine; a week later he was examined by Dr Halkett and Dr Dundas on an aphorism of Hippocrates; after a further week Dr Pitcairn and Dr Lauder examined him 'each on ane case in medicine'. The College minutes record that on 1 May 1705 'the examiners found him duly qualified to practise medicine and recommend to the President to make report to the Principal and Masters of the University of Edinburgh in order to have the degree of Doctor of Medicine conferred upon him, the said Dr Cockburn being always obliged to give his petition to be admitted a Licentiate of the College after he has got his degree to practise'. Between 1705 and 1726 candidates for the medical degrees at Edinburgh University continued to be examined in this way by Fellows nominated by the President of the College of Physicians.

During his years as Principal, Carstares made a number of important constitutional changes at Edinburgh University. He abolished the ancient system of regenting[15] and introduced teaching by specialist professors on the Dutch model. He established a faculty of arts with chairs of Humanity, Greek, Logic, Natural Philosophy and Moral Philosophy. In a new faculty of divinity he appointed a leading moderate Presbyterian, William Hamilton, as Professor of Divinity and revived the dormant chair of ecclesiastical history. However, during his term as Principal, progress toward the re-establishment of a faculty of medicine was haphazard and tentative. A small number of medical practitioners, who had achieved notable success teaching medicine at their own small private schools, were dignified by the Town Council with the title of professor and given some more or less close association with the university.[16] However, none of these ad hominem appointments was particularly distinguished and throughout the first quarter of the eighteenth century the teaching of medicine in Edinburgh continued outside the walls of the university and with only modest success.

15. As regent, a member of the university's teaching staff took charge of a class of new entrants to the university and continued to guide their studies while they continued at the university.

16. Sir A. Grant, *The Story of the University of Edinburgh* (London, 1884), Vol. 1, p. 296. The Town Council kept control of commercial activity in all its forms in Edinburgh, granting monopolies in everything from coach services to teaching ('professing'). Only a minority of those sanctioned by the Town Council as 'professors' held appointments at the university.

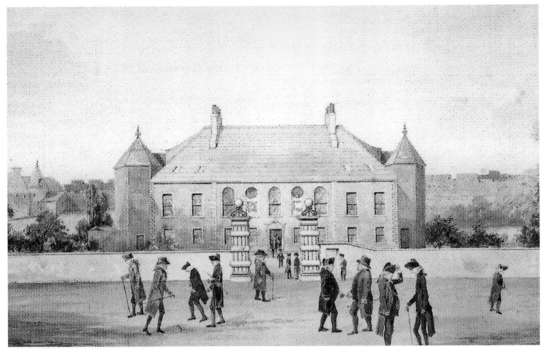

Old Surgeons' Hall (Royal College of Surgeons)

EDINBURGH'S SECOND FACULTY OF MEDICINE

From its foundation in 1505 the Incorporation of Surgeons had insisted on high standards of literacy (in Latin) among its apprentices and an elite among the apprentices had always been encouraged to travel abroad to study at the leading schools in Europe. In the later years of the seventeenth century, the Incorporation began to make progress in its ambition to become recognised as a learned society. From 1676, the twenty or twenty-five apprentices accepted on its roll each year were advised to attend the course of lectures and demonstrations of medicinal plants given by James Sutherland at Robert Sibbald's new physic garden (Chapter 1). Arrangements were also made that allowed apprentice surgeons to accompany Fellows of the College of Physicians when attending cases of 'uncommon interest'. After 1696, when a new Surgeons' Hall was built, the incorporation was able to extend its collection of books and go on to build a considerable library of its own. The teaching of anatomy was improved in 1697 on the installation of a new anatomy theatre at Surgeons' Hall. The Town Council gave permission for the bodies of prisoners who died in the town's prison to be used for dissection; when a body became available it was dissected over a period of eight or nine days, a different surgeon performing the dissection each day while a commentary was provided by a Fellow of the College of Physicians, Archibald Pitcairn.

The first of these dissections was carried out in 1702 but they continued in this way only for three years. In 1705 teaching at Surgeons' Hall was reorganised in response to an increasing demand for medical men to serve the British armies in Europe; the Duke of Marlborough was then continuing to make his reputation as a great general; the battles of Schellenberg and Blenheim had been won but causalities had been heavy and there were bloody campaigns still to come. Robert Elliot, a surgeon who had studied at Leiden, was appointed to take overall responsibility for instruction in anatomy and surgery at Surgeons' Hall. The Town Council gave its support, awarding Elliot an annual stipend of £15 and the title of Professor of Anatomy. Elliot died early in 1717 and, on 24 October, a surgeon-apothecary, Adam Drummond, was appointed to succeed him. Some months later Drummond agreed to share the office of professor and its emoluments with a surgeon, John McGill, 'a young man of enterprising temper' who later became Deacon of the Incorporation. However wild rumours and fierce accusations of grave robbing roused public hostility to the dissection of bodies and bodies became increasingly difficult to obtain. Between 1705 and 1720 dissections were carried out only once every two or three years.

Ventures in the education of physicians in Edinburgh in these years were even less successful. Sir Robert Sibbald, still denied the right to teach either within the College or within the university, made an ambitious, even grandiose, attempt to teach medicine on his own account. On 24 February 1706 the *Edinburgh Courant* carried his advertisement (in Latin):

> A good and favourable thing for his most dearly-loved country and lover of medicine in it: Sir Robert Sibbald M.D. will, God willing, begin to teach in private courses in the spring months of this year 1706 both natural history and the medical art which he hath with God's help successfully practised for forty-three years. But he thinks that young men interested in these matters should be warned that he is not going to enrol any but those who are versed in the Latin and Greek languages, the whole of philosophy and the fundamentals of mathematics; he wants this certified by the signatures of their teachers.[17]

Sibbald was now sixty-five years old. Still loyal to Galen and ever sceptical of all post-Newtonian theories, he had come to be regarded as a reactionary. His scheme, as advertised in the *Edinburgh Courier*, was also seen to make excessive demands of potential students. The entry qualifications were, in effect, the equivalent of a MA degree while the medical course itself was planned to occupy a further three years. Sibbald answered his critics in a pamphlet (again in Latin), *Commentaries on the law of Hippocrates and on his letter to his son Thessalus in which is shown what things are necessary for the future physician.*[18] Whether, in the end, any students ever answered Sibbald's advertisement is unknown but what is certain is that his scheme was abandoned before it was begun.

There was no further advance in medical education in Edinburgh until 1713. In November of that year the President of the College of Physicians received a letter from William Carstares, the Principal of the University, in which he:

17. Translated and quoted by A. Cunningham, *Clio Medica*, 1978, Vol. 13, No. 2, p. 135.
18. *In Hippoccrates legem, et inejus epistolam ad Thessalum Filium, Commentarii; in quibus ostenditur, quae Medico futuro, Necessaria sunt* (Edinburgh, 1706).

represented that it might be of public advantage to have a Professor of Medicine established in their university and that Dr James Crawford being mentioned to them as being peculiarly fitted for that post, the university thought it proper to acquaint the College of physicians with the affair that they might be favoured with character of that gentleman before they make application to their Patrons about it.[19]

The President, Matthew Sinclair, replied that the Fellows of the College were 'very well pleased' with the qualifications of James Crawford, a graduate of Leiden and a Fellow of the College since 1711. They considered him 'very fit for the post and gave him a very ample character'. They also 'gave thanks to the Principal and Masters of the university for their civility to the College'.

Crawford was appointed as Professor of Physic and Chemistry but with no salary. After his appointment, candidates for the degree of Doctor of Medicine were examined in the library of the university by Professor Crawford and two Fellows of the College of Physicians nominated by its President. However, Crawford made little commitment to teaching; he lectured only intermittently and then only on chemistry as it related to pharmacy. In 1719, he resigned on being appointed as Professor of Greek.

It was not until the 1720s that real progress was made towards the creation of the 'duly constituted faculty of medicine' that the College of Physicians had first advocated in 1685. The government of Britain was now firmly in the grip of the Whig 'Prime' Minister, Robert Walpole and Scotland was managed on his behalf by Archibald Campbell, the Earl of Ilay. He held the offices of Lord Privy Seal and Lord Justice General and when he visited Edinburgh he 'held court at Holyrood, waited on by the judges, magistrates and professors in their gowns'.[20] To many of his contemporaries he was the 'uncrowned King of Scotland'. His access to Walpole's great government patronage machine allowed him to determine the election of almost every Scottish Member of Parliament and to command every appointment of importance in the church and in local government. In Edinburgh, he controlled, the Town Council and, through the Town Council, the Town's university.

Ilay was a mathematician, a chemist who had studied under Boerhaave at Leiden and a Fellow of the Royal Society. He fully understood the importance of universities in shaping the religious and political culture of a modern state and he made sure that university chairs in Scotland were filled by the best scholars rather than by placemen, provided, of course, that those appointed were politically acceptable.[21] At Edinburgh, he was responsible for the appointment of William Wishart as Principal of Edinburgh University in 1716 and supported him as he continued the reforms begun by Carstares. He also gave his all-important approval to the initiatives of the Incorporation of Surgeons and, later, the College of Physicians that led ultimately to the re-establishing of the university's faculty of medicine.

19. College Minute, 23 November 1713.
20. Anderson et al., *An Illustrated History*, p. 63.
21. Ibid.

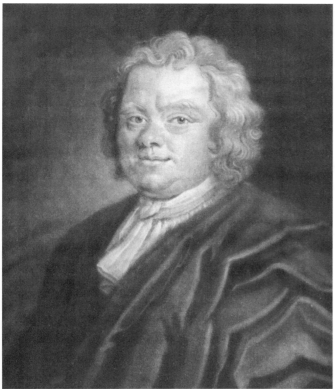

Herman Boerhaave

A FACULTY OF MEDICINE AT SURGEONS' HALL

In 1720, the Deacon of the Incorporation of Surgeons, John Monro, initiated a series of reforms at Surgeons' Hall. After completing his apprenticeship as a surgeon, John Monro had studied medicine at Leiden where he had been a fellow student of Boerhaave and had been taught by Archibald Pitcairn. Like Sibbald and other Scottish students before him, he had become inspired with an ambition to establish a medical school in Edinburgh on the model of Leiden. However, unlike Sibbald and Pitcairn, who had come to prominence under the Stuarts, John Monro was a Whig. His father, Sir Alexander Monro, had been convicted of treason in the last years of the reign of James II and had been lucky to escape with a pardon. In 1715, John Monro served as surgeon to the Hanoverian army that put an end to the Jacobite rebellion at Sheriffmuir. The Hanoverian army was commanded by Ilay's brother, the Duke of Argyll, and Ilay had been wounded in the battle; in the campaigns of the '15 Rebellion, Ilay had come to recognise Monro's professional abilities as well as his political loyalties. In 1720, John Monro could therefore be confident that his proposals for the reform of medical training in Edinburgh would be received sympathetically by Lord Ilay.

As Deacon of the Incorporation of Surgeons, John Monro required Adam Drummond and John McGill to relinquish their positions as Professors of Anatomy at Surgeons' Hall and proposed his son, Alexander, to replace them. In August 1720, Alexander informed the College

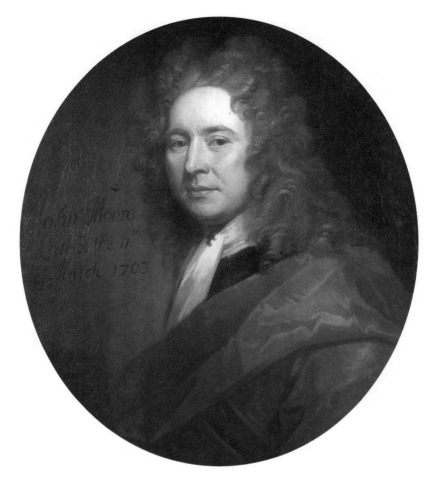

John Monro (Royal College of Surgeons)

of Physicians of his father's move to have him made Professor of Anatomy and 'craved a recommendation from them to the Magistrates of Edinburgh in his favour'. Alexander was well known to the College; he had been one of the surgical apprentices who had accompanied Fellows of the College in attending medical cases of 'uncommon interest'; when his surgical apprenticeship was completed he had gone on to study medicine at Leiden. The College readily agreed to his request. Recommended by the Incorporation of Surgeons and the College of Physicians and approved by Lord Ilay, Alexander was confirmed as the new Professor of Anatomy at Surgeons' Hall. In the following months, two further posts were created there. Charles Alston, the King's Botanist in Scotland and a Fellow of the College of Physicians, was recruited to teach botany and James Crawford, also a Fellow of the College of Physicians, was engaged to teach medical chemistry. By 1722, Surgeons' Hall had a school at which something approaching a comprehensive medical curriculum was taught by Fellows of the Royal College of Physicians and a medically trained member of the Incorporation of Surgeons.

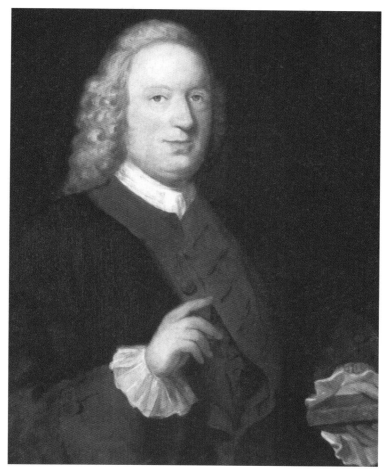

John Rutherford

In November 1723, William Porterfield, a graduate of Rheims and a Fellow of the College since 1721 asked the President and Council for their support in his application to be made a professor of medicine at Edinburgh University. In recommending Porterfield to the Town Council (as the governors of the university), John Drummond, the President of the College, took the occasion to present an argument for the creation of a faculty of medicine, an argument that had already been put forward several timers by Fellows of the College since 1705. Since Edinburgh had very recently been on the brink of bankruptcy it was an argument that was likely to carry weight with the Town Council in 1723. John Drummond drew their attention to:

> the great loss our youth sustain from not having medicine in all its parts taught
> in this place and the great advantage that would redound to such of the
> inhabitants of the good town of Edinburgh as have sons who are to follow

medicine by having them completely instructed in that science at home at no greater charge than a small gratification [remuneration] to the undertakers [instructors]; as also that, in the event, good numbers of students not only from all parts of our country but likewise from England and Ireland might be induced to come here for their improvement in medicine and spend money amongst us which otherwise they are obliged to carry abroad to foreign universities.

This argument, made again many times over the next twenty years, was to have great influence in the promotion of Edinburgh as a medical school to rival Leiden and the other leading medical schools of Europe.

A MEDICAL FACULTY AT THE UNIVERSITY

In August 1724 the Town Council duly granted Porterfield 'the powers, privileges and immunities' of a Professor. His appointment was not a success. The evidence suggests that he failed to attract any number of students. Certainly he gave no lectures and within months he had faded from the academic scene.[22] It seems probable that he succumbed to the competition offered by a private medical school set up only months after his appointment. In November 1724, John Rutherford, Andrew Sinclair, Andrew Plummer and John Innes, who had all recently studied at Leiden[23] and had all become Fellows of the College of Physicians only three weeks before, applied successfully to the Town Council for permission to take charge of the University's garden 'for furnishing the apothecaries shops with chemical medicines and instructing medical students in that part of the science'. They had already bought a house near the garden and equipped it for use as a laboratory. Their venture quickly proved successful and, in February 1726, they petitioned the Town Council 'to institute the professing of Medicine in the College of Edinburgh and appoint the petitioners to teach and profess the same'. The Town Council's Act of 1726 confirming their appointments is in effect the founding charter of the Medical Faculty of Edinburgh University. The Act stated:

> It would be of great advantage to this College, City and Country that Medicine in all its branches should be professed here by such number of professors of that science as may by themselves promote students to their degrees with as great a solemnity as is done in any other College or University at home or abroad. The Council does therefore unanimously constitute, nominate and appoint Doctors Andrew Sinclair and John Rutherford to be Professors of the Theory and Practice of Medicine, Doctors Andrew Plummer and John Innes to be Professors of Medicine and Chemistry in the College of Edinburgh; with full power to all of them to profess and teach Medicine in all its branches, to examine candidates and to do every other thing requisite and necessary to the graduation of doctors of medicine.

22. Grant, *The Story*, p. 307.
23. Only Plummer graduated at Leiden. Rutherford graduated at Reims, Sinclair at Angers and Innes at Padua.

In October 1726, Alexander Monro, the Professor of Anatomy, moved from Surgeons' Hall to teach within the University.[24] Later that month, the University informed the College of Physicians that 'there was now a sufficient number of professors to make a Faculty of Medicine'.[25] The Principal of the University thanked the College for its assistance in the past and expressed his determination that the University and the College would continue 'in good correspondence' in the future.

The College had reason to be well satisfied. From its foundation, it had advocated the creation of a school of medicine at Edinburgh. When the university medical school came into being in 1726, all but one of the members of the new Faculty of Medicine were Fellows of the College and the fifth, Alexander Monro, became a Fellow some years later. What had been established was a physicians' medical school but it could not have been founded without the exertions of the Deacon of the Incorporation of Surgeons, John Monro. Since his student years in the Netherlands, he had shared with the College of Physicians the ambition to create in Edinburgh a medical school to rival that at Leiden. But while the College of Physicians had been founded by a Stuart king and had continued to be tainted with Jacobitism, John Monro was a Whig and a loyal Hanoverian. In a Scotland managed by Lord Ilay in the interest of a Hanoverian king, John Monro had the standing and the political influence to accomplish what the College of Physicians alone could not.

25. Charles Alston continued to teach botany and, in September 1726, Joseph Gibson was appointed to teach midwifery. Both were 'city' Professors and neither was listed as a member of the new faculty of medicine in 1726. A. Dalzel, *History of the University of Edinburgh* (Edinburgh, 1862), p. 395.
26. College Minute, October 1726.

4

THE PHYSICIANS' HOSPITAL
Edinburgh Royal Infirmary

In 1714, Herman Boerhaave introduced the practice of teaching medical students at the bedside at the St Caecilia Hospital, a small charity hospital in Leiden. In 1721, a pamphlet was published advocating that Edinburgh should follow Leiden's example.[1] The author of this anonymous pamphlet reminded his readers that as 'Men and Christians' it was their duty 'to relieve our fellow creatures when in the utmost Distress from Pain and Trouble of Body and Anguish of Soul'. Great stress was also given to the economic arguments; first, that 'it is no less advantage to a nation, for as many as are recovered in an infirmary are so many working hands gained to the Country' and second, that 'students in physic and surgery might thereby have a rather better and easier opportunity of experience than they have hitherto had by studying abroad where such hospitals are at great charge to themselves and yearly loss to the Nation'. These economic arguments had been put forward before by the College of Physicians and would be again two years later. Although the pamphlet was published anonymously, it seems probable that it was written by a Fellow of the College.[2]

This appeal to the public at large attracted little or no response. In 1725 the College of Physicians tried a different approach. Fellows of the College appealed personally to likely donors among their friends and acquaintances. This proved to be very successful and on 1 February 1726, the President reported to the College that:

> he and several of the members had set on foot a subscription for erecting and maintaining an Infirmary or Hospital for the sick poor and had pretty good success and recommended to all members of the College to use their best endeavours to procure more subscriptions for accomplishing so good and charitable work.[3]

Nine months later, in November 1727 the President was able to inform the College the collection of 'the subscriptions for erecting the infirmary was complete' and that 'it was the members of the College that had set this charitable work on foot and had contributed for it themselves and procured contributions from other well disposed persons'.

---

1. The original document has been lost but it is quoted in full in A.L. Turner, *Story of A Great Hospital The Royal Infirmary of Edinburgh, 1729–1929* (Edinburgh, 1937), pp. 39–40.
2. It has been suggested by Sir Alexander Grant in *The Story of the History of the University of Edinburgh* (London, 1884), and repeated by A. L. Turner and other historians that the pamphlet was written by John Munro or his son Alexander but only on the unconvincing evidence that Alexander Munro later asked for the pamphlet to be re-issued.
3. College Minute.

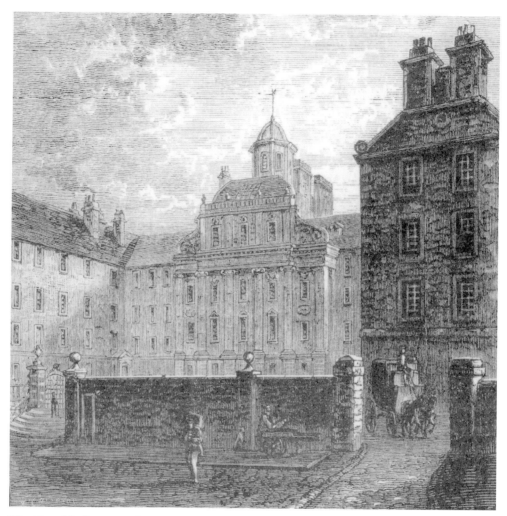

The Royal Infirmary of 1741

Responsibility for the project was now taken up by a new public body. On 19 February 1728 a meeting was called of all 'subscribers or contributors for erecting an infirmary or hospital for the sick poor' in the Burgh Room in Parliament Square. A minute of this meeting (the first minute of Edinburgh Royal Infirmary) records that 'the gentlemen of the Royal College of Physicians acquainted the meeting that the capital sum of £2000 designed for erecting the Infirmary was now subscribed'. A committee of twelve was formed to represent the Town Council, the Senators of the College of Justice, the Faculty of Advocates, the Royal College of Physicians, the Incorporation of Surgeons and the general body of subscribers; until 1742 this committee continued to meet in John's Coffee House in Parliament Close to manage the affairs of Edinburgh's new infirmary.

The infirmary ('Physicians' Hospital or Infirmary for the Sick Poor') was set up in a house in Robertson's Close in the Cowgate, near the College of Physicians' small garden at Fountain Close. Like the St Caecilia Hospital in Leiden, it had only six beds. The bedsteads were of wood and the mattresses of straw with cotton sheets and woollen blankets. The 'nursing' care of the patients was the responsibility of a housekeeper and one servant. The College arranged that all Fellows and Licentiates would 'attend the infirmary in their turn for the space of a fortnight until some more settled method be agreed on'. The Incorporation of Surgeons offered 'to furnish the sick and wounded in the infirmary with medicines and operations in society for two years'. However, it was later discovered that, by its Act of Incorporation, the Incorporation of Surgeons could not offer its services collectively ('in society') in this way. Six surgeons therefore agreed that, as individuals, they would 'divide the year equally among them; they would dispense gratis from their own shops the medicines prescribed by the physicians; and they would consult each other on all extra-ordinary surgical cases'.[4]

The infirmary was opened in 1729. The management committee ruled that the infirmary would admit as patients anyone 'residing in any county or burgh, or indeed in any country, provided they were true and worthy objects of charity and could produce, from a responsible person, a certificate of their honesty and poverty'.[5] With only six beds the new infirmary could be of only limited, even if very welcome, service to the sick poor. As a teaching hospital, it was an immediate success. John Rutherford, Professor of Medicine at Edinburgh University, became the first in Britain to teach clinical medicines at the bedside. Within eighteen months the number of students attending his clinical classes was threatening to become unmanageable. The establishment of a faculty of medicine in 1726 and the opening of a teaching hospital three years later had transformed the teaching of medicine in Edinburgh. After more than a quarter of a century, the College of Physicians had achieved one of its earliest objectives. Edinburgh had a medical school that could begin to compare with Europe's leading medical school at Leiden.

CARE FOR THE POOR

At its first meeting in 1681, the College had undertaken to provide medical aid for the poor. Scotland was then a poor country and, in the years that followed, the problems of poverty had become even more severe. In the 1690s disastrous harvest failures had caused widespread deprivation and, in several parts of Scotland, great loss of life from famine. The country had been slow to recover. Although harvests improved and there was no recurrence of famine, Scotland's economy remained depressed. Union with England in 1707 failed to produce the upturn in the country's economy that the people had been led to expect. The rebellion in Scotland in 1715 was as much an expression of discontent with the Union and a protest at Scotland's continuing poverty as a manifestation of support for the Jacobite cause.

In the 1740s, there were more years of failed harvests. Once again hunger and unemployment brought great numbers from the surrounding countryside flooding into

4. Turner, *The Story*, p. 57.
5. Ibid., p. 52.

Edinburgh in search of employment or simply to beg in the streets. Their arrival exacerbated the problems of an already overcrowded city. In 1700 the population of Edinburgh was less than 30,000; in the 1740s it had grown to over 50,000. Much of the fabric of the city was dilapidated. Most buildings were timbered, fires were common and in the economic depression of the time, repairs and restorations were often neglected. The water supply, piped in from springs at Comiston to a tank on Castle hill, was scarcely adequate and sewerage and refuse disposal were primitive in the extreme. Overcrowding, unhygienic living conditions and poverty led inevitably to a cruelly high infant mortality; typhus was endemic, increasing at times to almost epidemic proportions; but the diseases that did most to limit the expectation of life of the people of Edinburgh to thirty-seven years were tuberculosis, smallpox and dysentery.[6] In 1721, the College of Physicians had presented the Town Council with 'a plan to be put into execution to prevent and guard against pestilential infection'[7] but, whether from lack of will or from lack of funds, the plan had not been put into execution by the 1740s. Edinburgh remained overcrowded, disease-ridden and a place of refuge for great numbers of the poor and sick.

MEDICAL AID FOR THE POOR

It had long been the practice for the Town Council to employ a surgeon on a salary of '300 merks during the Council's pleasure'.[8] However, the Burgh Records indicate that the surgeon's time and energies were entirely given up to the care of the men of the Town Guard. The provision of medical aid for the poor of Edinburgh only began when the College of Physicians 'resolved that some persons be appointed by the College to be physicians to the poor'. From February 1682 two members of the College were appointed each year to make themselves available to attend the sick poor in their homes. In 1705, when the College had taken possession of its first College Hall at Fountain Close, the Fellows:

> unanimously agreed that two of their number shall attend at the place of meeting every Monday, Wednesday and Friday betwixt three and four in the afternoon for giving advice to the sick poor gratis and that the first day of their attendance shall be Wednesday the seventh day of November next.

This 'Dispensary' service continued at Fountain Close until 1729 when it was transferred to the new 'Physicians' Hospital or Infirmary for the Sick Poor'. The College also provided medical care at two later charitable institutions. In 1731, a Charity Workhouse was endowed jointly by the Town Council and the Kirk Sessions of Edinburgh. This first small house was later replaced by a building 'four stories in height, very spacious, but plain, massive and dingy';[9] an annexe contained twenty-one cells for the reception of lunatics. In 1733, an Orphan Hospital was founded for 'helpless orphans and distressed infants of indigent parents'; its Charter provided that two of its governors should be Fellows of College of Physicians.

6. T. Ferguson, *The Dawn of Scottish Social Welfare* (Edinburgh, 1948), p. 73.
7. College Minute, 31 October 1721.
8. H. Arnot, *The History of Edinburgh* (Edinburgh, 1779), p. 241.
9. W.S. Craig, *History of the Royal College of Physicians of Edinburgh* (Edinburgh, 1976), p. 496.

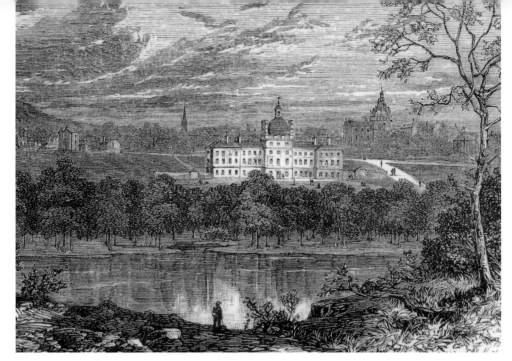

New Royal Infirmary

In 1736, the Incorporation of Surgeons, whose members played only a subsidiary role in the Infirmary, opened its own six-bed 'Surgeons' Hospital' for the poor. However the combined services of the College of Physicians and the Incorporation of Surgeons could not pretend to meet the needs of Edinburgh's sick poor. In 1748 their small institutions were superseded by the new Infirmary.

GEORGE DRUMMOND

The Edinburgh Royal Infirmary was the greatest of the charitable institutions founded in the city in the eighteenth century. It was planned as a much larger and finer successor to the 'Hospital or Infirmary for the Sick Poor' founded by the College of Physicians in 1729. For many years after the new Royal Infirmary was completed, it continued to be a physicians' hospital. However it was the creation, not of the physicians themselves, but of one of Edinburgh's most remarkable Lord Provosts.

George Drummond was born in 1687 at Newton Castle in Perthshire. His father, a member of the lesser landed gentry, supplemented his income as a merchant in Edinburgh. George was educated first at home and later in Edinburgh. As a schoolboy he was recognised as a considerable mathematician. At the age of seventeen he was employed as a secretary by Sir John Clerk of Penicuik, an influential Whig politician then campaigning for the Union of the English and Scottish Parliaments. He helped prepare Sir John Clerk's reports to Parliament and when, in 1705, Clerk became one of the Commissioners appointed to negotiate the terms of the Treaty of Union, George Drummond was entrusted by the Scottish Parliament with the calculation of the valuation of Scotland for tax and rating purposes. After the Union in 1707, in recognition of his services, he was made Accountant-General of Excise; ten years later he was promoted and made a Commissioner of Customs and, in 1723, a member of the Board of Customs, positions he resigned only a year before his death at the age of seventy-nine. While holding these offices he reported to the Whig government in London, keeping it informed of Jacobite activities in Scotland. At the same time he used what influence he had acquired with Walpole's government in London and with its representatives in Edinburgh to boost commerce, manufacturing and the fishing industry in Scotland.

In 1716, George Drummond had been appointed to Edinburgh's Town Council and a year later, when the town's finances were in great difficulty, he was elected as Treasurer. He succeeded in saving the city from bankruptcy and, in 1725, he became Lord Provost for the first time. He was an unconventional choice. He was not, as was customary, a wealthy merchant or an outstandingly successful craftsman but a salaried government official.[10] He qualified as a candidate for office only as the son of a merchant and as a partner in a small (and unsuccessful) business. However, his energy and his ambition to revive the fortunes of the city won the support of even the most conventional of the burgesses.

During his first terms of office his relationship with the Earl of Ilay, Walpole's agent in Scotland, was difficult. Drummond was a staunch and strictly orthodox Calvinist at a time when Lord Ilay, the most powerful political figure in Scotland, was intent on promoting those who supported the moderate faction in the Scottish church. In 1735, Drummond confided to his diary:

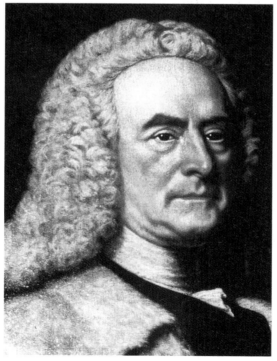

George Drummond
(Lothian Health Service Archive)

10. As the son of a burgess Drummond was allowed to trade. From 1712 he was a partner with James Nimmo and John Campbell in a trading company that ceased trading after only six years leaving him deeply in debt.

> My Lord Ilay has thrown the town's affairs into the hands of men void of
> religion, and little respected in the place. I am looked on as an enemy to their
> measures and have carefully avoided meddling with them. It is surely dangerous
> for me to speak my sentiments. May I have light from the Lord to be faithful
> and prudent, for I dwell among lions.

In private Drummond was timid and insecure but he could be physically brave in a crisis[11] and he was always resourceful and effective in office. In spite of their differences, Lord Ilay valued Drummond's financial expertise and his political skills. With the support of the burgesses and the backing of Ilay and successive Hanoverian governments in London, Drummond was to serve no fewer than six terms as Provost of Edinburgh. For over forty years he took the lead in rescuing Old Edinburgh from its dilapidation and in creating a New Town that, later in the century became the physical expression of the Scottish Enlightenment.

One of George Drummond's early ventures as Lord Provost was to prop up the small 'Physicians' Hospital or Infirmary for the Sick Poor'. The College of Physicians had raised sufficient funds to set up the hospital but not enough to provide for its maintenance. An appeal to the General Assembly of the Church of Scotland to 'recommend a voluntary contribution at the several parishes of this Kingdom for advancing this charitable work'[12] was made but met with only very modest success. As Lord Provost, George Drummond was a member of the new hospital's management committee. He suggested that the shareholders in a fishery company that he managed could be persuaded to sell and sign over their stock to a fund he had created to help maintain the hospital. He then persuaded the magistrates of Edinburgh and the Bank of Scotland to contribute the greater part of the purchase price. With this nucleus of funding and a number of smaller donations the hospital survived its first years.

In 1730, John Clerk, a Fellow of the College of Physicians, wrote to the Lord Advocate, his friend Duncan Forbes, that although the hospital had been successfully set up 'it would be impractical to carry it much further without public encouragement'; if the hospital were to be granted a Royal Charter this 'would establish the most charitable work that was ever projected in this country'. This personal appeal to the Lord Advocate was unsuccessful. A year later the managers of the hospital appointed George Drummond, John Drummond (Past President of the Royal College of Physicians), Charles Erskine (Solicitor General), and Thomas Pringle to draw up a petition for submission to George II. A Royal Charter was granted and in 1736 the Physicians' Hospital or Infirmary for the Sick Poor became the Edinburgh Royal Infirmary.

Drummond was now no longer Lord Provost and, in 1737, he fell foul of Lord Ilay. He remained out of favour with Ilay and the Whig administration until he distinguished himself by his vigorous opposition to the Jacobite Rebellion in 1745. It was during these eight years in the political wilderness that he was able to devote his energies to the building of a new Edinburgh Royal Infirmary.

11. In 1715 George Drummond raised his own Company of Volunteers and fought with distinction in the Duke of Argyll's army at Sheriffmuir.
12. College Minute, 7 May 1728.

The Infirmary's Charter 'erected … the Contributors and Donors into a Corporation with power to take donations, to purchase lands … to erect houses … and all other things that may tend to promote the said charitable Design'. Fund-raising pamphlets (possibly written by George Drummond and Alexander Monro[13]) distributed in Edinburgh in the following years stressed that, while the Infirmary would provide services for the poor, it would also bring great economic benefit to Edinburgh. The pamphlets claimed that, like charity hospitals elsewhere, the Infirmary would serve the town by getting people back to work. What was distinctive, even unique, was the proposition that Edinburgh Royal Infirmary would generate wealth by providing for the teaching of medical students.[14] Once Edinburgh's medical school could boast a large modern hospital it would attract Dissenters and Catholics from England and Ireland who were debarred from matriculating at Oxford, Cambridge or Trinity College, Dublin; it would also attract students from countries with no medical schools of their own. Edinburgh would become host to a population of young men who had nothing to do but study and spend money. (It was later estimated that in the thirty years that followed the establishment of the university's medical faculty, Edinburgh received over £300,000 from medical students.[15]) The author of the pamphlets also predicted that Edinburgh could expect to gain a further £100,000 annually when former students returned with the 'fortunes they had acquired abroad'.

The Royal Charter of the Infirmary laid down that there should be a governing body of twenty managers. The Lord Provost of Edinburgh, the President of the Royal College of Physicians, the Dean of Guild and the Professor of Anatomy were included *ex-officio*. The remaining sixteen were to be elected annually: four from the Royal College of Physicians (of whom two to be Professors of Medicine in the University), two from the Incorporation of Surgeons, one from the College of Justice, one from the Faculty of Advocates, one from the Society of the Clerks to the Senate, one Minister of the Gospel in Edinburgh and six from the contributors to the charity.

In November 1736, the trustees of George Watson's Hospital offered for sale a plot of land between the University and High School Yards; for the sum of £420 the land was bought as the site for a new Royal Infirmary and in 1738 the managers commissioned William Adam to design and build a hospital of some 200 beds 'which might be executed piecemeal' as funds and materials became available. They particularly required that there should be an 'anatomy theatre' or 'operating room' to accommodate two or three hundred students. George Drummond, Alexander Monro, representing the university, Andrew Sinclair of the College of Physicians and George Cunynghame of the Incorporation Surgeons were appointed as a Building Committee but there seems no doubt that Drummond, who personally carried out the day-to-day supervision of the work and paid the workmen with his 'own hands', was the true manager of the project.

The Royal Charter laid down that patients in the new Royal Infirmary would continue to be 'entertained and cared for by the Royal College of Physicians and some of the most skilful

13. Professor of Anatomy and later a Fellow of the Royal College of Physicians
14. C. Stevenson, *Medicine and Magnificence* (Yale, 2000), p. 113.
15. Ibid.

surgeons'. However, there was considerable dissatisfaction with the arrangements which had been in place since the original 'Hospital or Infirmary' was founded in 1729. The large number of Fellows and Licentiates of the College in the rota of attending physicians, the very short duration of each period of their attendance and the long intervals between each period tended to disrupt the continuity of patient care and detract from the teaching of students. And the Incorporation of Surgeons continued to resent its corporate exclusion from the Infirmary and the small number of individual attending surgeons felt they were being used 'more like hired servants than useful members and benefactors'.[16]

To meet the first of these objections, and in anticipation of the building of a much larger infirmary, new arrangements were agreed in 1738. The number of attending physicians was reduced by excluding Licentiates from the rota. To meet the discontent of the surgeons it was agreed that, when the new infirmary was opened, all master surgeons of the Incorporation who wished 'to oblige themselves to the Royal Infirmary' would be included in the rota of surgeons; on this understanding, the Incorporation of Surgeons transferred the financial stock of the Surgeons' Hospital (£500) to the Royal Infirmary and agreed that the services of the Surgeons' Hospital would be merged with those of the new Royal Infirmary.

Nevertheless, when the new Infirmary opened in 1741 it was still as a physician's hospital. Every Fellow of the College of Physicians was entitled to be included as an attending physician. The attendance and authority of the surgeons was to be carefully regulated by the Managers. Four surgeons (two for each floor of the Infirmary) from a list of participating surgeons drawn up by the Incorporation were to provide their services each month. But 'no operation of surgery by which the life of the patient is endangered shall be performed unless by the joint opinion of three surgeons and of the physician under whose care the patient is'.

The distinction intended by the managers of the Infirmary in 1741 was not that between the learned physician and the highly skilled surgeon; it was rather the emerging distinction between the recognised specialist and the general practitioner. The Fellows of the College of Physicians attending the Infirmary were university graduates whose learning and skills had been scrutinised by examination. The members of the Incorporation of Surgeons had all served an apprenticeship with masters who served the city as general practitioners; their experience of operative surgery during their apprenticeship was, in many cases, extremely limited and, in consequence, the practical skills of those offering their services to the Infirmary were very uncertain.

The caution of the managers of the Infirmary in allowing responsibility to individual surgeons continued into the second half of the century. In 1751, because of 'the increased number of patients and the expected further rise' the managers appointed 'two fixed physicians under the character of physicians-in-ordinary for the constant and daily attendance on the patients and requested the College to appoint some of their number monthly by rotation to visit the house once or twice a week to give advice and assistance to the two ordinary

16. H. Dingwall, *A Famous and Flourishing Society: The History of the Royal College of Surgeons of Edinburgh* (Edinburgh, 2005), p. 101.

physicians when they judge it necessary to apply to them for the same'.[17] The managers also decreed that 'in cases wholly internal the physicians are to be the judges of the patients ... and in like manner the surgeons in cases wholly external'.[18] However, in difficult cases the surgeons were still required to consult the relevant physician before operating and the physician could still require the attending surgeon to carry out post-mortems on their patients. The relative position of surgeons began to change in 1766 when 'surgeons-in-ordinary were appointed in line with the Infirmary's salaried physicians-in-ordinary. Equality of status within the Infirmary came only after the Incorporation of Surgeons became recognised as a learned and academic society and was reborn as the Royal College of Surgeons of Edinburgh in 1778.

When the first wards of the new Edinburgh Royal Infirmary opened in 1748, the managers were already confident that they had founded 'undoubtedly the most noble institution in Edinburgh reared by the hand of charity'.[19] When the building was completed it had grown to 'an aristocratic structure of stone and lime with all the pomp of capitals and quoins, friezes and architraves'.[20] Its 228 beds received over 1,600 patients every year. Its central amphitheatre could accommodate over three hundred students. It was the largest teaching hospital in Britain and an essential institution in what had become recognised as 'the pre-eminent centre of medical Education in the English speaking world'.[21]

17. College Minute, 5 February 1751.
18. Dingwall, *A Famouis*, p. 100.
19. Arnot, *The History*, p. 546.
20. G. B. Risse, *Hospital Life in Enlightenment Scotland* (Cambridge, 1986), p. 30.
21. C. Lawrence, Ornate Physicians and Learned Artisans in W.F. Bynum and R. Porter, *William Hunter and the Eighteenth-Century Medical World* (Cambridge, 1985), p. 153.

5

PRE-EMINENCE
Cullen and the Curriculum

Edinburgh's university medical school was founded in 1726 as a small provincial school on the model of the great school at Leiden. Before the end of the century it had become pre-eminent among the medical schools of Europe, offering a unique system of learning and a curriculum that included aspects of medicine that were taught nowhere else.

Those who brought about this transformation were the physicians, Robert Whytt, Alexander Monro, William Cullen, Joseph Black, John Gregory, James Gregory and Andrew Duncan, all presidents of Edinburgh's Royal College of Physicians. Each one made his own essential contribution but little would have been achieved without the vision and the organising genius of William Cullen. Cullen was one of the leaders of the intellectual life of Edinburgh, able to command the patronage of the most powerful men in Scotland; for almost half a century he dominated the College of Physicians, extending its library and housing it in a new prestigious College Hall in Edinburgh's New Town; during these same years he was a professor of medicine at Edinburgh University, occupying the most senior chair for the greater part of that time. It was from these positions of influence that he managed the transformation of Edinburgh University's medical school. The story of that transformation is the story of the College of Physicians in those years. It is also the story of William Cullen.

WILLIAM CULLEN

William Cullen was born in April 1710, the son of a landowner with an estate near Hamilton in Lanarkshire and farms in the parishes of Bothwell and Shotts. Cullen inherited the family lands in 1731 and later bought more farming property in the outskirts of Glasgow. Throughout his life Cullen maintained a passionate interest in agriculture and farming technology. It was his contribution to agricultural improvement that earned him his place among the landowning elite of the Scottish Enlightenment.

William Cullen was educated at the grammar school in Hamilton and at Glasgow University. While he was a student at Glasgow, the ancient regenting system was abolished and new chairs were created in logic and metaphysics, moral philosophy and natural philosophy. In addition to these core subjects Cullen studied mathematics and botany. At the age of seventeen he left university without taking a degree and was apprenticed to a Glasgow surgeon, John Paisley. Paisley owned a large library and Cullen read widely in philosophy and the new sciences of natural philosophy. He very soon abandoned all thought of becoming a surgeon and decided to make his career as a physician. After only two years he was released from his apprenticeship and, perhaps persuaded by the dictum that 'the best physicians travelled to the places where their drugs were bought to inform themselves concerning them',[1] he travelled to London where he joined a ship setting out on a voyage to the Spanish settlements in the West Indies. The ship was commanded by his cousin, Captain Cleland of Auchinlee. Since Cullen did not have a licence to practise as a surgeon, Captain Cleland entered him on the ships list as a surgeon's mate.

At Portobello, in Cuba, Cullen spent several months botanising and studying the effects of climate on health and disease. On his return to London, he spent some months improving his practical experience of *materia medica* as an assistant to an apothecary, William Murray.[2] While in London he attended the lectures at which interested members of the public could hear of the work of members of the Royal Society; it was probably in London that he first recognised the possibilities of philosophical chemistry.[3] A new branch of natural philosophy distinct from the force-mechanics of Isaac Newton, this new chemistry promised to be of importance not only in the understanding of health and disease but also in the advancement of agriculture and industry.

On his return to Scotland in 1732, Cullen lived for a time at Auchinlee, in Lanarkshire, to take care of Captain Cleland's son who was 'affected with a lingering disorder'[4] and to offer his medical skills to friends and acquaintances in the district. At Auchinlee, he was able to combine his undemanding medical duties with the management of the family estates he had recently inherited from his brother. He also continued to read widely on the new chemistry and the recent medical works of Stahl, Hoffman and Haller on the nervous system.

In 1734 he received a legacy that made it possible for him to give up practice and devote himself entirely to his studies. He spent the winter sessions of 1734–35 and 1735–36 in Edinburgh attending classes at the university medical school where 'the whole art of medicine was being taught in a systematic way'.[5] In the summer of 1736 he felt ready to set up as a general practitioner in Hamilton where, as a neighbour and a friend, he could expect to be consulted by 'all the families of any consideration in the neighbourhood'.[6] However, he was still determined to become recognised as a physician. In 1740 he took his MD degree at Glasgow and in 1741 he was at last able to give up general practice (with its embarrassing calls to practise surgery for which he had had no inclination) when he formed a partnership with Thomas Hamilton, a surgical Fellow of the Royal Faculty of Physicians and Surgeons of Glasgow. Three years later Cullen was elated a Fellow of the Faculty *qua physician*.

Practising as physician but with a practice limited to the 'families of consideration' at Hamilton, Cullen had ample time to add to his already considerable library and to continue with his chemical experiments in his private laboratory.[7] During these years in Hamilton, he

1. Sir Hans Sloane, quoted in A.L. Donovan, *Philosophical Chemistry in the Scottish Enlightenment* (Edinburgh, 1979) p. 4.
2. Murray corresponded with friends in Hamilton and must have been at least an acquaintance of the Cullen family.
3. Referred to at this time as philosophical chemistry to distinguish it from alchemy and the practices used in the preparation of medicines.
4. J. Thomson, *An Account of the Life Letters and Writings of William Cullen, MD*, (Edinburgh, 1856), Vol. I, p. 7.
5. *Dr Fothergill's Account of the Edinburgh School of Medicine* quoted in Thomson, *An Account*, Vol. I, pp. 523–5.
6. Thomson, *An Account*, Vol. I, p. 11.
7. The laboratory promised by the Duke of Hamilton was never completed.

was 'industriously employed in qualifying himself to occupy a position more favourable for the exercise of his talents'.[8] His aim was to establish a university school of medicine at Glasgow University on the model of school already flourishing at Edinburgh.

At Glasgow University, John Johnstoun had been appointed as Professor of Medicine in 1714 but he had few students, taught seldom and gave no formal lectures. In 1718, a new chair of anatomy and botany had been created but the first professor had died soon after his appointment and Thomas Brisbane had been appointed in his place. Brisbane was the most successful and most fashionable of Glasgow's physicians and had little time for teaching; he failed to provide any demonstrations of anatomy and gave few lectures on botany. In spite of repeated warnings and admonitions by the university's visitors neither Johnstoun or Brisbane could be persuaded to teach more effectively.[9] When Brisbane died in 1742, Robert Hamilton was appointed to the chair of Professor of Anatomy and Botany. There were now many calls for Cullen to take over Brisbane's practice. Cullen refused to be persuaded until, in 1744, Glasgow University offered him access to a lecture theatre where he might have 'full scope for the display of his knowledge and talents'.[10]

Cullen moved to Glasgow early in 1745. In September of that year Glasgow became embroiled in the Jacobite rebellion and it was not until the winter session of 1746 that he gave his first lectures on the practice and theory of medicine. In the summer of 1748, he gave his first course on botany and materia medica. In 1751 he succeeded John Johnstoun as Professor of Physic and thereafter he continued with these winter and summer courses for medical students until he gave up the chair in 1756. During his years in Glasgow, abandoning tradition, he 'laid aside the use of the Latin language' and lectured in the vernacular.[11] He did not read or dictate his lectures nor did he produce a textbook of his own; he provided his students with constantly updated abstracts of his lectures. He quickly gained a reputation as an excellent teacher. Nevertheless, the number of medical students attending his class continued to be very small.

The great success of Cullen's ten years in Glasgow came from his public lectures on chemistry. In 1748, a printed advertisement distributed by the university announced the first of his courses of 'Chemical Lectures and Experiments Directed Chiefly to the Improvement of Arts and Manufacturers'. Many years later, one of Cullen's students recalled that 'the number of students in [Cullen's] Physic classes and Materia Medica were very few, not above twenty. But in Chemistry the number was considerable, the lectures being calculated not only for medical students but for the general students of the university and for gentlemen engaged in any business connected with chemistry'.[12]

Cullen's lectures were not on chemistry as applied to the preparation of medicines but on the new philosophical chemistry. In his introductory lecture he thought it necessary to explain

8. Thomson, *An Account*, Vol. I, p. 18.
9. R. L. Emerson and P. Wood, Science and Enlightenment in Glasgow, 1690–1802 in C.W.J. Withers and P. Wood, *Science and Medicine in the Scottish Enlightenment* (East Linton, 2002), p. 96.
10. Thomson, *An Account*, Vol. I, p. 19.
11. The exception was in botany. Cullen could find no English alternatives for the Latin names used by botanists for the parts and classifications of plants so continued to lecture in Latin.
12. Letter from Robert Wallace to William Cullen, 1811, quoted by Thomson, *An Account*, p. 25

to the medical students in his audience the relevance of his philosophical chemistry to their studies.

> The human economy cannot be well understood unless we study also that of other animals. The study of animals therefore becomes necessarily a part of the study of physic … A physician must aim at finding the causes of the phenomena in the natural world. He must in short carefully study the principles of natural philosophy. Natural philosophy consists in two parts the one of which explains the general properties of bodies and is called the mathematical or mechanical part of Natural Philosophy. The other part explains the particular properties of bodies and is called the chemical branch of natural philosophy. The mechanical branch of natural philosophy is certainly necessary to a physician and I am afraid that it is not attended to at present so much as it deserves but I must own that the chemical philosophy is still more necessary.[13]

Cullen had no such need to proclaim the importance of chemistry to the 'gentlemen engaged in business'. The entrepreneurs of Scotland's new and expanding textile industry were vitally interested in the chemistry of bleaching. Industrialists looked for advances in the production of industrial alkali for the manufacture of soap and glass. Mine owners looked for guidance in the exploitation of mineral ores. Improving landowners understood that a knowledge of chemistry could assist them in increasing the productivity and profitability of their land. And James Watt, Mathematical Instrument Maker to Glasgow University and improver of the steam engine, had his own particular interest in Cullen's studies on heat and evaporation.[14]

Within a few years Cullen came to be valued by the 'practical' men who were then beginning the transformation of Glasgow from a small university town into a great industrial city. Even more important for the future of his career, he became accepted among the 'improving' landed gentry who were leading an agricultural revolution in Scotland. Through them he established long-lasting friendships with some of the leading figures of what was later recognised as the Scottish Enlightenment: Lord Kames, lawyer and agriculturalist; the economist Adam Smith, then Professor of Logic at Glasgow; the philosopher David Hume, whom he had tried to have appointed as Adam Smith's successor in that chair; the chemist and physician Joseph Black; the engineer James Watt. It was at this time too that he began regular international correspondence with Carl Linnaeus and other European leaders in the new sciences.

However, after some six years in Glasgow, Cullen was disappointed in the progress he had made in the medical world. He had been elected president of the Royal Faculty of Physicians and Surgeons of Glasgow and he had begun to form the network of medical colleagues and students that over the next forty years would spread his ideas throughout Britain.[15] But he had

---

13. W. Cullen, Lectures on Chemistry. MS, College Archive.
14. It was Cullen's student, Joseph Black, who introduced Watt to the concept of latent heat, the concept that led to the invention of the condenser and Watt's first successful steam engine.
15. J. Uglow, *The Lunar Men* (London, 2002), p. 29.

made little progress towards achieving his ambition to establish a faculty of medicine at Glasgow University and his medical practice had proved to be an unwelcome and financially unrewarding diversion from his teaching and research in chemistry. In August 1751 he wrote to William Hunter in London:

> I am quite tired of my present life; I have a good deal of country practice, which takes up a great deal of time and hardly even allows an hour's leisure. I get but little money for my labour; and indeed by country practice a man cannot make money as he cannot overtake a great deal of business. On this account I have some thoughts of acceding to a proposal that was lately made to me of removing to Edinburgh. Dr Plummer, Professor of Chemistry, a very rich man, has given up practice and had proposed to give up teaching in favour of Dr Elliot; but this gentleman died about six weeks ago and upon this event some friends of mine and along with some gentlemen concerned with the administration of the Town of Edinburgh have proposed to use their influence with Dr Plummer to induce him to resign in my favour.

Joseph Black

The 'friends' and 'gentlemen' of Cullen's letter were Lord Kames, David Hume and George Drummond the Lord Provost of Edinburgh and Chancellor of Edinburgh University. However, their efforts to secure the Edinburgh chair of chemistry for Cullen came to nothing.

Three years later, in 1754, Lord Kames suggested to Cullen that he should move to Edinburgh and 'give a private course of lectures on chemistry which will be successful and will make you a favourite with the College of Physicians';[16] meanwhile Kames and his friends would 'think of measures to treat with Plummer or Alston[17] about a resignation'. Cullen hesitated, having 'scarce the courage for so bold a step',[18] but a few months later Plummer suffered a stroke. Cullen now became a candidate to succeed him. His chief rival was Francis Home, a Fellow of the College of Physicians who had strong support within the College and among the members of the Town Council, the patrons of the University. However, Cullen had the backing not only of George Drummond but also, and even more crucially, the Duke of Argyll (the former Lord Ilay). Argyll, the Keeper of the Great Seal and the manager of government patronage in Scotland, had assumed control of appointments to the Scottish universities[19] he had met Cullen and been impressed by his chemical experiments, particularly his work on the purification of salt, an industrial process in which the Duke had a financial interest.[20] In November 1755 Cullen was duly appointed to be joint Professor of Chemistry during Plummer's lifetime and to succeed him on his death.

16. Letter, Lord Kames to William Cullen, 17 September 1754. College Archive.
17. Plummer was still Professor of Chemistry and Alston Professor of Botany.
18. Letter, Lord Kames to William Cullen, 30 September 1754. College Archive.
19. Argyll made over fifty university appointments and was largely responsible for the modernisation of Scotland's universities. R. Graham, *The Great Infidel* (Edinburgh, 2004), p. 15.
20. Argyll had a commercial interest in the production and marketing of salt.

CULLEN IN EDINBURGH

Cullen arrived in Edinburgh in January 1756. He received no salary from the university but he quickly built up a vast private practice extending far beyond Edinburgh and carried on in large part by correspondence. (His friend, James Watt, added to the efficiency of his correspondence by inventing and providing him with a copying machine.[21]) Almost from the moment of his arrival he began to dominate the medical scene in Edinburgh. In less than a year he had become Secretary of the Royal College of Physicians, an office he held for almost a decade; in 1773 he was elected President of the College; thereafter he continued as an influential member of Council until his death. At Edinburgh University, he became sole Professor of Chemistry following the death of Andrew Plummer in July 1756; he was appointed as Professor of the Theory of Physic in 1766 and from 1773 until 1789 he occupied the most prestigious of the medical chairs in the University as Professor of the Practice of Physic. In his early years at Edinburgh University he had the continuing support of the influential and long-serving Provost, George Drummond, the Chancellor of the University. Until 1760, he also continued to enjoy the patronage of the Duke of Argyll; when his friend and dining companion, Henry Dundas, became the political manager of Scotland in the 1770s he was once again assured of the support of the country's most powerful politician.

Dining played an important part in Cullen's life. He became a member of both the Rankenian Club and the smaller but even more distinguished Oyster Club; there and at other clubs and private dinners he debated and drank with his friends Adam Smith, David Hume, William Roberson, Adam Ferguson, Joseph Black, Lord Kames, Lord Mondobbo and James Hutton. Over dinner he met every distinguished visitor to Edinburgh from Sam Johnson to Benjamin Franklin. Cullen was one of the *virtuosi* who made Edinburgh the centre of intellectual life in eighteenth-century Britain

CULLEN, THE COLLEGE LIBRARY AND THE COLLEGE HALL

In March 1756 Cullen was elected a Fellow of the College of Physicians and, before the end of the year, he was appointed Secretary of the College. At the same time he became the 'keeper of the library' and he continued in that role until a librarian was appointed in 1772.

The College library had begun as 'a presse with three shelves of books' presented by Sir Robert Sibbald in 1681. These eighty-five books included 'Galen's works, five volumes in Greek and five in Latin and Hippocrates in Greek' with other sixteenth- and seventeenth-century works on medicine, surgery, botany, philosophy and history. In the College's first years there were donations of books from other Edinburgh libraries; John Hope of Hopetoun presented ten volumes of the works of Jerome Cardun, the sixteenth-century Professor of Medicine at Padua who had travelled to Scotland and successfully treated the Archbishop of St Andrews for asthma;[22] Sir George Mackenzie, the founder of the Advocates Library, gave five

---

21. Now in the Royal Scottish Museum in Edinburgh.
22. He ordered Archbishop Hamilton to avoid feathers, to amend his diet and to take more exercise.

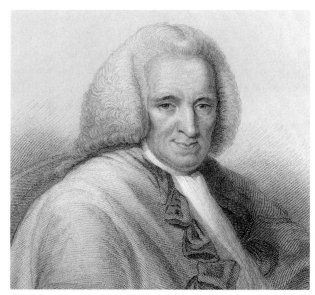

Lord Kames

manuscript volumes on alchemy;[23] John Drummond, the Treasurer of Scotland presented eleven volumes containing the works of his ancestor, the poet William Drummond of Hawthornden. Important contributions were made by friends of the founding members of the College; Archibald Pitcairn's fellow mathematicians, Sir Isaac Newton and David Gregory, Professor of Astronomy at Oxford, presented copies of their works; Thomas Burnet's brother Gilbert, the Bishop of Salisbury gave several volumes including a copy of his *History of the Reformation of the Church of England*; Andrew Balfour's old friend and fellow student, Sir Charles Scarborough, the King's physician, contributed books from his library. However, most additions to the library came from the Fellows themselves. In 1696, it was enacted by the College that every new Fellow must 'present a book to the library, one or more as they see fit'.

In the years before the College found a permanent home the number of books increased to over 500 and the 'presse' containing the library had to be transported, at some risk of damage to the books, from one temporary College meeting place to another. In the course of some twenty years several of the books became damaged and some may well have been lost.

In 1704 the College bought a house in Fountain Close, a lane running from the High Street to the Cowgate. In this, the first College Hall, the library was made more secure and more readily accessible to Fellows. The College began to 'spend lavishly on books'[24] and in the next fifty years the College also received many more generous donations. Sir Hans Sloane presented copies of his books including his *The Natural History of Jamaica*. In 1741, the bequest of the

23. Sir George, who became the Earl of Cromarty was the 'Bloody Mackenzie' of the Covenanting persecutions; one of his gifts included a method for discovering the philosopher's stone. The manuscripts given to the College had previously been owned by Napier of Merchiston.
24. L. Jolly, Medical Libraries of Great Britain: II Medical Libraries of Scotland, *British Medical Bulletin*, 1952, Vol. 8, No. 2, p. 256.

books collected by John Drummond, a former President of the College, more than doubled the size of the library. There were new important books by Fellows including Robert Whytt's *Essay on the Vital and Other Involuntary Motions of Animals* and Sir John Pringle's *Observations of the Diseases of the Army in Camp and in Garrison.*

When Cullen became 'keeper of the library' in 1756 the number of books had risen to well over 2,000 and the library had outgrown all the available space. The College was already discarding 'duplicates' and 'those not proper for making part of a medical library'. Cullen was asked to report on 'the present state of the library' and to advise on the 'measures that seem necessary for its better arrangement'. He reported that the library space was both inadequate and insecure; the roof of the College Hall leaked and the books were being damaged by rainwater. Cullen advised the College that there was now an urgent need to build a new hall, 'particularly for the purpose of the library'. A building committee was appointed with Cullen as its chairman.

The first task was to raise funds. Cullen's specification for 'a Hall, Library and Museum' was sent for his comment to Robert Adam, the leading architect of the time. Cullen and his committee were dismayed by his response; in his opinion Cullen's plan was 'quite unworthy of the body for which it was intended'. Adam submitted a plan of his own. Unfortunately the estimated cost of building the College Hall that Adam had in mind was £5,500, a sum 'much beyond the power of a society which has no funds beyond eight hundred pounds'. The project to build a new hall, library and museum was abandoned.

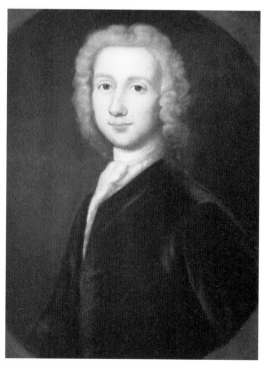

Robert Whytt

Cullen now received two proposals for the housing of the College's large and valuable collection of books. The Principal of the University, William Robertson, proposed that the College library should be united with the university's medical library to form a single medical library for Edinburgh. Robert Whytt suggested that the College library should simply be donated to the university. Both proposals were warmly supported but after much anxious discussion, both were rejected. Instead, it was decided to spend £600 on repairs to the existing Hall and on providing additional shelf space in the library.

In 1765 the plan to build a new College Hall and Library was revived. Since 1725 George Drummond, as Edinburgh's Lord Provost, had been promoting a scheme to build a new town on the slopes of Moutrie's Hill and Barefoot's Park on the north side of Edinburgh's Nor' Loch. In October 1763 he had at last been able to lay the foundation stone of the bridge that would link the Old Town with the New Town and, in 1765, negotiations had begun with the owners of the land on which the New Town was to be built. A member of Cullen's building committee suggested that the Town Council might be willing to grant the College a site for a new hall and library on the land being bought for the New Town. The Lord Provost and the Town Council agreed in principle but 'as there was no plan of the building intended to be made on Moutrie's Hill and Barefoot's Park yet determined on, they could not at present allocate any particular area' for a new College Hall.

The College's building plan was now once again on hold while the fabric of the hall at Fountain Close continued to deteriorate. In February 1766, the roof again began to leak and the books were once again at great risk of being damaged by rainwater. In this emergency the books were immediately transferred to an empty ward in the Royal Infirmary. The fabric of the College deteriorated still further and six months later all meetings and activities of the College were also transferred to the Royal Infirmary and the property at Fountain Close was offered for sale.[25]

Over the next few years the prospect of a home for the College on a new site on the north side of the Nor' Loch seemed to fade ever further into the distance. There had already been prolonged disputes over the layout of the New Town and delays in the allocation of a site for the new College when, in August 1769, progress was brought to a complete halt. At a very late stage in its construction, the bridge being built as the principal means of access to the site of the proposed New Town suddenly collapsed. It was immediately evident that a new College and Library in the new town could not be built, perhaps for some years. The building committee was disbanded and the College settled down for a prolonged stay at its temporary home. Housed at the Royal Infirmary, the library continued to grow; now assured that his gift could be kept safely, the Earl of Bute, recently King George III's first minister, presented the twenty-six magnificent volumes of Sir John Hill's *Vegetable System*. More donations followed and Fellows of the College continued to add their own works.

In 1773, Cullen became President of the College. He immediately began to 'forward the erection of a new hall'. He formed a new building committee with himself as chairman. Two

25. The College's first Hall was eventually sold in 1770 for 1,500 guineas.

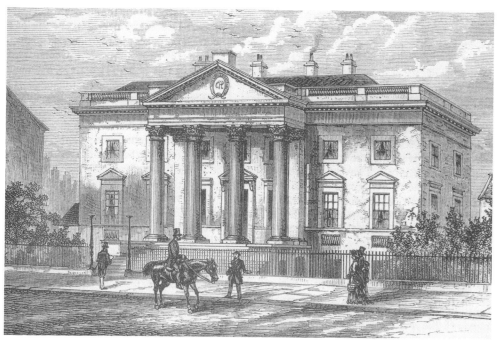

College in George Street

possible schemes were considered. The bridge connecting Edinburgh's High Street with the site of the new town had at last been completed; the plan to build in the New Town could be revived. Alternatively, the new College could be built on the south side of the town in George Square, then the most fashionable address in Edinburgh; there it would be near both the University and the Royal Infirmary. Before proceeding to a decision, Cullen made 'application to the Town Council to know what terms an area in the New Town may be procured'.[26] The Town Council offered a site at the east end of George Street on very generous terms and, in February 1775, their offer was accepted. Cullen drew up specifications for the new Hall and Library and James Craig, who had been responsible for the overall design of the New Town, was engaged as architect. In April 1779, Craig's plans were accepted and he was contracted to build the new hall and library at an estimated cost of £2,724 18s 5d. In a little over two years the work was completed.

On 7 August 1781 the College met for the first time in its new Hall. As its first item of business the College ordered that 'the books be immediately removed from the infirmary where they have hitherto been kept and put up in the best order possible in the ante-chamber until the great room shall be finished and fit for their reception'. Sir John Pringle marked the provision of the new and secure library space by presenting all ten manuscript volumes of his case notes and annotations for safekeeping and the widow of Dr James Mackenzie presented the seventy-nine volumes of the *Transactions* of the Academy of Sciences of Paris. Over the next

26. College Minute, 6 February 1775.

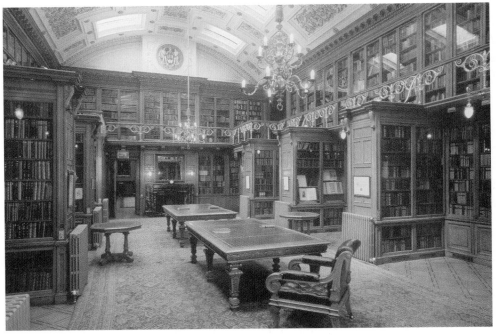

New Library

few years, at every meeting of the College new donations of books were acknowledged. Cullen drew up new regulations for the use and management of the library and ordered the preparation of a new catalogue.

When the interior of the new College Hall was completed in 1789 'the principal room' was occupied by the library. 'This room is upward of fifty feet long by thirty broad and twenty high. It is lighted by two rows of windows five in each row and on three sides surrounded by a gallery. Besides these, there are some smaller apartments where the members of the College may read or write when they borrow books from the library which they do not chose to carry home with them'.[27]

Before Cullen's death in 1790, the College library had acquired some of what have become its most treasured possessions: Galileo's *Discorsi e Dimonstazioni,* Vesalius' *De`Humani Corporis Fabrica*, Robert Hooke's *Micrographia*, Robert Boyle's *Sceptical Chemist*, Issac Newton's *Philosophiae Naturalis Principia Mathematica*, John Napier's *Mirifici Logorithmorum Canonis Descripto*. Readers had access to all the classical texts of Hippocrates and Galen and the canons of the Arabic physicians, Avicenna and Averroes; from the Renaissance there were books by Desiderius Erasmus (1466–1536), Andreas Vesalius (1514–1564), Gabriele Falloppio (1523–1563), Jacobus Sylvius (1478–1555), Jean Fernell (1497–1558) and Ambroise Pare (1510–1590); on the emergence of the 'new' science and the 'new' medicine they could find the complete works of all the leading figures – Paracelsus (1493–1542), Daniel Sennert

27. Hugh Arnot, quoted by J.P.S. Ferguson, The College Library, in R. Passmore (ed.), *Proceedings of the Royal College of Physicians of Edinburgh Tercentenary Congress 1981* (Edinburgh, 1982), p. 108.

(1572–1637), Francis Bacon (1561–1626), William Harvey (1578–1657), René Descartes (1596–1650), Isaac Newton (1642–1727), Linnaeus (1707–1778), Georg Stahl (1659–1734), Albrecht von Haller (1708–1777) and Herman Boerhaave (1668–1738). There was an excellent collection of works on mathematics by Newton, David Gregory (1659–1708) and Colin Maclaurin (1698–1746). The library of almost five thousand books and manuscripts also had many works on theology, history and philosophy.

At the Royal College of Physicians of Edinburgh, William Cullen had presided over the development and organisation of the most comprehensive medical and scientific library in Scotland. Over the same years in Edinburgh, his friends, the philosophers and historians David Hume and Adam Ferguson, had in turn presided over the expansion of the Advocates' Library.[28] Together these two were the most important libraries in Scotland during the years of the Enlightenment.

CULLEN AND MEDICAL EDUCATION

William Cullen's early training had been as an apprentice surgeon and then briefly as an assistant to an apothecary. His introduction to the theory and practice of physic had come two years later when he attended classes during two winter sessions at Edinburgh University. It may have been this experience together with some dissatisfaction with his own situation that fired his determination to reform medical education in Scotland.

At a meeting of the College of Physicians he set out the principle on which he justified the commanding and exclusive role that, under his leadership, physicians were to play in medical education in Edinburgh in the second half of the eighteenth century.

> It is everywhere understood that the doctor of medicine, as established by a diploma received from a university, is a person entitled to practise medicines in all its branches while the surgeon and the apothecary are confined to their respective branches and cannot practise on internal disease. It may be considered whether, by allowing physicians imbued with general knowledge and following their inclinations and talents for the practice of surgery, we may not have persons more generally excelling in that art than by confining the practice of surgery to persons who study it as a mechanical art and seldom go far in acquiring the science that should constantly govern them. If a physician be determined to the practice of surgery no harm can ensue to the public. On the contrary such a physician is likely to become more excellent in surgery than any man who from the beginning was determined to be a surgeon only.

On this principle, Fellows of the Royal College of Physicians of Edinburgh were not to be excluded from the practice and teaching of surgery or midwifery. It also followed that the medical education of students at Edinburgh University should be entirely in the hands of physicians.

---

28. Established in 1689, the Advocates' Library had grown rapidly after the Copyright Act of 1709 made it a library of legal deposit whereby it received thereafter a copy of every book published in the United Kingdom.

TABLE 5.1 Medical Faculty of Edinburgh University, 1756–1800

Chair	Professor	University Degree (MD)	Fellow of RCPE
Anatomy	Alexander Monro I	Edinburgh 1765	1756
	Alexander Monro II[a] (1758)	Edinburgh 1755	1758
Anatomy and Surgery	Alexander Monro II	Edinburgh 1797	1797
	Alexander Monro III (1798)		
Botany	Charles Alston	Glasgow 1719	1721
	John Hope (1761)	Glasgow 1750	1762
	Daniel Rutherford (1786)	Edinburgh 1772	1777
Chemistry	William Cullen	Glasgow 1740	1756
	Joseph Black (1766)	Edinburgh 1754	1769
	Thomas Hope (1795)	Edinburgh 1784	1795
Theory of Medicine	Robert Whytt	Rheims 1736	1738
	William Cullen (1766)	Glasgow 1740	
	James Gregory (1776)	Edinburgh 1776	1777
Practice of Medicine	John Rutherford		
	John Gregory (1766)	Rheims 1719	1724
	William Cullen (1773)	Aberdeen 1746	1765
Midwifery	Thomas Young	Edinburgh 1761	1762
	Alexander Hamilton (1780)	St Andrews 1783	1789
Materia Medica	Francis Home (1768)	Edinburgh 1750	1752
	James Home (1798)	Edinburgh 1781	1791
Institutes of Medicine	Andrew Duncan (1789)	Edinburgh 1769	1771

Notes

[a] Alexander Monro *secundus* assumed his father's duties in 1754, three years before his father died.

When Cullen came to Edinburgh University as Professor of Chemistry, the Professors of Botany, the Theory of Medicine and the Practice of Medicine were all Fellows of the College of Physicians. The Professor of Anatomy, Alexander Monro *primus*, who had trained as a surgeon but had also studied at Leyden, became a Fellow of the College later that year. By the summer of 1756 every member of the University Faculty of Medicine was a physician. In the years that followed Cullen used his influence, particularly his influence with his patron the Duke of Argyll and his friend Henry Dundas (the politician whose recommendation was enough to secure appointment to a chair at Edinburgh University[29]) to ensure that only

29. R. Emerson. Medical Men, Politicians and the Medical School, in A. Doig, J. Ferguson, I. Milne and R. Passmore, *William Cullen and the Eighteenth Century Medical World* (Edinburgh, 1993) pp. 204–5.

physicians were appointed to teach at Edinburgh's expanding medical school (Table 5.1). From 1754, four years before Alexander Munro *primus* resigned as Professor of Anatomy, surgery had been taught by his son, a physician who, unlike his father, had never been a surgeon. When Alexander Monro *secundus* succeeded to his father's chair in 1758, he successfully excluded members of the Incorporation of Surgeons from taking any part in the teaching of surgery at the university's medical school.[30] His place in the teaching of surgery was formally recognised by the University in 1777, when the title of his chair was changed to Professor of Anatomy and Surgery.

During the years in which Edinburgh became recognised as the pre-eminent medical school in Europe and the English speaking world, medical teaching at Edinburgh University was, as Cullen had determined, entirely the province of the Fellows of the Royal College of Physicians.

CHEMISTRY AND MEDICINE

In Edinburgh, Cullen continued his successful promotion of the new science of philosophical chemistry. Only seventeen students enrolled for his first series of lectures in January 1756 but within a very few years that number had risen to almost a hundred and fifty. Every session he described new experiments and introduced new ideas; some students attended the course five or even six times. As in Glasgow, he lectured to numbers of 'gentlemen of business' whose interest in chemistry was practical and commercial. But in Edinburgh he lectured to even larger numbers whose interest was in knowledge for its own sake; mathematics, physics, geology, moral philosophy, medicine and chemistry were all the subjects of informed discourse in the intellectual clubs and salons of mid-eighteenth-century Edinburgh. Cullen, it was said, 'succeeded in taking chemistry out of the hands of the artists [artisans], metallurgists and pharmaceutists and exhibited it as a liberal science, the study of a gentleman'.[31]

On chemistry as it applied to medicine, Cullen took his lead from Boerhaave. At Leiden, Boerhaave had lectured on chemistry to medical students for twenty-four years, taking a position somewhere between that of one of his early predecessors at Leiden, Francois de le Boe (Franciscus Sylvius) and that of his German contemporary, Georg Stahl. Sylvius, the leading exponent of the iatrochemical or chemiatric school in the late seventeenth century, had tried to explain all physiological and pathological processes in the body in analogy with processes he was able to demonstrate in the laboratory. On the other hand, Stahl, one of the leading chemists of his century, was convinced that chemistry could throw no light at all on the vital function of the body and was of no value in the study of medicine.[32]

In line with Archibald Pitcairn, his predecessor as Professor of Physic at Leyden, Boerhaave's concept of human physiology was essentially mechanistic; the body was a machine subject to the laws of physics and hydraulics. But unlike Pitcairn, Boerhaave was

30. C. Lawrence, Ornate Physicians and Learned Artisans, in W. F. Bynum and R. Porter, *William Hunter and the Eighteenth Century Medical World* (Cambridge, 1985), p. 163.
31. John Robinson, Professor of Natural Philosophy at Edinburgh quoted by Thomson, *An Account*, p. 46.
32. G.A. Lindeboom, Boerhaave's Impact on the Relation between Chemistry and Medicine, *Cleo Medica*, 1972, Vol. 7 , p. 273.

open to the possibility that chemistry might provide answers to at least some of the great mysteries of health and disease. Cullen also believed that chemistry could be of the greatest importance to medicine

> but the facts lie scattered in many different books, involved in obscure terms mixed with many falsehoods and joined to a great deal of false philosophy… The art should have been put into form and a system of it attempted, the scattered facts collected and arranged in a proper order.[33]

Cullen made his own additions to the 'facts' in books on chemistry. He presented an *Essay Towards Ascertaining the Different Species of Salts* to the Philosophical Society. He published an *Essay on the Cold Produced by Evaporating Fluids*. He carried out a great many experiments in an attempt to establish the laws governing the 'changes of temperature occasioned by the combinations of various substances; by the solution in water of certain salts in their crystalline state; and by the addition of water to the same salts'.

However, his greatest contribution to chemistry was in gathering the 'scattered facts', arranging and presenting them in a proper order.[34] His lectures, in English, were carefully planned; he made great use of tables, diagrams and algebraic symbols; he may have been the first to represent diagrammatically 'the double elective attraction' between substances. Above all he introduced the system that Boerhaave's teaching had lacked. Cullen had read Linnaeus's *Systema Natura* soon after it was published in 1735 and he had continued to correspond with Linnaeus for several years. Linnaeus's system had become 'as familiar as [his] mother-tongue' and Cullen had made it the model for his lectures on chemistry. His system was kept under review; year after year, he assured his students that 'I am yet far from satisfied with the perfection of my plan. It will only be when age shall restrain me that I shall cease to make some corrections'.

Cullen's successor as Professor of Chemistry, Joseph Black, is remembered as Scotland's most eminent chemist of the eighteenth century but it was Cullen who established the place of philosophical chemistry in the teaching of medicine at Edinburgh.

CLINICAL TEACHING

As a Fellow of the Royal College of Physicians, Cullen was, by right, an Extraordinary-Physician at Edinburgh Royal Infirmary. Within a year he had revived and reorganised the system of clinical teaching.

At the old Infirmary at Robertson's Close, medical students had been able to buy, for two guineas, a pass that allowed them access to the wards. There they could interview and examine patients and follow the physicians and their clinical clerks on their rounds. In 1748, as the final phase in the construction of the new infirmary building was nearing completion, John Rutherford proposed that provision should be made for clinical teaching in the form that Boerhaave had made famous at the teaching hospital at Leiden and that he had introduced at

33. W. Cullen, Lectures on Chemistry, MS, College Archive.
34. Ibid.

Edinburgh's first physician's Infirmary in 1729. The managers of the Infirmary agreed that this would be 'of very great service to the students and the house'.[35] Permission was granted for the university's medical professors to give clinical lectures in the new Infirmary's amphitheatre and, in 1750, a clinical teaching ward of ten beds was opened in the new Infirmary. The teaching was to be open, during the six months of the academic year, in the charge of the professors of medicine, each serving in rotation for a fixed period in sole charge; during his term the professor was to be free to select the patients for admission to the teaching ward.

This new venture achieved only modest success. Rutherford's colleagues declined to take part. With Rutherford as the only professor admitting patients to the ward, the variety of cases presented to the students was somewhat limited and the teaching ward was open for less than half the year. In the summer months of the vacation, many of Edinburgh's medical students continued to look elsewhere for clinical experience.

In the 1750s Rutherford became unwell and his clinical teaching became increasingly burdensome and, in 1757, he willingly gave way to Cullen. Cullen reintroduced and expanded the scheme that had been put in place by the managers of the Infirmary in 1748. The clinical course was extended to six months. The teaching ward was enlarged to a total of twenty beds, in two separate rooms for equal numbers male and female patients.[36] Robert Whytt and Alexander Munro *secundus* agreed to share responsibility for the teaching ward and to give clinical lectures twice weekly for five of the weeks of the six month course. The fee paid by students for a ticket for access to the Infirmary was increased to seven and a half guineas but, without any additional fee, students could now attend a professor's round in the teaching unit each day at noon and his evening lectures on Tuesdays and Fridays.

The teaching ward now offered the students much wider clinical experience:

> The best marked diseases, the most singular in nature and the greatest variety of acute as well as chronic are chosen. Regular and circumstantial reports of every symptom belonging to the disease and every effect produced by the remedies exhibited are taken in the presence of the students.[37]

The patients that the students saw in the teaching ward reflected to some degree the different interests and practices of the professors who had arranged their admission. The variety of interests and philosophies of the professors was even more evident at their evening clinical lectures when one or more of their patients was presented for more open discussion of their management and prognosis than was possible at the bedside.

At various times over the next several years Cullen shared the course of clinical medicine with Alexander Monro, Robert Whytt and John Gregory. By 1772, Monro and Gregory had retired from the course and Whytt had died. Cullen took sole charge until he was joined by James Gregory in 1774. In 1775 Cullen withdrew and was succeeded by Francis Home.

35. Minutes, Board of Management RIE, 1 February 1748 quoted by G. B. Risse, *Hospital Life in Enlightenment Scotland* (Cambridge, 1986), p. 243.
36. By 1790 the total number of beds had risen to 100.
37. F. Home, *Clinical Experiments, Histories and Dissections* (London, 1783), p 6. Francis Home was one of the professors who had charge of the Teaching Ward.

Over these twenty-seven years, Cullen treated large numbers of charity patients in the teaching ward. For the most part these were young people (average age, males 26.5, females 23.7[38]) suffering from common and acute diseases and 'admit[ting] of frequent trial of practice'. At the same time, in his private practice, he was consulted principally by older and more wealthy patients, typically suffering from chronic 'constitutional' illnesses perhaps influenced by long-term environmental factors or injudicious lifestyle. Based on this wide experience Cullen introduced what was originally designed as an aid for students being introduced to clinical medicine in the teaching ward. This was his *Nosology* which set out the clinical signs that distinguished each particular disease, a nomenclature for these recognisable diseases and a classification of these diseases in a 'methodic and convenient order' modelled on Linnaeus's classification of plants. Cullen allotted diseases into four classes – Pyrexiae, Neuroses, Cachexiae and Locales and these were subdivided into a total of 19 orders which included, in all, 132 genera.

Many experienced physicians regarded the attempt to draw up such a nosology as 'a frivolous and unobtainable pursuit'.[39] Even Sir John Pringle who had co-operated with Cullen in revising the *Edinburgh Pharmacopoeia* thought the *Synopsis Nosologiae Methodicae* was fanciful and useless. Nevertheless, its first edition, published in 1769, sold well among the medical profession and revised and expanded editions were published in 1771, 1780 and 1785. The nosology was well received by medical students and valued particularly by those attending ward rounds at the Infirmary's teaching unit.

By 1790 the number of beds in the teaching unit had been increased to a hundred. The number of students enrolled for the clinical course had risen to ninety-five and attendance at the clinical lecture course at Edinburgh Royal Infirmary had become a requirement for candidates for a medical degree from Edinburgh University.

THE THEORY OF MEDICINE

In 1764, John Rutherford, who had been Professor of the Practice of Medicine for over thirty-five years, let it be known that he wished to retire. It became widely expected, not least by Cullen himself, that Cullen would be appointed as his successor. However, Rutherford would only give up his chair to a successor who would could be relied upon to follow the 'system' of Boerhaave, the 'system' that Rutherford had learned at Leiden and had taught at Edinburgh for almost forty years. Cullen, who had often drawn attention to the 'imperfections and even the errors'[40] in that system, was not acceptable; in 1766 Rutherford retired in favour of John Gregory, who had been his pupil at Edinburgh in 1742 and had later studied at Leiden. Gregory, fourteen years younger than Cullen, had been Professor of Medicine at Aberdeen for ten years but had never been called on to teach. The student body protested vigorously at the failure to appoint Cullen as Professor of the Practice of Medicine and when Robert Whytt died later that year, Cullen was appointed unopposed as Professor of the Theory of Medicine.

38. G.H. Risse, Cullen as Clinician. in Doig et al., *William Cullen*, p. 140.
39. Thomson, *An Account*, p. 6.
40. Ibid, p. 119.

Pressure from the students continued and in 1769 it was agreed that Cullen and Gregory would share responsibilities, each lecturing, on alternate years, on both the Theory and the Practice of Medicine. On Gregory's death in 1773, Cullen became Professor of the Practice of Medicine but continued to lecture on both the Theory and Practice of Medicine until James Gregory was able to take up his appointment as Professor of the Institutes of Medicine (the new name for what had been the chair of the Theory of Medicine) in 1776. Thereafter Cullen lectured only on the Practice of Medicine almost until his death in 1790.

In his lectures in Edinburgh over the long period of thirty-six years and in his books published between 1769 and 1784[41] Cullen promoted his own 'clear order and method' or 'system'. He taught that any attempt to base the study and practice of medicine simply on 'facts' as they were gathered from observation and experience was an attempt 'to form a rope of sand;' such empiricism in medicine was 'fallacious if not impossible'.[42] Facts were best taught and most effectively used if, by inductive reasoning, they were developed as the basis of a coherent theoretical model or system. Once the true facts had been separated from the false they could be perceived as parts of 'one harmonious whole'.

'Systems' or models of the overall human economy in health and disease had been put forward and widely accepted for centuries but they had been based on metaphysical or imaginary concepts. Aristotle had proposed that man's functions of nutrition and generation were subject to a vegetative soul, his senses and voluntary motions to a sentient soul and his intellectual powers to a rational soul; Galen, in 'perfecting' the legacy of Hippocrates[43] had perpetuated the notion that health and disease were determined by the balance of the four 'humours', yellow bile, black bile, phlegm and blood. For Cullen, such systems based on reasoning alone 'had not the least effect or influence in explaining anything'. (He was perhaps influenced by his friend the philosopher, David Hume, who had written that all metaphysical books were 'nothing but sophistry and illusion' and should be burned.) A 'system' that would be useful as an aid to the understanding of health and disease could only be achieved by observing the principles of natural philosophy.[44] Cullen accepted that the system devised by Boerhaave in the first years of the eighteenth century was 'as perfect as the state of science in his time would permit of'. In his *Physiology*, Boerhaave had discounted the metaphysical spirits and the mythical humours in favour of a Newtonian concept:

> All the functions of the human economy depend on innumerable physical causes so combined into one organic body by the First Mind that the body can preserve and restore itself; nor does it stand more in need of any subordinate mover than a clock after it is once set in motion.

Boerhaave based his system on the demonstration of capillaries by the early microscopists and on the assumption that, in time, ever finer and finer networks of vessels would be

---

41. *Synopsis Nosologiae Medicae*, 1769; *Lectures on Materia Medica*, 1772; *Institutes of Medicine: Physiology*, 1772; *First Lines of the Practice of Medicine*, Vols I–IV, 1777–84.
42. M. Barfoot, Philosophy and Method in Cullen's Medical Teaching in Doig et al., *William Cullen*, p. 122.
43. R. Porter, *The Greatest Benefit to Mankind* (London, 1999), p. 75.
44. W. Cullen, Lectures on Chemistry, MS, College Archive.

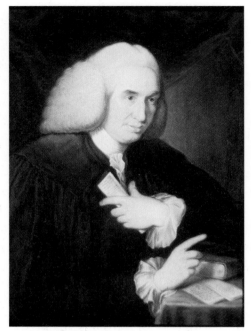

William Cullen

discovered. In Boerhhaave's system the human body was made up entirely of vessels and their fluid contents, the 'solid' organs being no more than elaborate vascular differentiations;[45] the body functioned according to the laws of mechanics and hydraulics and the all-important function was movement; life itself being the movement of fluid through the vessels. Boerhaave could only speculate on the role of the nervous system or chemical factors in the regulation of bodily functions. Cullen's re-shaping of Boerhaave's system was determined by recent work on the nerves and brain by Albrecht von Haller and Robert Whytt; in Cullen's system the body functioned on an 'animated nervous frame'. His system was also much less mechanical in that it proposed a pervasive role for the operation of the mind upon the body.[46]

Cullen's modification of Boerhaave's system was to be of little lasting value. This was also true of the systems that Cullen devised for the didactic teaching of every topic he covered in the medical curriculum. However, in the open market of university teaching, his method was preferred by students over the teaching methods offered by his rivals. From year to year, Cullen kept his lectures under review, discarding 'false' facts and substituting the 'true'. The dogmatism Cullen promoted during his years in Edinburgh was therefore a sceptical dogmatism and his sceptical dogmatism became characteristic not only of medical education at Edinburgh but of Scottish medical education in general. This was in sharp contrast with medical education in England where empiricism continued to prevail. This difference became the basis of the two contrasting medical traditions that grew up north and south of the border

45. G.A. Lindeboom, Boerhaave's Concept of the Basic Structure of the Body, *Clio Medica*, 1970, Vol. 5, p 203.
46. Barfoot, Philosophy, p. 123.

and continued into the middle years of the twentieth century. As late as 1936 Lord Horder was to write that while he respected the dogmatic Scottish tradition of Cullen he was proud to belong to a very different tradition, the empiric English tradition of Sydenham.[47]

THE CURRICULUM

In the 1750s, students studying at Edinburgh University were invited at the beginning of each winter term to attend a ceremony in the library at which they signed the matriculation album, gave notice of the courses they intended to take that year; on matriculation they were required to pay a fee of half a crown that allowed them access to the library. Since the university library had few medical books, medical students often did not matriculate but enrolled directly with the professor of each course they wished to attend and paid him a fee of three guineas for a ticket for his classes.

To help students choose the courses they should attend, it was the custom for each professor to set out the scope of his course in a free introductory lecture. Students could also buy a *Guide for Gentlemen Studying Medicine at Edinburgh University*[48] which described the content and assessed the value of each course. In the years between 1756 and 1790 courses were given by the Professors of Botany, Anatomy, Anatomy and Surgery, Chemistry, Theory of Medicine, Practice of Medicine, Midwifery,[49] Materia Medica and the Institutes of Medicine. However these titles do not exactly define the limits or the emphasis of their lectures. Robert Whytt gave great attention to neurology, Alexander Monro taught physiology as well as anatomy and surgery, William Cullen extended his course to include military medicine and public health, John Gregory introduced the teaching of medical ethics, Andrew Duncan taught students at the Public Dispensary and in the homes of the poor. In the late eighteenth century Edinburgh was recognised as the only 'university where every branch of medicine is taught'.[50]

For almost half a century after its faculty of medicine was created, Edinburgh University did not require candidates for the MD degree to show which courses they attended or indeed that they had completed any course; candidates were obliged only to satisfy the examiners of their medical knowledge. In 1767, a regulation was introduced that demanded that candidates must have attended 'a course of study in all the branches of medicine at this or some other university'. Cullen now received complaints from a number of his former students practising in England that the failure of the other Scottish universities to introduce similar regulations was calling in question the value of all Scottish medical degrees including those granted by Edinburgh. At that time St Andrews and Aberdeen granted degrees on the recommendation of two physicians, without examination and without the candidate having studied at a university; Glasgow granted very few medical degrees and none without examination but did not require candidates to provide evidence of the courses of study they had completed at a university.

47. M. McCrae, *The National Health Service in Scotland* (East Lothian, 2003), p. 43.
48. L. Rosner, *Medical Education in the Age of Improvement* (Edinburgh, 1991), p. 47.
49. The Professor of Midwifery was not a member of Faculty.
50. Rosner, *Medical Education*, p. 47.

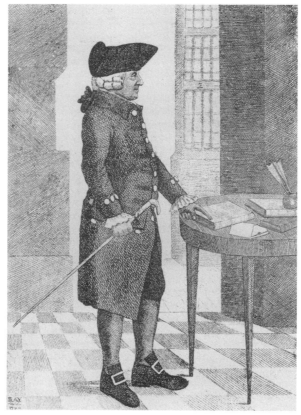

Adam Smith

In 1774, Cullen took what seemed an excellent opportunity to draw the attention of the government to this continuing problem. Cullen was then President of the Edinburgh College of Physicians and during his term of office the Duke of Buccleuch, then the most influential politician in Scotland, was made an Honorary Fellow of the College. In his letter of acceptance Buccleuch asked 'if it is true that in any of the Scottish Universities degrees in physic are given on paying certain fees without due examination and previous attendance at the Universities; if it is so it is truly a matter of reproach to the country he would wish to have remedied if he had information how it can be done'. In reply, Cullen sent a memorandum setting out the evidence that there was indeed 'a shameful traffic of degrees in physic at some of the Universities of Scotland' and proposing that a degree should only be granted after proper examination and that before being examined every candidate should produce a 'certificate of his having resided for two years at least in a University wherein physic is regularly taught and of his having applied to all the branches of medical study'.[51]

Buccleuch passed Cullen's memorandum to his former tutor, the economist Adam Smith, for his comment and advice. In a lengthy document Adam Smith, the great advocate of free

51. Thomson, *An Account*, Vol. I, pp. 468–72.

trade, argued that universities should not be given a monopoly in medical education or in granting licences to practise. Buccleuch accepted his view, Cullen's petition was not passed on to government and practices remained unchanged at St Andrews, Glasgow and Aberdeen. At Edinburgh however, Cullen had the regulations of 1767 clarified and strengthened; no student would be admitted as a candidate for a medical degree unless he could show that he had attended courses in Anatomy and Surgery, Chemistry, Botany, Materia Medica and Pharmacy, Medical Theory and Practice and had attended the clinical lectures at the Royal Infirmary.[52]

When William Cullen died in 1790, the Edinburgh University medical school was at the height of its fame. Over 600 students were attending medical courses in the city; 510 had matriculated at the university,[53] almost as many had not matriculated ('auditors') but had paid fees directly to the professors teaching the medical subjects in which they had a particular interest; 323 had enrolled for clinical instruction at Edinburgh Royal Infirmary.[54] Those graduating *Doctoratus in Arte Medica* at Edinburgh University at that time came from every part of the English-speaking world (Table 5.2). At Edinburgh, they had been offered a more comprehensive curriculum than could then be found anywhere else in the world. They had received clinical instruction and experience at the largest teaching hospital in Britain. In contrast with the empiricism that prevailed in the teaching and practice of medicine in England, medical students at Edinburgh had been taught an orderly and methodical ('systematic') understanding of medicine but taught to temper this useful dogmatism with scepticism. The transformation of Edinburgh's university medical school in the middle years of the eighteenth century led to the establishment of a peculiarly Scottish tradition of medicine and medical practice that survived for more than two centuries. That tradition was shaped by William Cullen and Fellows of the Royal College of Physicians. At the end of the eighteenth century the overwhelming majority of medical graduates practising in Britain had been trained in that tradition (Table 5.3).

TABLE 5.2 Country of origin of Edinburgh medical graduates, 1726–1799

Country	Number	%
Ireland	280	24.7
England	254	22.4
Scotland	237	20.9
North America & West Indies	195	17.2
'Britain' or otherwise unspecified	143	12.6
Europe	26	2.3

Source: M.H. Kaufman, *Medical Teaching in Edinburgh* (Edinburgh, 2003).

52. Rosner, *Medical Education*, p. 63.
53. Sir John Sinclair, *The First Statistical Account of Scotland*.
54. Ibid.

Table 5.3 Place of graduation of physicians practising in Britain 1650–1800

Period	Oxford and Cambridge (%)		Europe (%)		Scotland (%)	
1650-1700	933	(79.9)	197	(16.9)	38	(3.3)
1700-1750	617	(43.8)	385	(27.3)	406	(28.8)
1750-1800	246	(8.1)	194	(6.4)	2,594	(85.3)

Source: M. H. Kaufman, *Medical Teaching in Edinburgh* (Edinburgh, 2003).

6

THE INVENTION OF MEDICAL ETHICS
The Legacy of John Gregory

In the middle years of the eighteenth century, John Gregory, a Fellow of the College, invented medical ethics and set the disciplines that made the practice of medicine a profession rather than a trade.[1] Gregory was born in 1724 into a distinguished academic family. His father, James, was Professor of Medicine (Mediciner) at King's College, Aberdeen; his grandfather, also James, was a mathematician, a Fellow of the Royal Society and the inventor of the reflecting microscope; an uncle, David, also a Fellow of the Royal Society, was Professor of Astronomy at Oxford; one of a large number of academic cousins was the philosopher, Thomas Reid.

John Gregory was educated at Aberdeen Grammar School and at King's College, Aberdeen, where his paternal grandfather was Principal. In 1742, he began his medical studies at Edinburgh University[2] where he was taught by Alexander Monro *primus*, John Rutherford, Andrew Sinclair and Andrew Plummer. In 1745, like many other Scottish medical students at that time, he travelled abroad to complete his medical education. In March 1746, while still a student at Leiden, he was awarded an MD by King's College, Aberdeen,[3] a distinction he had not sought and for which he had neither submitted a thesis nor suffered any examination. Three months later he was appointed Professor of Philosophy at King's College, the appointment to be effective on his return to Aberdeen.

At King's College from 1747, he lectured on mathematics and on moral and natural philosophy; he also tried to introduce a regular course of lectures on medicine but that project failed because of the very small number of students at King's College interested in medicine at that time. While still Professor of Philosophy he joined his brother James in practising as a physician in Aberdeen. He very soon found that his obligations at King's were distracting him from what promised to become a very successful medical practice and in September 1749 he resigned his chair. In 1752, he married he married Elizabeth, the younger daughter of Lord Forbes. In 1753, the first of his three sons and three daughters was born. It may have been his new family commitments that persuaded him to leave his Aberdeen medical practice in the hands of his brother James and 'try his fortunes in London. Thither he accordingly went in 1754 and being already known by reputation as a man of genius, he found an easy introduction to many persons of distinction both in the literary and polite world'.[4] In London he made

1. L.B. McCullough, *John Gregory and the Invention of Professional Medical Ethics and the Profession of Medicine* (Dordrecht, 1998).
2. Both his half-brother James and his brother George had earlier decided on medical careers; George had died while still a student.
3. McCullough, *John Gregory*, p. 53.
4. A.F. Tytler, An Account of the Life and Writings of Dr. John Gregory, in W. Creech (ed.), *The Works of the Late John Gregory MD* (Edinburgh, 1788), p. 34.

some progress towards establishing a fashionable medical practice but it was in the literary and intellectual life of the capital that he made his name and it was for the exercise of his intellectual gifts and for his philosophy rather than for his contribution to medical science that he was made a Fellow of the Royal Society in 1754.

In November 1755 his father died and John Gregory was invited to succeed him as Mediciner (Professor of Medicine) at King's College, Aberdeen. In 1756, he returned to Scotland and 'took upon him the duties of that office to which he had been elected in his absence'. There were in fact no such duties. At King's there was still no medical school and the office of Mediciner was a sinecure. Gregory was therefore able to divide his time between his practice as a physician and the interests of the Aberdeen Philosophical Society.

> To Gregory, the society of Aberdeen had many attractions. There he had formed his most cordial friendships. These had been contracted chiefly with a few persons of distinguished abilities and learning who it was now his fortune to find attached to the same place and engaged in pursuits similar to his own. The animosities and mean jealousies, which so often disgrace the characters of literary men, were unknown to friends of Gregory who, educated in one school, professing no opposite tenets, or contending principles, seem to have united themselves as in a common cause, the defence of virtue of religion and of truth.[5]

For a time Gregory seemed content to remain in Aberdeen but, after a few years, he let it be known that he would welcome an opportunity to join the already prestigious faculty of medicine at Edinburgh University.[6] John Rutherford, the Professor of Medicine at Edinburgh, had, for some time, been hoping to retire. To many in Edinburgh, and certainly to the student body, William Cullen seemed the obvious and most worthy candidate to succeed him. However, Rutherford was determined not to surrender his chair to Cullen whom he regarded as a medical heretic, a physician who dared to question the teachings of Boerhaave. Rutherford, with the support of the conservative faction within the University, contrived that John Gregory would be invited to succeed him and on that understanding Rutherford resigned from his chair; in 1766 Gregory became Professor of Medicine at Edinburgh.

On his arrival in Edinburgh, Gregory was immediately made a Fellow of the College of Physicians and, later that year, he succeeded Robert Whytt as First Physician to the King in Scotland. Gregory was not made so readily welcome by the student body at Edinburgh University who continued to resent his appointment despite the proven merits and greater accomplishments of their favoured candidate, William Cullen. Their protests only subsided when, later in 1766, Cullen was made Professor of the Institutes of Medicine in succession to Robert Whytt.

---

5. Ibid., p. 37.
6. E. Climenson, *Elizabeth Montague: The Queen of the Blue Stockings. Her Correspondence, 1720-1761* (London, 1906), Vol. II, p. 226.

THE LECTURES

Gregory's lectures always attracted large numbers of students[7] and for sixteen years he gave to each new body of medical students at Edinburgh University an introductory course of 'Lectures on the Duties and Qualifications of a Physician':

> The design of the profession which I have the honour to hold in this university is to explain the practice of medicine, by which I understand the art of preserving health, of prolonging life and of curing diseases. But before I enter this course, I shall give some preliminary lectures in which I shall lay before you some considerations which deserve the attention of all those who would practise medicine. It is needless to dwell on the utility and dignity of the medical art. Its utility was never seriously called in question; every man who suffers pain or sickness will very gratefully acknowledge the usefulness of an art which gives him relief. People may dispute whether physic, on the whole, does more good or harm to mankind … The reasons for this [are] sufficiently obvious. Physicians, considered as a body of men who live by the practice of medicine, have an interest separate and distinct from the honour of the science.

The regrettable 'interest' that so often distracted physicians from the honourable practice of their profession took three closely related forms: the pursuit of reputation, the pursuit of power and status and the pursuit of financial reward. In the eighteenth century there were many practitioners – university educated physicians, apprentice trained surgeons, apothecaries, midwives and quacks – all eager to sell their services. Gregory conceded that in this fiercely competitive medical market, some physicians:

> impelled by necessity, some stimulated by vanity and others anxious to conceal ignorance have recourse to various mean and unworthy arts to raise their importance among the ignorant who are always the most numerous part of mankind. Some of these arts have been an affectation of mystery in all their conversations relating to their profession; an affectation of knowledge inscrutable to all except adepts in the science; an air of perfect confidence in their own skill and abilities and a demeanour solemn, contemptuous and highly expressive of self-sufficiency.

Physicians advertised themselves not only in their manners and conversations but also in their writings. While they published the peculiar merits of their own nostrums and skills in booklets and pamphlets, they also vigorously denigrated each other.[8] Patients therefore had good reason to be uncertain of the knowledge and competence of those they could choose to consult. Wealthy patients, as a matter of course, took care to consult more than one physician; but patients who could afford to consult only one had to be guided by nothing more reliable than the popular reputations of the physicians who offered their services.

7. R. Passmore, *Fellows of Edinburgh's College of Physicians during the Enlightenment* (Edinburgh, 2001), p. 57.
8. L. B. McCullough, John Gregory's Medical Ethics and the Reform of Medical Practice in Eighteenth Century Edinburgh, *Journal of the Royal College of Physicians of Edinburgh*, 2006, Vol. 36, 1, p. 87.

Gregory deplored the part that Edinburgh's Royal Infirmary (and other leading public hospitals) could be made to play in the creation of medical reputations. From the Infirmary's foundation, Edinburgh's most eminent physicians, as an act of charity had freely given their services in the care of the sick poor; but for a physician at an early stage in his career, an appointment to the staff of the infirmary was coveted as a public mark of distinction likely to confer advantage in the competition to attract paying patients. The patients admitted to the infirmary were the poor and sick in need of free medical care. But it was not unknown for these vulnerable and dependent patients to be used; without their knowledge they could be included in some clinical experiment being carried out principally to boost an ambitious physician's reputation as a master of medical science.[9]

Gregory believed that it was the untested and fanciful 'notions' of certain well-meaning physicians and the blatantly self-serving activities of others in the pursuit of reputation, status and financial gain that caused all physicians to be exposed to the 'censure of the judicious' and the practice of medicine to be seen as a trade no different from any other. Gregory believed that the disreputable and damaging pursuit of interest would cease if it were only possible to restrict the ranks of the profession to men of independent means.[10] Since, regrettably, this could not be done Gregory offered his students an acceptable compromise:

> Medicine may be considered as an art the most beneficial and important to mankind or as a trade by which a considerable body of men gain their subsistence. These two views, though distinct, are far from being incompatible though in fact they are often made so. I shall endeavour to set this matter in such a light as may show that the system of conduct in a physician, which tends most to the advancement of his art is such as will most efficiently maintain the true dignity and honour of the profession and even promote the private interest of such of its members as are of real capacity and merit.

'Conscious of their own worth, physicians should disdain every artifice and depend for their success on their real merit.' Above all, they must 'act with candour, with honour, with the ingenuous and liberal manners of gentlemen'. For Gregory, candour was the essential discipline of both the medical scientist and the practising physician. A lack of candour would inevitably corrupt all the intellectual and moral qualities required in a physician.

Gregory discussed in detail the qualities that 'naturally fit a man for being a physician'.

Francis Bacon

9. Ibid.
10. Ibid., p. 91.

BACON AND EVIDENCE-BASED MEDICINE

Among the essential qualifications of a physician was the adoption of a systematic scientific methodology for inquiry into the nature of disease and the assessment of the measures to be used in its relief.

> Perhaps no profession requires so comprehensive a mind as medicine. In the other learned professions, considered as sciences, there is a certain established standard, certain fixed laws and statutes, to which every question must constantly refer. And by which it must be determined. A knowledge of this established authority may be attained by assiduous application and a good memory. There is little room left for the display of genius where invention cannot add nor judgement improve because the laws, whether right or wrong, must be submitted to. The case is very different in medicine. There is no established authority to which we can refer in doubtful cases. Every physician must rely on his own judgement which appeals for its rectitude to nature and experience alone. Among the infinite variety of facts and theories with which his memory has been filled in the course of a liberal education, it is his business to make judicial separation between those founded in nature and experience and those which own their birth to ignorance, fraud or the capricious systems of a deluded imagination.[11]

Gregory advised his students to follow 'the whole plan laid down by Bacon for prosecuting enquiries into nature and many branches of natural philosophy'.[12] Bacon's method combined well ordered observation and experience with inductive reasoning.

> Experience if taken as it comes is called 'accident', if sought for 'experiment'. But this kind of experience is a mere groping as of men in the dark that feel all around them for the chance of finding their way when they had much better light a candle and then go on. The true method of experience first lights the candle and by means of the candle shows the way; commencing as it does with experience duly ordered and digested and from it educing axioms and from established axioms again new experiments.[13]

In 1757, Gregory was already introducing Edinburgh medical students to what, more than two centuries later, was to become generally known as evidence-based medicine:

> In teaching a system of the practice of physic every disease must be considered separately and as existing by itself. But, in fact, diseases are found complicated in endless varieties which no system is able to comprehend. This occasions an embarrassment to a young practitioner which nothing can remove but a habit of nice discernment and quickness of apprehension which enables him to

11. J. Gregory, *Lectures on the Duties and Qualification of a Physician* (London, 1772), p. 14.
12. J. Gregory, Medical Notes, Aberdeen University Library, MSS 2206/45, quoted by McCullough, *John Gregory*, p. 92.
13. J. Spalding, R. Ellis and D. Heath (eds), *The Works of Francis Bacon* (New York, 1875) Vol. IV, p

perceive real analogies and a solidity of judgement which secures him from being deceived by imaginary ones. A student of much fancy and some learning has no idea of this difficulty. In the pride of his heart he fancies every disease must fly before him. He thinks he not only knows the proximate causes and indications of cure in all distempers but also a variety of remedies that will exactly answer them. It will be unfortunate for his patients if a little experience does not humble his pride and satisfy him that in many cases he neither knows the proximate causes nor the indications of cure nor how to fulfil these indications when he does know them or show him that the indications are different and contradictory. In this situation his boasted science must stoop perhaps for some time to be an idle spectator or to palliate the violence of particular symptoms or to proceed with the utmost fear and diffidence with such lights as he can receive from a precarious analogy. Such are the difficulties which a physician has to encounter in his early practice; to conquer which is required, besides the qualifications of a proper education, the concurrence of a penetrating genius and a solid judgement and of a quickness of apprehension instantly to perceive where the greatest probability of success lies and to act accordingly.

Talents of another kind are also required. A physician has not only for an object the improvement of his own mind but he must study the temper and struggle with the prejudices of the patient, of the relations and of the world in general. Hence appears the necessity of a physician's having a large share of good sense and a knowledge of the world as well as medical genius and learning.

HUME AND HUMANITY

Gregory gave great weight to the moral qualities required in a physician, the most important of which was humanity, 'that sensibility which makes us feel for the distresses of our fellow creatures and which of consequence incites us in the most powerful manner to relieve them'. This was a concept that Gregory had taken from David Hume. In his *Treatise of Human Nature*, Hume had written that when someone is in the presence of another, injured and in pain, he is given the idea of pain and 'this idea is presently converted into an impression and acquires such a degree of force and vivacity as to become the very passion itself'. This sharing of the pain, this human sympathy, makes the witness suffer as the injured suffers and moved to remove the suffering.

SYMPATHY

Gregory taught that, in the humane physician,

> sympathy produces an anxious attention to a thousand little circumstances that
> may tend to relieve the patient; an attention which money can never purchase;

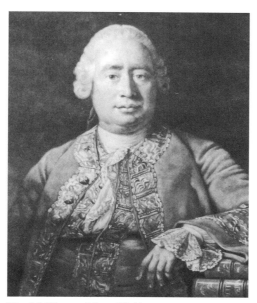

David Hume (New Club)

hence the inexpressible comfort of having a friend for a physician. Sympathy naturally engages the affection and confidence of a patient, which, in many cases, is of the utmost consequence to his recovery. If the physician possesses gentleness of manners and a compassionate heart and what Shakespeare so emphatically calls 'the milk of human kindness', the patient feels his approach like of a guardian angel ministering to his relief while every visit of a physician who is unfeeling and rough in his manners makes the heart sink within him as the presence of one who comes to pronounce his doom. Men of the most compassionate tempers, by being in daily conversant with scenes of distress, acquire in process of time that composure and firmness of mind so necessary in the practice of physic. They can feel whatever is amiable in pity without suffering it to enervate or unman them. Such physicians as are callous to sentiments of humanity treat this sympathy with ridicule and represent it either as hypocrisy or the indication of a feeble mind. That sympathy is often affected, I am afraid, is true; but this affectation can be easily seen through. Real sympathy is never ostentatious; on the contrary it rather strives to conceal itself. But what most effectively detects this hypocrisy is a physician's different manner of behaving to people in high and people in low life, to those who reward him handsomely and those who have not the means to do so. A generous and elevated mind is even more shy in expressing sympathy with those of high rank than those in humbler life, being jealous of the unworthy construction so usually annexed to it. The insinuation that a compassionate and feeling heart is commonly accompanied with weak understanding and feeble mind is malignant and false. Experience demonstrates that a gentle and humane temper, so far from being inconsistent with vigour of mind, is its usual attendant and that rough and blustering manners generally accompany a weak understanding and mean souls and are indeed frequently affected by men void of magnanimity and personal courage to conceal their natural defects.

PATIENCE AND FLEXIBILITY

There is a specious of good humour which is amiable in a physician. It consists in a certain gentleness and flexibility which makes him suffer with patience and even apparent cheerfulness the many contradictions and disappointments he is subjected to in his practice. If he is rigid and too minute in his directions about regimen he may be assured they will not be strictly followed. And, if he is severe in his manners, the deviations from his rules will as certainly be concealed from him; the consequence is that he is kept in ignorance of the true state of the patient, he ascribes to the consequences of the disease what is merely owning to irregularities in the diet and attributes effects to medicines which were perhaps never taken. The errors which, in this way, he may be led into might easily be prevented by a prudent relaxation of rules that could not well be obeyed. The government of a physician over his patients should undoubtedly be great but an absolute government very few patients will submit to. A prudent physician should therefore prescribe such laws as, though not the best, are yet the best that will be obeyed ... However, this indulgence which I am pleading for must be managed with judgement and discretion as it is very necessary that a physician should support a proper dignity and authority with his patients for their sakes as well as his own.

MANNERS

We sometimes see a remarkable difference between the behaviour of a physician at his first setting out and afterwards when he is fully established in reputation and practice. In the beginning he is affable, polite, humane and assiduously attentive to his patients. But afterwards when he has reaped the fruits of such behaviour and finds himself independent he assumes a very different tone; he becomes haughty, rapacious and somewhat brutal in his manners. Conscious of the ascendancy he has acquired he acts a despotic part and takes a most ungenerous advantage of the confidence which people have in his abilities.

DISCRETION AND SECRECY

A physician, by the nature of his profession, has many opportunities of knowing the private characters and concerns of the families in which he is employed. Bedsides what he may know from his own observations, he is often admitted to the confidence of those who perhaps think they owe their life to his care. He sees people in the most disadvantageous circumstances, very different from those in which the world views them – oppressed with pain, sickness and low spirits. In their humiliating situations, instead of wonted cheerfulness, evenness of temper and vigour of mind he meets with peevishness, impatience and timidity. Hence it appears how much the characters of individuals and the credit of families may sometimes depend on the discretion, secrecy and honour of the physician.

TEMPERANCE AND SOBRIETY

In the course of an extensive practice difficult cases frequently occur which demand the most vigorous exertion of memory and judgement. I have heard it said of some eminent physicians that they prescribe as justly when intoxicated as when sober. If there was any truth in the report it contains severe reflection against their abilities in their profession. It shows that they practise by rote or prescribe some of the more obvious symptoms without attending to those nice peculiar circumstances a knowledge of which constitutes the great difference between a physician who has genius and one who has none. Intoxication implies a defect in the memory and judgement; it implies confusion of ideas, perplexity and unsteadiness and must therefore unfit a man for every business that requires the lively and vigorous use of his understanding.

THE LEGACY

John Gregory published his *Lectures on the Duties and Qualifications of a Physician* in 1772. His *Lectures* were translated into French in 1787, into German in 1788 and into Italian in 1789. Benjamin Rush, who, as a student, had attended Gregory's lectures in Edinburgh, published an Americanised version, *Observations on the Duties and Offices of a Physician and Methods of Improving Medicine: Accommodated to the Present State of Society and Manners in the United States* in 1805; an American edition of Gregory's own Lectures followed in 1817.

Gregory's work, like that of his contemporaries in Edinburgh – Francis Hutchison, David Hume, Adam Smith, Lord Kames, Robert Adam, Adam Ferguson and William Robertson – was a product of the Scottish Enlightenment. It helped to shape the modern world and, in particular, the modern world of medicine.

7

AN INDUSTRIAL SOCIETY
Andrew Duncan and Medical Police

In the middle years of the eighteenth century, the College was faced by the problems of a changing society. Less than one in ten of the people of Scotland still lived in a town[1] but that proportion was increasing rapidly. Manufacturers had found that by setting up in town they were closer to their markets and to their sources of of providing accommodation and other support for their workers. Most of those who left the countryside to work in the workshops and businesses of the towns were young adults attracted by the prospect of betters paid jobs, 'a wider diversity of social contacts and infinitively greater colour and excitement in their lives'.[2] But prospering towns also attracted the idle, the disaffected and the vagrants who came to beg. Over rapid expansion of the towns led to the overcrowding of decaying ancient housing, the overwhelming of primitive systems of sanitation, disease and a constantly rising mortality. Belligerent relationships within an increasingly competitive urban society led to violence and crime.

These problems of urbanisation had already occurred elsewhere in Europe. In the German-speaking world, both Frederick the Great of Prussia and Franz Joseph II of Austria had deprived the church of its role in the promotion of health and the regulation of society in favour of strong central 'rational' lay administrations. In both countries medicine and the law became 'sister professions, serving the ruler and benefiting the nation'.[3] The policy adopted for the management of 'the urban problem' was based on the ideas of Johann Peter Frank, Professor of Medicine at Vienna.

Like the great majority of his German contemporaries, Frank believed that a nation's greatest wealth was its people and that, in the interest of the state, the people should be as numerous, healthy and productive as possible. In his six-volume *System Einer Vollstandigen Medicinischen Polizey (A Complete System of Medical Police)* he stressed the importance of social factors (public cleanliness, proper ventilation of houses, adequate loose clothing, affectionate marriages, breastfeeding and the vaccination of children). He advocated active intervention by the state to regulate all environmental and social factors believed to have an influence on health. He proposed that central governments should assume cradle-to-grave responsibility for the health of their people and, guided by medical experts, legislate on such factors as nutrition, wages, housing, marriage, pregnancy and prostitution, quarantine and vaccination. The state was also to regulate the activities of all the caring services – hospitals and dispensaries,

1. T.D. Devine, Urbanisation, in T.D. Devine and R. Mitchison, *People and Society in Scotland Vol. I* (Edinburgh, 1988), p. 28.
2. A.S. Wohl, *Endangered Lives* (London, 1983), p. 80.
3. R. Porter, *The Greatest Gift to Mankind* (London, 1999), p. 293.

maternity services, poorhouses and pharmacies – and take responsibility for medical education and the licensing of medical practitioners. Frank's proposals derived from the philosophy of Christian Wolff (1679–1754) who held that, as individuals, the people had no personal intrinsic rights in relation to health but, as citizens, must accept that they were 'objects of governmental care'[4] and that the state had an absolute right of guardianship over their health.

Elsewhere in Europe moral philosophers and political economists rejected Wolff's concept of the proper relationship between the state and its people. In France, where the process of urbanisation had proceeded almost twice as far as in Germany, the policy advocated for management was based on the works of Rousseau. Rousseau, in his *Du Contrat Social ou Principes Politique*, claimed that man must be free to form a society based on equality. Since the physical degeneration and disease suffered by the poor was ultimately the result of the gross inequality in contemporary society, Rousseau proposed that the first duty of the medical profession should be to rescue the people from the ill-effects of inequality. In the years leading up to the Revolution, French *philosophes* demanded that this should be done by ensuring that all citizens had equal access to health care, free for those unable to pay. Poverty, in this context, was to be recognised as a socio-economic problem with no moral or religious overtones. The aid provided by religious, philanthropic and municipal charities was to be coordinated and directed by the state and redefined as poor relief ('bienfaisance') which the poor had a right to receive and which the state had a duty to deliver. The French Academy of Science and the Royal Society of Medicine in Paris were called on to draw up schemes for the reform of the country's hospitals, poor houses and dispensaries to improve their therapeutic efficiency, to make them more accessible and to relieve what had become unacceptable levels of overcrowding and squalor. The Royal Society of Medicine in Paris was to act as the centre for the active promotion of new ideas on hygiene and the control of epidemics. Practical schemes were to be drawn up for the improvement of public drainage and water supply and for the education of the people on hygiene. The essential characteristic of health policy proposed for France was the massive intervention by the state in the medical care of the whole population. The system was to be demand led, ready to respond to the individual needs presented by every citizen.

ELEGANCE AND SQUALOR IN EDINBURGH

In Scotland urbanisation had begun much later and had progressed much faster than in Germany or France. The consequences of urbanisation were to be seen at their most extreme in the industrial towns of west and central Scotland but, by the 1790s, Edinburgh had also been both socially and physically transformed. Those who had been greatly rewarded by change had become separated geographically as well as socially from those who had been its victims, making the contrast all the more starkly visible.

In 1763, Edinburgh had been confined almost entirely within the city walls. The town consisted of two long parallel streets with a maze of wynds and closes leading off from both.

---

4. S.M.K. Martin, 'William P. Alison: Active Philanthropist and Pioneer of Social Medicine' (PhD thesis, St Andrews University, 1997).

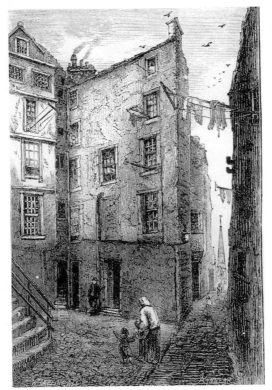

Flesh Market Close with High Street 'landes' in the background

Every space that had once been occupied by a garden had long been built over. For lack of space the town had grown vertically. People of every rank lived cheek by jowl in flats in the city's multi-storied 'landes'. Even 'persons of quality' who could command the most desirable residences in these ancient high tenements still lived in 'mean and dirty abodes … where there was little cleanliness or comfort'.[5]

But by the 1790s, Edinburgh was displaying impressive and visible evidence of a new prosperity. The aristocracy and landed magnates had given up their town houses in the insalubrious confines of the Old Town and bought spacious, comfortable and elegant houses in George Square, the fashionable new suburb on the south side of the city or in the even more elegant terraces of the New Town to the north; the lesser gentry who came to Edinburgh only for the winter months and in the past had rented a flat in the High Street or the Canongate for £8 or £10 could now well afford to rent a house in the New Town for £100. There they no longer rubbed shoulders with the whole gamut of Edinburgh's citizens as their families had done for generations. Their neighbours in their new surroundings were members of their own kindred who, with little inheritance other than family influence, had made successful careers in the army, in the navy, in government or in learned professions with perhaps the addition of one or two of Edinburgh's most successful merchants or entrepreneurs. In 1763, few of these

5. Sir Walter Scott, quoted by H.G. Graham, *The Social Life of Scotland in the Eighteenth Century* (London, 1928), p. 125.

families could have thought of employing a male servant; in 1790 no genteel family could be without a manservant employed on a salary of £10 to £20 per annum and numbers of maid-servants who were now dressed as well as their mistresses had been in 1763. In 1763, one stage-coach each month had connected Edinburgh and London, taking twelve to sixteen days on the journey. In 1790 fifteen stage-coaches left Edinburgh every week reaching London within three days. This frequent and easy traffic with polite society in London, carried to Edinburgh a new and more extravagant lifestyle. Perfumers, never before known in Edinburgh, opened their splendid shops in every principal street (some kept bears that were killed to provide the fat that was then fashionable for the management of ladies' hair). Many thousands of pounds of starch were sold as hair powder. Carriages replaced sedan chairs, carrying their passengers to dine with friends, to balls in the new Assembly Rooms in George Street or to performances at Edinburgh's two new theatres. Edinburgh now had a decorative and decorous polite society of its own.

This new elite society owed its prosperity to advances in Scotland's trade, agriculture, and industry that had begun much earlier in the century. Merchants in Glasgow and the West of Scotland had exploited the legal access to trade with the (formerly English) colonies in America and the West Indies that had come with the Act of Union in 1707. In the middle years of the century Scotland was importing 13 million pounds of tobacco from Virginia; by 1775 that amount had increased to 21,000 tons. The very handsome profits from this trade in tobacco and from the importation of sugar from the West Indies provided capital for investment in new industries. The first industries to benefit were the manufacture of linen in small towns across Fife and the central belt and the production of woollens in the Borders and Ayrshire but by the end of the century cotton manufacture, concentrated in the growing industrial towns in the west, had become the dominant industry in Scotland.

As early as the 1720s and 1730s, a number of landlords had invested in draining and liming their fields and had introduced new crops and systems of crop rotation. But although they had increased the productivity of their estates most had lost money and a few had made themselves bankrupt. Later in the century, however the growth of the textile towns provided lucrative markets and new roads and improvements in the transport made the exploitation of these markets possible. By the 1790s, the landed gentry who were at the centre of Edinburgh's new polite society were enjoying the benefits of increased productivity, steadily rising farm prices and higher rents from their tenants. Some had also invested parts of their profits in the new industries. A few become extravagantly wealthy and were able to commission the architects Robert Adam or Robert Mylne to build great country houses; Inverary (for the Duke of Argyll), Mellerstain (for George Baillie) and Culzean (for the Earl of Cassillis) were the finest examples.

But those enjoying the full benefits of this upturn in the economy formed only a tiny minority of the people of Scotland. The modernisation of farming practices enriched the landlords and led to an increase in the wages of skilled workers. But it severely reduced the need for the services of the unskilled. There was now a surplus of labour and that surplus was made worse by a sudden and unprecedented increase in the population. Between 1755 and the end of the century the population of Scotland increased by 27 per cent. During these years there was a steady drift of people from the country to towns which offered some hope of employment. Some found work in their county towns where the commercialisation of farming had increased the volume of business; the population of Perth, Ayr and other county towns doubled. But many more flocked to the growing centres of industry and commerce. The textile town of Paisley more than trebled in size; Greenock, which was both a trading port and a manufacturing town, quadrupled. Glasgow had new chemical works and thousands of new textile looms and was at the heart of all the commercial activities of the West of Scotland.

In Edinburgh there were no new major industries to attract the unemployed. Nevertheless, Edinburgh was the administrative, legal and banking centre of a nation growing more commercially aggressive and more litigious. The number of paper mills increased from three to twelve, six printing-and-publishing houses became sixteen. the production of glass and crystal in the city had quintupled. And there were a number of new small concerns – glass and crystal factories, coach builders and button makers – catering for the luxury market. In half a century Edinburgh's population increased from 57,000 to 82,000. The overcrowded Old Town became even more overcrowded. In the 1760s the people of the Old Town had lived in 'dwellings where fetid air brought sickness and death to young lives, where infectious diseases passed like wild fire through the inmates of a crowded common stair bringing havoc to many a household'.[6] These same dwellings were now subdivided to accommodate ever larger numbers of families. The fabric of the Old Town was allowed to deteriorate. The water supply and the sewerage and public cleansing arrangements, already primitive, became dangerously inadequate. For skilled workers, although their living conditions were still miserably inadequate, wages had increased to between ten shillings and thirty shillings a week and there was a degree of security. At most times, food was cheap and plentiful; in 1781 a fleet of 600 ships and 30,000 men anchored in the Forth for seven weeks was provisioned from Edinburgh without causing any rise in prices. However, day-labourers, who made up a much higher proportion of the population, earned no more than one or two shillings a day; at low points in the trade cycle they could suffer long periods of unemployment and when harvests were poor and food prices rose they could go hungry; in the great dearth of 1795 one in eight of Edinburgh's population was fed by charity. Tuberculosis, typhus, scarlet fever and measles, diseases that were to become major causes of death in Britain's town and cities in the nineteenth century, were already on the increase in Edinburgh.

It was popularly believed that such diseases were carried by the noxious urban miasma. Many came to believe that the same urban miasma also brought criminality. In the 1760s house breaking was rare, street robbery and pick-pocketing were unknown and 'a person could walk the length of the city without being accosted by a single street walker'. By the end of the century, house breaking, theft and robbery had become 'astonishingly frequent',[7] the number of brothels had increased from five to over a hundred and there were street prostitutes to be seen in every part of the city. Capital crimes had also increased alarmingly; at the middle of the

6. Sir Walter Scott, *Provincial Antiquities and Picturesque Scenery of Scotland* (Edinburgh, 1826).
7. *The Statistical Account of Scotland; Letters to Sir John Sinclair Bt; Letter Second* (Edinburgh, 1791).

century there were, on average, only three executions in Scotland each year. In one autumn circuit in Edinburgh in 1783, thirty-seven criminals were sentenced to death.

In the last years of the eighteenth century, Edinburgh was a flourishing and picturesque city. Its New Town was the elegant setting for a wealthy and polite society. It was home to the largest and most modern university in Britain. Its medical school was the leading such institution in Europe. For more than two generations its philosophers, historians and natural scientists influenced the thinking of the world. But, in the mean streets of its Old Town, Edinburgh already harboured the urban problems of overcrowding, squalor, poverty, disease and public disorder that would afflict all the industrial towns of Britain as they continued to grow throughout the nineteenth century.

As the industrialisation and urbanisation of Britain continued and intensified into the nineteenth century, doctors in every part of the country found themselves called upon to provide new medical services for the poor and professional advice for local and central government authorities. But for the greater part of the nineteenth century in Britain, it was only graduates of Scottish universities who had formal instruction on the promotion of the health of the public and on the medical aspects of the maintenance of law and order. These subjects had been introduced to the Scottish medical curriculum in the last years of the eighteenth century by Andrew Duncan, twice President of the Royal College of Physicians of Edinburgh.

ANDREW DUNCAN

Andrew Duncan was born into a family without wealth or influence in 1744. His father was a merchant in Crail, a small fishing town ten miles south of St Andrews, a port once thriving but now in decline. Although Duncan's mother was distantly related to families of the lesser landed gentry of Fife his parents were far from rich. Nevertheless they were able to invest in their son's education. As a child he was taught by Sandy Con and by Richard Dick who both had considerable reputations as scholars and tutors; at the age of fourteen he became a student at St Andrews University taking his MA degree in 1762. He then moved to Edinburgh University to study medicine, paying his class fees of three guineas to attend the courses given by Alexander Monro *secundus*, Joseph Black, John Hope John Gregory and William Cullen. While in Edinburgh, he also became strongly influenced by the philosophy, economics and sociology of David Hume, Adam Smith and Adam Ferguson, then at the height of their powers as the leaders of intellectual life in Edinburgh.

THE ROYAL MEDICAL SOCIETY

As a student at Edinburgh, Duncan became president of the university's Medical Society (later the Royal Medical Society). The Society had been founded in 1734 by Edinburgh's medical students to provide a forum for their own independent efforts to advance their medical education. The Society met to discuss matters of current medical interest and to hear and criticise dissertations presented by the students themselves; it bought cadavers for anatomical dissection; and it built up its own excellent library. The Medical Society also gave Edinburgh

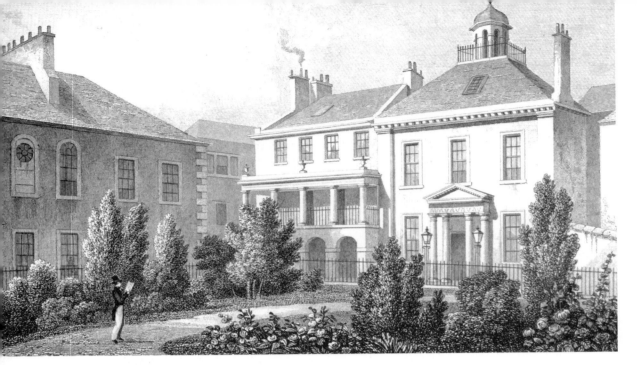

Surgeons' Hall and Royal Medical Society

students a voice in shaping their formal training. The Medical Society had become the recognised channel thought which the views, demands and protests of the student body were presented to the dean and faculty. As we shall see, the Medical Society was to play an important part in furthering Duncan's career in Edinburgh.

In 1768, Duncan left Edinburgh without taking a degree. He enlisted as surgeon on the East India Company's ship *Asia* then engaged in the company's immensely lucrative trade with India and in carrying opium from India to China. Duncan did not travel, as William Cullen had done, to study the medicinal plants of foreign climates but to gather enough money to support him while he established himself in an academic career in Scotland. His plan was even more successful than he had hoped. After only one voyage he could afford to refuse the offer of 500 guineas to make a second voyage and to return to Scotland and marry Mary Knox, the daughter of a surgeon.

SHAPING A CAREER

In October 1769, Duncan obtained his diploma as a Doctor of Medicine from St Andrews and in May 1770 he became a licentiate of the Royal College of Physicians of Edinburgh. Only weeks later he applied to be appointed as Professor of Medicine at St Andrews. His application was rejected but his confidence and his academic ambitions remained undiminished. He set up in practice in Edinburgh, supplementing his income by giving private extra-mural lectures on Materia Medica. He also renewed his association with the Royal Medical Society becoming its president for the second time; in the following years he was to serve a further four terms as its president. In 1775 he organised the fundraising campaign that enabled the Society first to furnish and equip the rooms provided for its use by the university and, later, to build a Hall of its own in 1786. He was also the prime mover in securing the Society's Royal Charter in 1778. On many occasions Duncan acted as spokesman for the students in negotiations and confrontations with faculty. Towards the end of his life, he frequently claimed that it was he who had established the Royal Medical Society as `an essential part of the medical school of Edinburgh'. It is certainly true that it was the Royal Medical Society that gave him his first opportunity to demonstrate his persuasive skills as a reformer and innovator and to make his mark in the community of Edinburgh medicine.

THE OUTSIDER

In a long career Duncan received many honours. He was twice elected president of the Royal College of Physicians. For thirty-eight years he held the chair of the Institutes of Medicine at Edinburgh University. He became First Physician to the King. He was made a freeman of the City of Edinburgh. He was elected to the Danish Philosophical Society, the Royal Society of Medicine of Paris, the American Philosophical Society of Philadelphia and the Medical Society of London. He was elected the first president of the Medico-chirurgical Society of Edinburgh. He was a genial and clubbable man with a great number of friends outside the world of medicine and Fellows of both the Royal College of Physicians and the Royal College of Surgeons were more than ready to join him in founding his dining club, the Aescalapian Society.

However he was not without his detractors and his enemies. Lord Cockburn wrote of him:

> He was so simple that even those who were suffering under his interminable projects checked their impatience and submitted. Scientific ambition, charitable restlessness and social cheerfulness made him thrust himself into everything ... His patronage was generally dangerous and his talk always wearisome.[8]

Duncan's most powerful opponent was William Cullen. In 1769, Duncan had paid the required fee at St Andrew's University and had been granted a medical degree without examination. As a graduate of a Scottish university, he was then accepted as a licentiate of the Royal College of Physicians of Edinburgh, again without examination (Chapter 1). William Cullen was at that time 'extremely desirous that the practice of conferring medical degrees on unqualified persons should be effectively checked by the universities being prevented from granting these to persons who had not submitted themselves to examination'.[9] That Duncan should have chosen to take advantage of this regrettable practice to gain entry to Edinburgh medicine made his presence in Edinburgh most unwelcome to Cullen. As the direction of Duncan's ambitions became clear in the years that followed, Cullen came to regard him as not only unwelcome but also dangerous.

From his arrival in Edinburgh in 1755, Cullen had contested the teachings of Boerhaave that had been unchallenged in Edinburgh for half a century and had introduced new concepts

8. Lord Cockburn, *Memorials of His Time* (Edinburgh, 1854), p. 273.
9. J. Thomson, *An Account of the Life, Lectures and Writings of William Cullen* (Edinburgh, 1859).

of his own. In the years that followed he was always ready to amend his ideas in the light of new advances in medical science. But he believed that the future of medicine lay in applying the discoveries of medical science to the care of individual patients. The management of the well-being of the public at large, the focus of Duncan's emerging ambitions, did not appeal to Cullen as a proper field of activity for the medical profession. Cullen was warm in his hospitality and generous in his support for generations of new men in the profession but he lent his support only to those who were ready to follow the direction he had set. He was also authoritarian. Until illness forced him to retire in 1789, Cullen used his very considerable influence to prevent Duncan from receiving the imprimatur of the College of Physicians or of Edinburgh University.

For eighteen years until Cullen retired, Duncan attended almost every meeting of the College but in these many years he was never appointed to any office or invited to play any real part in College affairs. When, at a meeting of the College in 1781, Duncan ventured to put forward a proposal for 'a general inoculation for the smallpox at certain fixed periods' in Edinburgh the project was quietly and purposely allowed to die. Nevertheless, Duncan continued to make his frequent donations of books and copies of all his own publications to the College library and there is no evidence that he ever expressed any resentment at the coolness of his reception by the College. He was more deeply distressed by his rejection by the University.

Since setting up practice in Edinburgh in 1770, Duncan had been successful as an extramural lecturer. In 1772, with the backing of the publishers John Murray in London and William Creech in Edinburgh, he had launched the world's first English-language medical journal. His *Medical and Philosophical Commentaries* was based on the model of the Leipzig journal, *Commentarii de Remus in Scientio Natirali et Medicina Gestis*. In the Introduction to the first issue of his new journal Duncan explained:

> No one, who wishes to practise medicine, with safety to others or credit to himself, will incline to remain ignorant of any discovery which time or attention has brought to light. But it is well known that the greatest part of those who are engaged in the actual prosecution of this art, have neither the leisure nor opportunity for very extensive reading

Medical and Philosophical Commentaries was published quarterly. Each issue was in four sections: reviews of the 'best new books on medicine and those branches of philosophy most intimately connected with it'; medical cases and observations; medical news; and a list of new medical publications. In its first month, the *Commentaries* reviewed works from Vienna, Paris, Petersburg, Leyden, London, Philadelphia, Gottigen, Bologna, Turin, Dublin, Zurich and Tubingen. More than 1,000 copies of each quarterly issue were published simultaneously in Edinburgh, London and Dublin. From the beginning the journal was well received by all types of medical practitioners – university-trained physicians, barber surgeons and apothecaries – and its reputation soon justified its translation into several other languages.

Within a very few years Duncan's publications had earned him an international reputation;

his services to the Royal Medical Society had brought him to notice within the university; and the success of his extramural lectures had demonstrated his abilities as a teacher. In 1773, when John Gregory, the Professor of the Institutes of Medicine, died at the age of 49, Duncan was among the five applicants to succeed him. The patrons of the University, guided by Cullen, appointed Dr Alexander Munro Drummond, a relative of Edinburgh's provost and the university's Chancellor, George Drummond and a closer relative of Professor Alexander Monro *primus*. Alexander Munro Drummond was then physician to the King of Naples and unable to take up the chair immediately. Andrew Duncan was invited to fill what was expected to be a temporary vacancy.

Duncan acted as locum Professor of the Institutes of Medicine during the sessions 1774–75 and 1775–76. Then, in the continuing absence of Dr Drummond, the University decided that it must make a new substantive appointment. The competition was intense. Duncan's most formidable rivals for the appointment were William Small and James Gregory. Small was a former protégé of John Gregory, a friend of David Hume, Lord Kames and Joseph Black, a former professor at the College of William and Mary at Williamsburg and a Fellow of the Royal Society; he also had the strong support of Joseph Priestly and Benjamin Franklin. James Gregory was still a very young man, but he was the son of the previous professor; he was also the favoured candidate of William Cullen who was not only the most powerful member of the medical faculty but had also undertaken to pay the salary of the person appointed.[10] In spite of this very formidable competition, Andrew Duncan assumed that, having successfully occupied the post for two years, his appointment would be automatic.

When the Town Council elected James Gregory to follow his father as Professor of the Institutes of Medicine, Duncan's disappointment was intense. He attributed his failure, in part to his politics (he was known to be a Whig of decidedly progressive views) but principally to his lack of patronage or family interest. He made this clear to students he had been teaching since 1774:

> I have the satisfaction of being able to retire from this arduous task with ease in my own mind, and I hope not without some additional credit in your estimation. My academic labours have not indeed in other respects been attended with equal advantage ... I had no hesitation in offering myself a candidate for the Chair recently vacant [but] in that competition I had no powerful connection, no political interest to aid my cause ... I can no longer act in an equally conspicuous capacity, yet I hope I may hereafter be employed as a teacher in one not less useful. It is my intention to dedicate my lab to the service of students of medicine. The present disappointment may yet afford me strongest instance of the favour of heaven.[11]

Rejected by the university, Duncan decided to teach on his own account. In 1776, his advertisement for an 'Independent Course of Lectures on the Theory and Practice of

10. A. Dalzel, *History of the University of Edinburgh* (Edinburgh, 1862), p. 443.
11. *Medical and Philosophical Commentaries*, 1776, Vol. IV, p. 103.

Medicine without the walls of the university' attracted over a hundred students to his classes at 10 Surgeons' Square.[12] Building on this success, in 1777 he added a course on Materia Medica. He also established a Dispensary in Edinburgh's Old Town.

A Dispensary for the Infant Poor had already been established in London in 1769. That first Dispensary had not survived but the idea had been taken up and expanded. By 1776, Dispensaries providing out-patient care and home visiting for the poor of all ages had been established in a number of towns in England. Duncan's dispensary was established and financed as a public charity but from the beginning, and unlike the dispensaries elsewhere, it was planned as an extension of Duncan's extramural teaching programme. Students paying a fee of one guinea for each of his two lecture courses were also required to contribute half a guinea towards the expenses of the dispensary. Patients attending the Dispensary received free medicines and advice and in return agreed to be demonstrated to classes of medical students by Duncan or his assistant, Charles Webster.

The poor and the sick came in unexpectedly large numbers, revealing the full extent of the disease, the disability and physical deterioration suffered by the urban poor. Duncan's students became familiar with chronic diseases that were rarely if ever to be seen in the Royal Infirmary. And, since dispensary patients were also visited in their homes, the students were also introduced to a form of clinical practice not taught by the university school. Duncan's extramural medical school continued to flourish for thirteen years.

WILLIAM BUCHAN, MEDICINE AND THE INDIVIDUAL.

During these thirteen years, Duncan found it impossible to challenge Cullen's authority within both the College and the University or Cullen's negative view of the part the medical profession should play in promoting the health of the general public. However, a challenge was attempted by William Buchan.

Buchan had studied medicine at Edinburgh for nine years. In 1758, without taking a degree, he left Edinburgh to practise in Yorkshire. A year later he was appointed as medical officer to the Foundling Hospital at Ackworth and, from there, he wrote his MD thesis on 'De Infantum Vita Conservanda'. In 1771, he obtained his licence to practise from the College and returned to Edinburgh, becoming a Fellow of the College in 1772.

Buchan believed that the health of the nation could best be improved by enabling every literate member of the public to take charge of his own health, the health of his family and the health of his dependants as far as that could be done without the intervention of the medical profession. While in Yorkshire he had corresponded with his friend, the Edinburgh publisher and polymath William Creech. Creech had studied theology at Edinburgh but, as he explained to his friends, he had moved from theology to medicine because he believed that he should not devote himself to the saving of souls while so many lived in physical misery.

In 1769, in partnership with Creech, Buchan published his book *Domestic Medicine: A Treatise on the Prevention and Cure of Diseases by Regimen and Simple Medicines*. The book was

12. M. Kaufman, *Medical Teaching in Edinburgh during the Eighteenth and Nineteenth Century* (Edinburgh, 2003), p. 6.

greatly influenced by the 'common sense' doctrines of Buchan's friend, the Aberdeen philosopher, Thomas Reid. An advertisement for the book published in the *Edinburgh Weekly Journal* explained that it had been written 'to show how far it is in the power of every man to preserve his own health by proper conduct or restore it when it is lost'. In an Introduction to the first edition of *Domestic Medicine* the author (probably Creech) wrote:

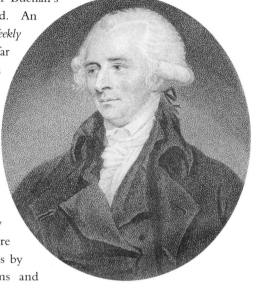

William Buchan

> Medicine has been studied by few except those who intend to live by it as a trade. Such, either from a mistaken zeal or to raise their own importance, have endeavoured to disguise and conceal the art. Medical authors have generally written in a foreign language and those who are unequal to this task have even valued themselves by couching at least their prescriptions in terms and characters unintelligible to the rest of mankind ...

> We do not mean that every man should become a physician. That would be an attempt as ridiculous as it is impossible. All we plead for is that men of sense and learning should be so far acquainted with the general principles of medicine as to be in a condition to derive from it some of those advantaged with which it is fraught and at the same time to guard against the destructive influences of ignorance, superstition and quackery.

The book proved to be immensely popular and for many years *Domestic Medicine* came second only to the Bible as the book most likely to be found in Scottish households. In all it ran to nineteen editions in Britain with further editions in North America and translations into all the main languages of Europe. In over 700 pages, Buchan set out simple advice on the care of infants and young children, on diet, on clothing, on fresh air, on exercise, on sleep, on travel and on the 'passions' and gave guidance on the management of the common medical and surgical conditions of the time.

The book was not well received by Cullen and the medical establishment in Edinburgh. *Domestic Medicine* was not immediately added to the library of the College of Physicians in 1769 and was not to be found there until Cullen was dead. In 1773, Buchan, like Duncan, applied for the Chair of the Institutes of Medicine at Edinburgh. When Cullen's protégé, Alexander Munro Drummond – a young man not yet licensed to practise in Edinburgh – was appointed, Buchan was furious. He attacked Cullen in print and, it has been said, had to be restrained by his friends from calling him out 'on the field of honour'. Cullen was unmoved and in 1778, Buchan left for London where he built up a successful practice and continued to publish works such as On the Offices and Duties of a Mother and Advice to Mothers on the Subject of their own Health. When he died in 1805 he was buried in Westminster Abbey.

ANDREW DUNCAN, MEDICINE AND THE STATE

Duncan's approach to the promotion of the well-being of the population was in sharp contrast with that promoted by Buchan. As editor of his *Medical and Philosophical Commentaries*, Duncan had become involved in an international discourse on public health policy. In other countries in Western Europe the urbanisation of the population had been less abrupt than in Scotland but had continued over a much longer period. There were many towns in Europe larger and more crowded than any in Scotland and, on the Continent, concern for the health of urbanised populations had a much longer history.

Duncan studied the German and French models and concluded, correctly, that neither was likely to succeed. The full elaborate bureaucratic structure required for the scheme envisioned for Germany was found to be impractical and was soon abandoned for more modest schemes. The idealistic concept of equal and universal health, tentatively put in place in Revolutionary France, soon ran into trouble; as the Revolutionary Wars continued, the depletion of Treasury funds put an end to expensive public health schemes and a demand-led system providing equal healthcare for every citizen proved to be impossibly expensive.

Duncan envisaged a quite different relationship between the state and the medical profession. He proposed that, while the profession should not act as an instrument of the state, it should be ready to assist the state in combating the social evils of crime and squalor. It should advise the state in the formulation of legislation that would protect the health and safety of the people and provide medical expertise in support of the law. At the end of the eighteenth century the medical profession in Britain did not have the expertise to assist the state in either of these ways. As soon as it became possible for him to mend what he had come to see as a lamentable deficiency in medical education in Britain, Duncan introduced instruction of Medical Police and Medical Jurisprudence at Edinburgh.

ANDREW DUNCAN AND THE *INSTITUTES MEDICINAE LEGALIS*

In February 1789 William Cullen, now aged 79, became unwell and unable to take any further part in the affairs of the College; in November, Andrew Duncan was elected to the Council. In December, Cullen resigned as Professor of Medicine and James Gregory was appointed to succeed him. In Gregory's place, Duncan at last became Professor of the Institutes of Medicine (and the only medical professor at Edinburgh who had not succeeded his father in office). From the beginning his course on the Institutes of Medicine included a few lectures on what he called the *Institutes Medicinae Legalis*. After a few years these lectures had come to occupy so much of the time allotted to his weekday statutory course on the traditional *Institutes of Medicine* that, in 1792, he launched a separate course of lectures on his *Institutes Medicinae Legalis* at two o'clock on Saturday afternoons. The course was open to medical and law students and to members of the lay public. In the summer the lectures were on medical police in the winter on forensic medicine. Although these were disciplines that had been taught for some years at leading European universities they had not, until then, been taught in Britain.

In a letter to the senate of the university he explained that traditionally the Institutes of

Medicine had been presented as 'five inferior brands' – physiology, pathology, symptomatolgy, hygiene and therapeutics. He had re-grouped these five topics together under two headings, pathological physiology and general therapeutics and had added two new subjects: medical jurisprudence and medical police. Duncan insisted that the inclusion of these new subjects was more than justified since they were 'of considerably greater consequence both to the profession and to the public' than many of the traditional subjects taught at the medical school since they concerned 'not merely the welfare of individuals but 'the prosperity of nations'. In 1792 and again in 1795, he published the subjects to be covered in his lectures on medical police and medical jurisprudence in a pamphlet subtitled *Institutiones Medicinae Legalis.*[13]

MEDICAL POLICE

Duncan's teaching on the promotion of the public health was based on the concept of 'Medical Police' set out by Frank in his System *Einer Vollstandigen Medicinischen Polizey*. He published his Heads of Lectures:

- *Insalubritas aeris* (temperature, humidity and foreign impregnations of the air)
- *Insalubritas aquae* (purity, smell, temperature and supply of water)
- *Insalubritas victus et potus* (price, quality and preparation of food and drink)
- *Consuetudines salutare et noxiae* (exercise conducive or adverse to health)
- *Morbi contagiosi* (prevention of infectious diseases
- *Carceres* (abuses and defects of jails)
- *Nosocomia* (regulation of hospitals)
- *Sepultura cadaveum* (proper burial of the dead).

MEDICAL JURISPRUDENCE

On medical jurisprudence Duncan looked to the expertise that had been built up over many years in Germany and France. It was an experience that was in sharp contrast to that in Scotland and England. In British courts it was the function of the jury to assess the value of evidence and to take the final judgment on the facts as they had been presented. Any medical man with knowledge of facts or circumstances relevant to the case could be called as a witness and was expected to do so as his civic duty, without payment and at whatever inconvenience. Forensic medicine had therefore not developed as a lucrative or prestigious from of expert professional practice.[14] In Germany and France there were no juries. Judges interrogated the witnesses, established the facts and decided the verdict. The judges were, however, expected to be guided by a code that laid down what evidence should be sought, how it should be obtained and how its value should be assessed. The judge's verdict was always open to review by a higher court and in the course of that review the medical evidence could be re-examined – in France by recognised (usually free-lance) medico-legal experts and in Germany usually by

---

13. A. Duncan, *Heads of Lectures on Medical Jurisprudence or the Institutiones Medicinae Legalis* (Edinburgh, 1795).
14. C. Crawford, Legalising Medicine, in M. Clark and C. Crawford (eds), *Legal Medicine in History* (Cambridge, 1994), p. 93.

medical professors at the country's leading universities. In both France and Germany these medico-legal experts formed a prestigious and well-paid elite. They produced their own body of literature and published works on forensic medicine which gave instructions on how medico-legal inspections should be conducted, what observations should be made and what conclusions might be drawn. Duncan's lectures on Medical Jurisprudence were based on this published work.

Lectures on Medical Jurisprudence - Questions before Criminal Courts

The inspection and reporting on:

- *Inspectio cadaverum legalis* (dead bodies)
- *Homicidum per vulnus* (nature and causes of wounds)
- *Homicidium per contusionem* (deaths from contusions)
- *Homicidiun per suspensionem* (deaths from hanging)
- *Homcidium per submersionem* (deaths from drowning)
- *Homicidium per siffocationem* (deaths from suffocation)
- *Homicicium per toxicationem* (deaths from poisons)
- *Infanticidilum* (child murder)
- *Abortus procuratus* (the circumstances giving rise to abortion)

Questions before Civil Courts: circumstances, evidence and proof of:

- *Mania* (insanity)
- *Melancholia* (depression)
- *Fatuitas* (idiocy)
- *Graviditas simulate* (feigned pregnancy)
- *Graviditas celeta* (concealed pregnancy)
- *Partus celatus* (previous delivery)
- *Partus simulatus* (previous deliveries)
- *Partus sertinu* (legitimacy of children)
- *Morbi simulate* (feigned illness)
- *Morby celati* (concealed disease)
- *Morbu imputati* (accusations of dotage, insanity, venereal disease)

Questions before Consistorial Courts: evidence relating to:

- *Impotentia virilis* (male impotence)
- *Sterilitas muliebris* (female sterility)
- *Sexus dubius* (hermaphrodites)
- *Syphilis* (venereal disease.)

In 1795 Duncan submitted a memorial to the patrons of the University setting out the case for the creation of a chair of Medical Police and Medical Jurisprudence. His proposal was rejected on the grounds that such a chair would not contribute to the dignity or prosperity of the university. Undaunted, Duncan continued his campaign to reform the medical curriculum to give greater emphasis to the protection and welfare of the public in general and the lower orders in society in particular. The political climate, however, had turned against reform. These were the years of the French Revolution and the Revolutionary Wars. In Scotland, as in much of Europe, the years of Enlightenment had given way to years of counter-Enlightenment.

Since 1775, when he became Lord Advocate, Henry Dundas had been the country's chief officer of government and thereafter made himself the supreme manipulator of political power and influence in Scotland; no one had exercised such control over the affairs of Scotland since Lord Ilay had fallen from power in 1763. While Dundas continued to hold high office under the Crown – in the Cabinet as Home Secretary later as Secretary of State for War and still later First Lord of the Admiralty and also as President of the Board of Control of the East India Company and Lord Privy Seal of Scotland – his command of patronage had made his authority complete. Although the office had been officially abolished after the '45 Rebellion, Dundas was the de facto Secretary of State for Scotland. For twenty years he had been amenable to measures of reform provided they were sufficiently supported in the country and were sure to bring practical benefits to Scotland.[15] In 1789, he was undisturbed by the Revolution in France since it seemed to be no more than a change in the nature of the monarchy akin to the Glorious Revolution in Britain in 1688. But within a few years it seemed to him that it had become 'not a limitation of the ancient and monarchical form of government but a conspiracy of the most profligate and ignorant people in the nation, against all the principals of society and religion, against all property, landed or commercial'. It had 'taken an aspect so formidable to neighboring nation that every man of a sober and deliberating mind had taken alarm'. In Scotland, he saw 'signs of a very turbulent and pernicious spirit having pervaded numerous and various descriptions of persons in this country'. There were riots in Edinburgh against the social order and against Dundas in particular; in 1792, his house in George Square was stoned and he was burned in effigy. Over the next two years, Dundas employed spies to gather intelligence of possible insurrection and soon earned a reputation as the representative of a repressive and tyrannical government. Whigs became suspect and Andrew Duncan was not only a Whig but also a close friend of Henry Erskine, Dundas's leading Whig opponent in Scotland. When Andrew Duncan submitted his proposals for reform of the medical curriculum at the university he was already tainted with radicalism. His proposal therefore found no favour with Dundas or with the university authorities who were firmly of Dundas's party.

NO LONGER AN OUTSIDER
Andrew Duncan's attempt to establish a Chair of Medical Jurisprudence and Medical Police had failed in 1795. At the height of the Revolutionary Wars with France such radical social reforms were almost bound to fail. But Duncan was no longer an outsider. He had been

---

15. M. Fry, *The Dundas Despotism* (Edinburgh, 2004), p. 159.

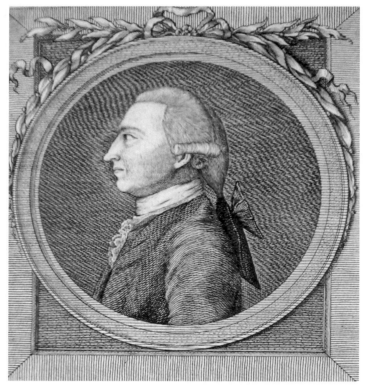

Andrew Duncan

President of the Royal College of Physicians of Edinburgh and was established as a Professor in the Faculty of Medicine at Edinburgh University. He had many friends and correspondents in Europe ready to support him and help groom his son as his successor. His son, also Andrew, had graduated MD at Edinburgh in 1792. It had twice been arranged for him to travel to Europe to study medical practice in the leading medical schools of Germany, France and Italy. There he had been befriended by J.P. Frank and other exponents of medical police and medical jurisprudence. He had reported regularly to his father on his European experience and had sent several consignments of European textbooks back to Edinburgh. In 1796 he returned to Edinburgh to become a Fellow of the Royal College of Physicians and Physician to the Royal Public Dispensary and to assist his father in editing his journal, now the *Annals of Medicine*. By 1806 there was no one in Scotland so well qualified to occupy a chair of Medical Police and Medical Jurisprudence when a chair could be created.

The occasion came in 1806. William Pitt, the Prime Minister who for more than twenty years had been the ultimate source of Dundas's power, was dead. Dundas was out of office and, as he wrote to a friend, 'in the hands of my enemies'. In Scotland the new Whig Lord Advocate was Andrew Duncan's friend, Henry Erskine. Erskine arranged for the creation of a Regius Chair of Medical Police and Medical Jurisprudence. As a Crown appointment the university could not refuse its creation but they could refuse to include the holder of the chair as one of the professors of medicine. The new chair was therefore established within the Faculty of Law. With Erskine's support Andrew Duncan junior was appointed and occupied the chair until 1820 when he was succeed by William Pultney Alison. Alison, the grandson of John Gregory, was welcomed by the medical establishment and Jurisprudence and Medical Police had become recognised as important subjects of study for medical students and the chair was transferred to the Faculty of Medicine. In the 1820s, the universities of Glasgow and Aberdeen also introduced instruction in Jurisprudence and Medical Police and in the 1830s competence in these subjects became mandatory for all graduates of Scottish universities and for all licentiates of the Scottish Royal Corporations. These were subjects that were not introduced at English medical schools until 1878.

Following Andrew Duncan's initiatives, the College made two new commitments to society in Britain. In the first half of the nineteenth century, the College campaigned to ensure that appropriate legislation was introduced for the promotion of public health and safety in Scotland. It also campaigned to ensure that graduates of Scottish universities, who made up the great majority of medical graduates in Britain and were the only graduates trained in medical police and medical jurisprudence, were able to practise in England.

8

CERTAIN MEASURES FOR THE PUBLIC GOOD
Inoculation against Smallpox, Sea Bathing, Care of the Insane

At the end of the eighteenth century Scotland was still without a central government body with responsibility for the health of its people. In England the protection of the health of the people was the responsibility of the Privy Council. But in Scotland, the Privy Council had been abolished in 1708 and, after the Jacobite Rebellion of 1745, the British Government had not allowed any principal department of government to be established north of the border.[1] In London the office of Secretary of State for Scotland had been allowed to lapse in 1746. Until late in the nineteenth century, Scotland was not represented in Cabinet and, in Parliament, Scottish business was usually ignored.[2] In the absence of an appropriate and interested central government body, either in Edinburgh in London, Duncan believed that it fell to the College to take the initiative in protecting and promoting the health of the public in Scotland.

On his first election as President, Andrew Duncan immediately appointed committees 'for the consideration of various subjects of a public nature to which the College seems in some measure called upon to attend'. These six committees, all chaired by Duncan himself, presented their reports in May 1791.

INOCULATION AGAINST SMALLPOX

For centuries smallpox had been endemic among the peoples of Asia, Arabia, Africa and Europe. It was a common disease of infants and young children and for those infected in childhood it was a mild illness causing little if any lasting damage. For those who did not contract the disease until adult life, smallpox was often fatal and the survivors were inevitably left disfigured by pockmarks and, in many cases, blind. Those who had suffered in the mild disease of childhood were recognised as having been fortunate and in different parts of the world folk customs evolved in which infants were deliberately exposed to infection. In China the custom was to 'open the pustules of one who has the small pox ripe upon him, drying up the matter with a little cotton and afterward put it up the nostrils of those that they would infect'. In Turkey, matter from 'the best sort of smallpox' was introduced under the skin on the point of 'a needle which gives no more than a scratch'. In some parts of the Highlands of Scotland, parents whose children had not yet had the smallpox would watch out for any other child 'having a good mild smallpox that they may communicate the disease to their children

1. I. Levitt (ed.), *Government and Social Conditions in Scotland* (Edinburgh, 1988), p. xi.
2. B.P. Lenman, *Integration and Enlightenment: Scotland 1746–1832* (Edinburgh, 1981); M. Lynch, *Scotland: A New History* (London, 1992), pp. 320, 325; T.M. Devine *The Scottish Nation* (London, 1999), pp. 5 and 18.

by making them bed fellows to those in it and by tying worsted threads with the pocking material around their wrists.[3]

> In England in the middle of the seventeenth century, Sydenham had followed a similar practice; when visiting patients with 'a favourable sort of smallpox' he taken with him the children of his friends and relations, hoping that they too would have the advantage of contracting the disease at an early age and in its mild form.

In Britain in the last years of the seventeenth century, smallpox became much more virulent. In the cities and larger towns there were severe epidemics and over time the interval between epidemics became shorter. In England the epidemic of 1681 was the most severe on record and others followed in 1710, 1714, 1716 and 1719. In London in 1721, Lady Mary Wortley Montague, the wife of the British Ambassador at Constantinople, famously had her daughter inoculated against the disease using the Turkish technique which a previous ambassador, Sir Robert Sutton, had found successful when he had his son inoculated at Constantinople. Sir Hans Sloane, the King's physician became persuaded of the merits of the procedure and, on his advice, George II had his daughters inoculated in 1722.[4] By the end of that year over 182 inoculations had been performed in England. But already there had been a number of deaths. Over the next few years the procedure became increasingly controversial and by 1728 it had been largely abandoned in England. The epidemics of small pox continued and by the middle and later years of the century, although still controversial, programmes of inoculation were introduced in Liverpool, Chester and a few other provincial centres in England.

In Scotland inoculation against smallpox was first introduced at Aberdeen in 1726 but was soon abandoned because of some early fatalities. It was introduced at Dumfries in 1733 and there it was continued in spite of a death rate of 1.5 per cent.[5] In a number of Highland parishes the landowner had the whole population inoculated at his expense, the procedure being carried out by the landowner himself, the parish minister or, in some parishes, by the blacksmith. In Edinburgh in 1754, the College pronounced that inoculation was proving 'highly salutary to the human race' and William Cullen advocated the procedure in his *First Lines of the Practice of Physic*. In Scotland, the value of inoculation, as carried out on an individual basis in private practice, was not disputed. But carried out in this limited way, inoculation had done nothing to control the recurring epidemics of smallpox. In the outbreak in 1742–44 in Edinburgh, 2,700 had died of smallpox and in the next twenty years epidemics continued to occur every three or four years. Nevertheless, whether it could be safely offered to the public at large was still as hotly disputed in Scotland as it was in England.

In 1781 a review was published of the results of the inoculation programmes that had been tried in Chester and other provincial towns in England.[6] The issues raised in the book were

---

3. A. Munro, *An Account of the Inoculation of Smallpox in Scotland* (Edinburgh, 1765); D. Hamilton, *The Healers* (Edinburgh, 1981), p. 96.
4. G. Miller, *The Adoption of Inoculation for Smallpox in England and France* (Pennsylvania, 1957), p. 96.
5. T. Ferguson, *The Dawn of Social Welfare in Scotland* (Edinburgh, 1948), p. 111.
6. W. Black, *Observations, Medical and Political on the Smallpox and the Advantages and Disadvantages of General Inoculation* (London, 1781).

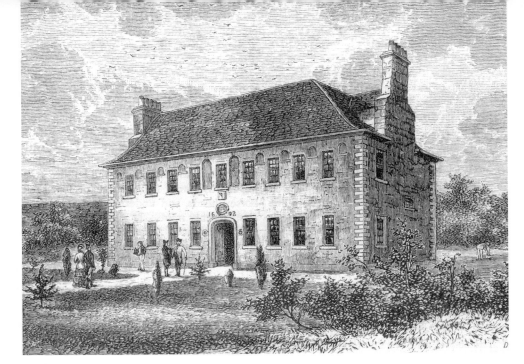

Darien House

discussed at length by Andrew Duncan in his journal *Medical Commentaries*.[7] Those opposed to general inoculation argued that, although there was little loss of life among those inoculated, the spreading of the disease, even in its mild form, by the inoculation of the whole population would inevitably lead to an increase in the numbers acquiring the disease 'in the natural way' later in life and in its severe form thus increasing the total number of deaths. They also argued that the inoculation of the children of the poor would prove to be dangerous since:

> the poor from being miserably lodged, their houses being in close lanes, courts and alleys; from their being often in want of necessities; from the father and mother being so constantly being abroad as would put it out of their power to give proper attention to their children under inoculation and such articles of medicine and diet as might be thought proper by the physician would never be regularly administered.[8]

On the other hand, proponents of inoculation argued that the bad air, deprivation and lack of parental and medical care suffered by the poor would 'surely prove more hurtful in the natural and malignant smallpox than in the mild artificial disease'. It was also claimed that it had been shown that in towns where a few hundred children had been inoculated 'as an experiment' there had been a significant fall in the total number of deaths from smallpox.

It was following the publication of this review in 1781 that Duncan had first proposed the introduction of 'general inoculation' in Scotland. That proposal, as we have seen, found no support at that time. In 1791 the College Committee on inoculation, which Duncan chaired, put forward a scheme for the 'Practice of Inoculation among the Lower Ranks':

7. A. Duncan, *Medical Commentaries*, 1783, Vol. 8, pp. 141–50.
8. Ibid., p.144.

1. The College of Physicians should insert an advertisement in the newspapers stating their sentiments of the great advantage which may be derived from the practice of inoculation becoming more general among the lower ranks and of the influence it might have in preserving many lives.

2. That this advertisement should make an offer of giving **gratis** attendance to the children of the lower ranks under inoculation during the months of September and October annually.

3. That they should recommend it to the managers of the Royal Infirmary and Public Dispensary to offer **gratis** inoculation during the same months.

4. That they should address a letter to every clergyman in Edinburgh informing him of these particulars and recommending it to him to take such methods as he may think best for convincing the people at large that by delaying to have their children inoculated in a populous town where they are constantly exposed to infection they neglect the means which providence has furnished them for preserving the lives of their offspring.

HOUSES OR ASYLUMS FOR LUNATICS

On 17 October 1774, the poet, Robert Fergusson, died in squalor in Darien House once the headquarters of the commercial company responsible for the disastrous Darien Expedition but now one of the two 'melancholy and desolate' buildings that housed Edinburgh's public asylum.[9] Andrew Duncan later wrote that 'at that time, 'no large town in Britain had worse accommodation for the cure or comfort of the insane than the city of Edinburgh, notwithstanding its excellent charitable establishments for other purposes'.

In medieval times in Scotland, as elsewhere in Europe 'madness' or 'lunacy' of any kind was attributed to witchcraft or demonic possession and, if it could not be relieved by healing wells or other mystical devices, the victim was persecuted or even put to death as the community attempted to purge itself of the attentions of the devil. From early in the sixteenth century madness was secularised and the victims became subject to social control; when control within the family failed, the victim was controlled by the same methods that were used to control criminals – stocks, prisons or madhouses that were little different from prisons.

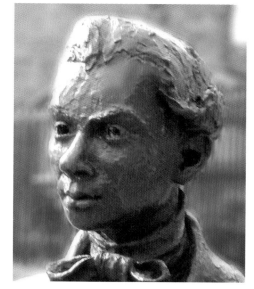

Robert Fergusson

9. H. Coghill, *Lost Edinburgh* (Edinburgh, 2005), p. 124.

Robert Fergusson, along with Alan Ramsay and Robert Burns, was one of Scotland's greatest poets of the eighteenth century. Since his late childhood he had suffered recurring and alternating periods of mania and depression. In July 1774 he was 'seized by a very dangerous illness'. During one of his periods of mental disturbance 'he had the misfortune to tangle with a rod-knob at the head of the staircase and fell from it striking his head violently against the lower steps. When lifted up and taken home he was utterly insensible'.[10] At home he regained consciousness but his behaviour became uncontrollable and his mother had him committed to the public asylum, known generally in Edinburgh as the 'Bedlam'. There he was visited by Andrew Duncan and the surgeon, Alexander Wood. They 'found him in a very deplorable condition subject to furious insanity'.[11] Fergusson remained incarcerated for over three months. In October, the surgeon, John Aitken, 'found Robert lying in his clothes, stretched upon a bed of loose uncovered straw. The moment he heard my voice he instantly rose, got me in his arms and wept and pleaded for his liberty'. Aitken thought him 'in a reasonable mental state and promised that he would soon be sent home'. However, a few days later Fergusson was dead.

Andrew Duncan had continued to visit Fergusson throughout his last illness and the memory of the appalling misery of the poet's many weeks in Edinburgh's 'Bedlam' remained with Duncan and inspired his determination to make better provision for the care of the insane. Duncan later wrote:

> Of all the calamities to which human nature is subjected insanity may justly be considered as the most deplorable. It not only deprives the unhappy individual who is affected with it of all the superiority derived from his rational faculties but reduces him to a state endangering his own life and that of others particularly of his best friends. The removal of insanity, therefore, should certainly call forth the united exertions of all who are not deprived of understanding and not void of humanity. It has accordingly been a common observation that among the different enlightened States of Europe in proportion to the degree of civilisation at which they have arrived means have been furnished for the accommodation and cure of those subject to mental derangement.[12]

When the Royal Infirmary was built in 1741 provision had been made for 'the proper restraint of patients labouring under mental derangement' in cells in the basement. Andrew Duncan records that it was soon found that these cells afforded 'neither proper convenience for the cure or comfort of the unhappy maniac' and the plan to accommodate mentally ill patients in the Infirmary had been abandoned. Since then 'the want of a proper building for the cure of insanity was felt by almost all the medical practitioners of Edinburgh'.

Duncan had in mind not only a new building but also a new regime of care. He hoped to

10. A.B. Grossart (ed.), *The Poetical Works of Robert Fergusson* (Edinburgh, 1840), p. 20.
11. D. Daiches, *Robert Fergusson* (Edinburgh, 1982), p.107.
12. A. Duncan, *Short Account of the Rise, Progress and present State of the Lunatic Asylum at Edinburgh* (Edinburgh, 1812), p. 5.

introduce the style of treatment that had first been devised by Jean-Baptiste Pussin and Philipe Pinel at the Bicentre in Paris in the 1780s and had since been further developed at the Retreat, a Quaker establishment at York. The immediate objective of this new mode of management was to control the patient but not by means of chains, strait-jackets and corporal punishment. The aim was to school the patients in self-control. The treatment regime was modelled on the ideal of family life. Patients were housed, as far as possible, in quiet and comfort with careful attention to 'diet, air, drink, exercise and other circumstances'.[13] Staff maintained contact with the patients throughout the day to encourage a return to acceptable behaviour by persuasion, by praise and blame, by reward and correction.[14]

In August 1791 the College Committee on Lunatic Asylums, chaired by Andrew Duncan, recommended:

- That houses for the reception of lunatics kept by private persons in the city and neighbourhood of Edinburgh be subject to visitation of Commissioners appointed by the College of Physicians.

- That the establishment in the neighbourhood of Edinburgh of a Lunatic Asylum similar to that of York would be of the utmost advantage to those who have the misfortune to be deprived of their reason.

- That considerable funds both in the way of donations and legacy might be obtained for this purpose provided a respectable set of Trustees were appointed for receiving the money and for superintending the building of a lunatic asylum after sufficient fund has been procured.

- That the Lord Provost of Edinburgh, the Lord President of the Court of Session, the Lord Chief Baron of Exchequer, the Lord Advocate of Scotland, the Dean of the Faculty of Advocates, the Principal of the University of Edinburgh, the Keeper of His Majesty's Signet, the President of the College of Physicians and the Deacon of the Incorporation of Surgeons would form a committee in whom the public could not fail of placing the highest degree of confidence.

- That the money appointed by the Trustees of the late Mr Watson to be employed in the building of a Foundling Hospital, a species of charity to which there are many strong objections, would be much more usefully employed in building a lunatic asylum and that if the Keeper of His Majesty's Signet and the other gentlemen to whom the administration of the money is entrusted were to get the whole or at least a part of it appropriated by Act of Parliament to the purpose of a Lunatic Asylum they would do an essential service to the Community.

APOTHECARY SHOPS

In 1790 there were twelve apothecary shops in Edinburgh. All the complex processes required in the preparation of contemporary medicaments were carried out on their premises. Herbs

13. Ibid., p. 19.
14. R. Porter, *The Greatest Benefit to Mankind* (London, 1999) p. 498.

were bought in from local herb gatherers; drugs imported from the West and East Indies could be purchased from a shop in the High Street. Forty-nine ingredients were included in the preparation of Mithridatum Damocratis, sixty-one for Andromanche and forty for the most popular medicament of the time, Anderson's Scots Pill (Pil. Aloes et Myrrhae) which took four days to prepare.[15] Powders were packed in scraps of paper and mussel shells were used as containers for ointments.

By its Charter the College was required, twice a year, to visit and inspect 'all Apothecarys Shops and Chambers within Edinburgh suburbs and libertys thereof calling to their assistance one or two of the eldest or ablest of the Brotherhood [Fraternity] of Apothecarys and also one of the Baillies of Edinburgh or Magistrates of the place where the shops to be visited do lye'. This duty followed from a decision of the Court of Session in 1684 when, with the assistance of the College of Physicians, the Fraternity of Apothcaries had successfully appealed to the Court to end the Apothecaries' association with the Incorporation of Surgeons. (Chapter I). Unfortunately the Court of Session failed to set aside an Act of the Town Council of 1657 that had ruled that apothecary shops should be inspected by members of the Incorporation of Surgeons. The resulting confusion continued for ten years. Then, in 1694, the duties and responsibilities of the College of Physicians became even more uncertain in 1694 when the Incorporation of Surgeons obtained a royal patent from William and Mary that restored all the original rights and privileges of the Incorporation including its responsibilities in the supervision of Edinburgh's apothecary shops. Efforts by the College of Physicians to fulfil the obligation to visit apothecary shops enshrined in its Charter became hesitant and ineffective and in time this 'distasteful inspectorial function' was abandoned.

However, the College of Physicians did not surrender the teaching of pharmacy to the surgeons. From 1668, when Edinburgh's great physic garden was established by Robert Sibbald and Andrew Balfour, apprentice surgeons and apothecaries had paid a fee of one guinea to attend the classes given by the garden's Keeper, James Sutherland. Then, in 1694, when the College of Surgeons moved into its first purpose-built Hall, it opened a laboratory in which apprentices were given practical training in pharmacy.

In 1723, the College of Physicians offered 'in an amicable way to consort with the [College of Surgeons] what method would be the most proper for improving and regulating pharmacy'.[16] The offer was refused but it stimulated the College of Surgeons to include more works on Materia Medica in its library, to extend its systematic teaching in pharmacy and introduce examinations in the subject for its apprentice apothecaries. Nevertheless, many apprentice apothecaries continued to look elsewhere for instruction.

In 1776, Andrew Duncan instituted classes in pharmacy at the Royal Public Dispensary that were to expand into a School of Pharmacy (which in turn became part of Heriot-Watt University in the twentieth century). By 1790, Andrew Duncan's school was already the principal school of pharmacy in Edinburgh and it was no doubt on this basis that Duncan felt justified when he proposed that the full 'powers of the College relative to the visiting of

15. J.P. Gilmour, Phases of Pharmacy in Edinburgh, *Quarterly Journal of Pharmacy and Pharmacology*, 1928, Vol. 11, pp. 351–62.
16. Minutes of the Incorporation of Surgeons, 23 May 1723.

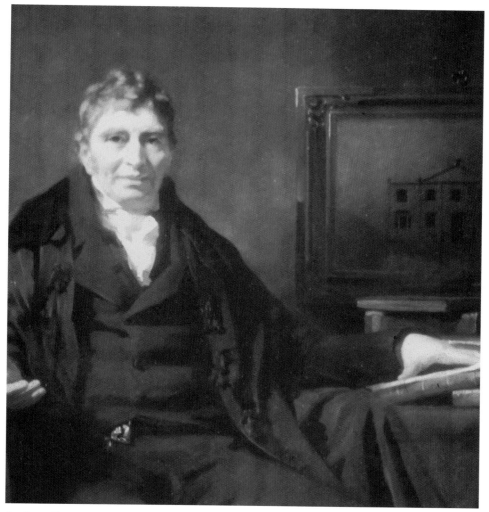

Andrew Duncan

apothecary's Shops' should once again be 'put in force'.

A committee was formed to consider how far Duncan's proposal was 'expedient'. Although the committee was chaired by Duncan himself it proved reluctant to revive the old disputes with the College of Surgeons and to risk damaging the College's congenial relationship with the Fraternity of Apothecaries. The committee reported that it was 'of the opinion that any formal visitation of the shops of apothecaries might be attended with many bad effects and could be productive of little benefit to the public'. The committee also recommended that any apothecaries coming more informally to the attention of the Censors and Procurator Fiscal of the College as in some way 'delinquent' should be prosecuted only when 'admonitions had not been productive of the desired effect'.

SEA BATHING

In 1769 in his Domestic Medicine William Buchan, Andrew Duncan's fellow advocate of improved healthcare for the common people, wrote of the benefits of sea bathing.

> By it the body is braced and strengthened, the circulation and secretions promoted and, were it conducted with prudence, many diseases might be thereby be prevented … A class who stand in particular need of the bracing qualities of cold water includes a great number of the male and nearly all the female inhabitants of great cities … To young people and particularly to children cold bathing is of the last importance. It promotes their growth, increases their strength and prevents a variety of diseases incident to childhood.

This message was repeated in all the nineteen later editions of *Domestic Medicine*.

In 1787 a Mr Alexander Stenhouse wrote soliciting the countenance and sanction of the College to a plan to establish a set of seawater baths at Leith. At a meeting on 1 May 1787 the College acknowledged benefits that could be gained from 'the salutary practice of sea bathing' but refused to offer an opinion on the merits of the scheme put forward by Mr Stenhouse. Unhelpfully, Mr Stenhouse was informed that he must be 'the proper judge of his own matters'. However, in February 1791 Andrew Duncan appointed a committee 'to consider whether any improvements or additional conveniences could with ease be introduced into the practice of sea bathing at Edinburgh'. In August it was reported that:

- The Committee are of the opinion that although the conveniences for sea bathing in the neighbourhood of Leith be much greater than formerly yet they may admit of further improvement.

- A large pond or basin to be filled with sea water every tide might be formed on a spot of ground at the east of Leith Links which is at present of almost no value. In this basin bathing might be carried on with convenience and advantage at all times of the tide and in all weathers. It might be divided in two, one half for women and children the other for men and boys each half being provided with a few dressing closets

- The committee think that this work could be executed at no great expense and that the money obtained for permission to bathe in it though that permission were granted at a very moderate rate might be considerable. They therefore beg leave to propose that the College should recommend it to the Town Council who are proprietors of the ground either to carry that plan into execution themselves or to feu out the ground to some individual under condition that it be applied to the above purpose and to no other and under obligation to permit bathing at rates to be fixed by the council.

The College approved the report and directed the President to communicate with the Lord Provost, Magistrates and Town Council requesting that 'they take steps in this business as may seem to them most conducive to the convenience of the public'.

VAPOUR BATHS

In 1783 Andrew Duncan, in the eighth volume of his *Medical Commentaries*, reviewed the report of a case in which a 'Vapour Bath' had been used in the treatment of hydrocephalus. The treatment had been given by Dr Hunter, a physician in York and its success had been published in an open letter addressed to the Queen's physician, Dr Will. The child patient had been secured in a 'fumigation chair' in a steam room for seven minutes each day for over three months. 'The Vapour Baths, when highly impregnated with stimulating aromatic, occasioned a sudden redness of the skin, a temporary fever and a copious perspiration which usually terminated as soon as the patient is dressed'.[17] Before treatment the child had 'lost its speech, its eyes wandered without design its apprehension almost annihilated'. The treatment had been given 'not from any just reasoning but from a desire to cultivate a forlorn hope'. After only one treatment the child had become fully conscious and able to walk.

In 1783, Duncan commented that 'this being a solitary case let it therefore only be considered as fair ground for experiment'. In 1791, he appointed a committee to consider whether vapour baths should be made available in Edinburgh. The committee decided that since vapour baths were already 'employed with advantage in London and in most of the large towns of England it should be the endeavour of the College of Physicians to get this defect at Edinburgh supplied as soon as possible'. The Committee recommended that the Managers should be asked to add a vapour bath to the hot and cold baths already open to the public at the Royal Infirmary

DELAY, FRUSTRATION AND COMPROMISE

In 1791, it was almost inevitable that Andrew Duncan's initiatives would fail. Their success depended on the goodwill of a tiny and corrupt ruling elite and, in 1791, that good will did not exist. The ruling elite was already reacting with some severity to what it feared were the stirrings of rebellion among those that Duncan's measures were intended to help, the ordinary people of Scotland.

Scotland then elected sixty Members of Parliament to represent the nation in Westminster. Fifteen represented the burghs and were chosen by the self-perpetuating oligarchies that made up the burgh councils; in Edinburgh, of a population of over 80,000, only the thirty-three people from whom the Town Council was drawn had the right to vote. In the counties, where the ownership of property alone gave the right to vote, even the middling lairds and minor landowners were excluded from a total franchise that numbered less than 2,600. Each tiny electorate, whether in town or county, was open to corruption and Henry Dundas, the Keeper of the Signet and the controller of government patronage in Scotland, freely acknowledged that almost every electorate could be controlled by 'a discriminating distribution of loaves and fishes'. In London, Dundas could marshal and deliver the Scottish vote in Parliament and at home he controlled the appointment of the Lord Advocate, the Solicitor General, the Lord Justice Clerk and the senior judges who formed the executive government in Scotland.

17. Duncan, 1783, pp. 106-9.

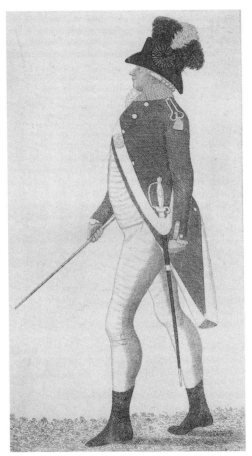

Henry Dundas

Resistance to this grossly hegemonic regime had been encouraged by events in America and France. A great many people in Scotland had been excited by the democratic ideals that had inspired the American colonies to declare their independence in 1776 and had later motivated the French Revolution in 1789. In Britain, the first volume of Tom Paine's *Rights of Man* had been published in February 1791 and had been widely read among the generally literate people of Scotland. Without legitimate political means to express their discontent, it had become normal for the unfranchised masses in Scotland to resort to riot. In 1706, Daniel Defoe had famously described the Scots as 'a refectory and terrible people' and the Scottish mobs as 'the worst of their kind'. In 1709, 1710, 1720, 1727, 1740, 1756, 1757, 1763, 1767, 1771, 1772, 1773, 1774, 1778 and 1778 there had been serious rioting in Scotland, usually in protest over food prices; now in 1790 the riots were more specifically political. In Edinburgh the most serious riots were in May and June of 1792 when the houses of Henry Dundas, his nephew the Lord Advocate and the Lord Provost of Edinburgh were attacked and their effigies thrown on bonfires in George Square. The propertied and political classes were now in fear of the mass of the people and of the growing prospect of revolution. Tension increased further in 1793 when war broke out with Revolutionary France. There were fears that if the French were to invade they would choose to land in Scotland in the expectation of support from a disaffected people. To strengthen the defences in Scotland a Corps of Gentlemen Volunteers was raised from among those who could provide their own uniforms and equipment. A Bill was also published with the intention of conscripting Militia Regiments in Scotland but the plan was quickly abandoned because it was thought that unwise 'to trust arms in the hands of the lower classes of people'. Lords Lieutenants and Deputy Lieutenants were appointed in all the counties of Scotland to form the framework of an intelligence network for the collection of evidence of sedition.[18] When, in 1797, the scheme to conscript a militia was revived there was a new outbreak of rioting and 1400 regular troops were withdrawn from England and stationed in Scotland.

In these years of division and conflicting interests, those that Duncan looked to to implement his public health schemes – the Lord Provost and Town Council of Edinburgh; the Sheriffs in the Counties; the judges, advocates, town councillors, university professors and prosperous citizens who dominated the Board of Management of the Royal Infirmary; and the leaders of the Church in Scotland – were all loyal to government and suspicious if not hostile to schemes intended to benefit what was believed to be a disaffected and potentially rebellious public. Duncan's schemes remained in abeyance until the Revolutionary Wars with France were over, the people of Scotland had become united in support of the wars against Napoleon and the years of civil unrest in Scotland had come to an end. After varying periods of delay, they were all then put into effect but in somewhat modified form.

The scheme of free inoculation against smallpox had been implemented with some success in September and October on 1791 and again in the autumn of 1792 but had then been abandoned. The scheme was not revived when civil harmony was restored after 1805. By then inoculation had been generally abandoned in Britain in favour of the much safer vaccination. Since vaccination, unlike inoculation, caused 'effects so inconsiderable and slight the aid of a physician was never required' it was performed in Edinburgh by surgeons and was no longer seen as the province of Edinburgh's physicians. In 1805, a seawater pool was opened, not at Leith but at Portobello. The proposed reform of the preparation and publication of Bills of Mortality made no progress even after 1805; from 1810, Andrew Duncan drew up his own quarterly reports of deaths and 'epidemics' in Edinburgh for presentation to the College. From 1822, a vapour bath owned and operated by a private contactor, provided treatments for patients attending the Old Town Dispensary.

The most celebrated of Andrew Duncan's schemes was the founding of a lunatic asylum. A public appeal was launched by the College in 1792. Every Fellow of the College of Physicians made a donation but there were only four subscribers from the general public and the sum collected amounted to only £119 11s. The project to found an asylum was then left in abeyance until the years of civil unrest came to an end and fears of invasion by the French had evaporated.

18. K.J. Logue, *Popular Disturbances in Scotland* 1780-1815 (Edinburgh, 1979).

In 1806, a Parliamentary Committee chaired by Sir John Sinclair and persuaded by Duncan's friend Henry Erskine, now the Lord Advocate, voted to contribute £2,000 from the proceeds of the sale of the estates forfeited by landowners who had taken the wrong part in the Jacobite Rebellion of 1745. For a period of two years fines paid at Edinburgh Sheriff Court were also allocated to the Asylum fund. In 1887, a Royal Charter was granted, trustees were appointed and a new appeal was made to the public in the expectation that several thousand subscribers would contribute at least 'one guinea or upwards'. In the event there were only 185 subscribers but they contributed over £2,000 and in the next few years £1,000 was received from expatriates in Madras with smaller sums from Bombay, Ceylon, the West Indies and America. In 1812, the funds amounted to £7,446 and the construction of the asylum began. The building was designed to accommodate three classes of patients:

> It is proposed that pauper or criminal lunatics, supported by parishes or other charitable funds shall be received at the rate of seven shillings per week; that a second class, furnished with better accommodation and a more expensive diet tea, coffee etc. shall pay one guinea per week; and that a third class, each having a servant to attend him and provided with apartments much better suited to his condition than can be had in any private house, shall pay at the rate of three guineas a week.[19]

The first patient was admitted to the new asylum on 19 July 1813.

DUNCAN, COLLEGE AND PARLIAMENT

In June 1808, Parliament passed an *Act for the Better Care and Maintenance of Lunatics, being Paupers or Criminals in England*. In June 1811, Parliament passed a further *Act to Amend the Act of the 48th Year of his present Majesty for the Better Care and Maintenance of Lunatics being Paupers or Criminals in England*. These Acts did not apply in Scotland. In 1812 and again in 1818 in an open letter addressed to the Sheriffs-Depute of all the counties in Scotland, Andrew Duncan put forward a scheme for Scotland.[20] He argued that 'if the kingdom of Scotland be still deficient in proper accommodation for the cure of pauper lunatics it is even much more deficient in the necessary prisons for criminal lunatics'. Duncan proposed that a National Asylum for the reception of criminal and pauper lunatics and should be built as special annexe of each of the asylums that had recently been opened in Edinburgh, Glasgow, Aberdeen and Dumfries. These National Asylums would serve respectively the counties of the East, West, North and South of Scotland and the Sheriff-Deputes of the relevant counties would act *ex officio* as their managers. The Sheriff-Deputes were asked to rally support in their counties and, together, to find an appropriate influential spokesman to put the proposed scheme to Parliament.

Duncan's proposal for the establishment of National Asylums came to nothing. The indirect approach to Parliament through Scotland's Sheriffs-Depute had proved ineffective. There after, in its various campaigns to promote improvements in medical services in

19. Duncan, *Short Account*, p. 14.
20. A. Duncan. *A Letter to Her Majesty's Sheriffs-Deput in Scotland* (Edinburgh, 1818).

Scotland, the College adopted more direct methods to make its views known at Westminster.

In 1813 a Bill was introduced to Parliament to amend provision of the Act of 1777 the 'regulation of Mad Houses' in England. A College committee proposed that the Bill should be amended to make its provisions applicable to Scotland. The proposed amendments were drawn up as a petition to be presented to the House of Commons by the Lord Advocate. When the Act was later passed in the House of Commons not all the 'material additions necessary to make the operation of it fully beneficial to Scotland' had been included. Henry Dundas, now Viscount Melville, was therefore asked to present the College's case to the House of Lords. Dundas's intervention resulted in a new *Act to Regulate Madhouses in Scotland* being passed by Parliament in June 1815.

In 1817 a Bill was introduced by the Attorney General of England for the Regulation of Surgery throughout the United Kingdom. The College found that a number of the clauses in the Bill were 'injurious' to its interests and decided that such steps should be taken 'as might be necessary to prevent the progress of the Bill through Parliament in its present state'. The College drew up its objections to the Bill in a lengthy and detailed petition to Attorney General. Some months later an appropriately amended Act was passed by Parliament.

In these early decades of the nineteenth century, Andrew Duncan's Presidency was one of the most remarkable in the history of the College. When he was first elected in 1790 there was no government body in Scotland charged with a responsibility for health policy. In the absence of such a body Andrew Duncan led the College to become an agency through which otherwise neglected health concerns in Scotland were brought to the attention of the British Government in London. By the end of his second term as President in 1825, the Royal College of Physicians of Edinburgh had begun to assume an obligation to intervene with government in the shaping of health policy in Scotland. This was an obligation that was to occupy the College for much of the nineteenth century.

9

CHOLERA AND ITS LEGACY

W. P. Alison and the Management of the Poor

On 2 March 1820, the College received from the Secretary of the East India Company copies of its reports on the progress of the epidemic of cholera then ravaging populations across India. The first cases had been reported in Calcutta in May 1817; three months later 3,000 of the Company's 10,000 strong army in Bengal died from the disease. By July 1818, the disease had spread to the Presidency of Madras and by August it had reached the third of the Company's Presidencies at Bombay. An Assistant Surgeon at Bombay, on seeing his first cases, wrote:

> I never saw a disease where the debility came so soon or so suddenly and with such violence. It is common to find patients one hour after the first attack perfectly cold with no pulsation at the wrist.

The cause of the disease was unknown. Unable to discover any 'assignable connection between source and diffusion' of the disease, the medical staff of the East India Company 'rejected at once the agency of contagion and ascribe it to the operation of a more general source'. That general source was assumed to be the weather; the case reports sent to the College were accompanied by full reports of local meteorological conditions and the phases of the moon.

As the epidemic began to subside in India it broke out in an even more virulent form in the Volga basin on the Caspian Sea and from there it spread into Russia. In 1830, it reached Moscow and spread west to Riga on the Baltic coast and then to Hamburg, only a few hours sailing time from the English coast. When the first cases were diagnosed in Sunderland in October 1831 its arrival in Britain had long been expected and dreaded. As the disease spread through England and Scotland there was widespread bewilderment, terror and panic.

> To see a number of our fellow creatures, in a good state of health, in the full possession of their wonted strength and in the midst of their years, suddenly seized with the most violent spasms and in a few hours cast into the tomb is calculated to inspire dread in the stoutest heart.

Communities across both countries reacted as they had done in past centuries to the Black Death or the worst outbreaks of plague.

This, the first epidemic of cholera in Britain, lasted for nine months. Those who suffered most severely were the malnourished poor, living in overcrowded squalor in mining villages that had suddenly grown into shanty townships or in the rapidly growing industrial cities

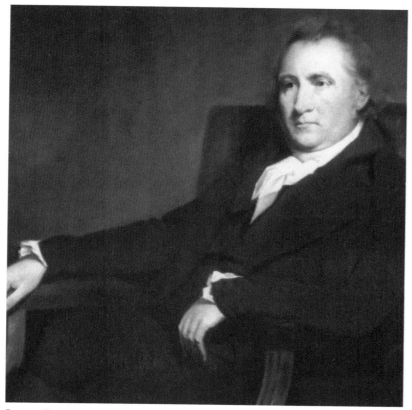

James Gregory

where every factory created its neighbourhood slum of houses run up with little or no proper attention to water supply or drainage. The workers, obliged to live within walking distance of their employment, had no escape. Over 30,000 people are known to have died. The majority were adults in their middle years and many had been the essential providers for their families. Their deaths added many more thousands to the already alarming numbers that had become dependent for their sustenance on the meagre provisions of Britain's Poor Laws since the wars with France ended in 1815. The epidemic therefore added a new sense of urgency to a drive for social reform that already begun.

The visible physical degeneration of the ever-growing numbers of the urban poor and the associated increase in crime, alcoholism and prostitution in Britain's industrial towns was the great Social Problem of the middle decades of the nineteenth century. In these years Parliament introduced legislation to reform the systems in place for the maintenance of the poor and to safeguard the health of the whole population. The College played the leading role in ensuring that the relevant legislation conformed to the problems as they existed in Scotland. In all its effort the College was inspired by the concepts and the commitment of William Alison.

WILLIAM PULTENEY ALISON

William Pulteney Alison was born in 1790 at Boroughmuirhead, a small estate to the south of Edinburgh. His father, the Rev. Archibald Alison was the son of a Lord Provost of Edinburgh who was remembered by Lord Cockburn as 'the most distinguished of the Episcopal clergy of Edinburgh, and so far as I know, of Scotland; a great associate of all the eminent among us'. His mother, Dorothea, was the daughter of John Gregory, the Professor of the Practice of Physic at Edinburgh in 1766–73 and the brother of James Gregory who was appointed to the same chair in 1790 and was later elected President of the College. Before her marriage in 1784 Dorothea Gregory had lived for a time in Paris where she had been welcomed at the literary salons and had mixed with the leading *philosophes* of pre-Revolutionary France.[1]

While William was still an infant, his father, the Rev. Archibald Alison, was appointed to a living in England in the gift of Sir William Pulteney. Sir William (then William Johnstone) had been an advocate in Edinburgh before inheriting, through his wife, the vast fortune and Shropshire estates of the Earl of Bath. The Alisons the Johnstones and the Pulteneys became friends. In all, the Rev Alison was appointed to three livings in Sir William's gift and his infant son became Sir William Pulteney's godson.

William Pulteney Alison's childhood was spent on his godfather's Kenley estate in Shropshire where he received his education from his father and from private tutors. In 1800, his father was invited to return to Edinburgh to become minister to the fashionable Episcopal congregation that was about to build a new modern church in York Place. The family move back to Boroughmuirhead where the Rev Alison became 'the centre of a select social circle' that included some of the most prominent men in Scotland at that time. As they grew up, William and his younger brother Archibald (later Sir Archibald) were introduced to the political economist, Francis Horner, the writer and judge, Francis Jeffrey, the writer, Sir Henry Mackenzie, the poet and novelist, Sir Walter Scott; the philosopher, Dugald Stewart; the engineer, Thomas Telford and the lawyer and writer Alexander Fraser Tytler (later Lord Woodhouselee). Of those that he came to know at his father's house at Edinburgh, those who were to have the greatest influence in shaping his philosophy and his career were Dugald Stewart and his uncle, James Gregory.[2]

At the age of twelve, William was enrolled at Edinburgh University where, for five years, he studied Latin, Greek, logic, mathematics and natural philosophy. But his chief interest was in moral philosophy, taught by his father's friend Dugald Stewart. Then in 1896, no doubt influenced by his uncle, James Gregory, he enrolled once again at Edinburgh to study medicine. For four years he attended all the classes of the medical curriculum (some more than once), graduating MD in September 1811. In October he became a licentiate of the College and a year later he was elected as a Fellow.

From 1811 until 1814, Alison was formally engaged to assist his uncle James Gregory in

1. C. Hamlin, William Pulteney Alison, the Scottish Philosophy and the Making of Political Medicine, *Journal of the History of Medicine,* 2006, Vol. 61, p. 151.
2. Ibid., p. 152; S.M.K. Martin, William Pulteney Alison: Activist Philanthropist and Pioneer of Social Medicine, PhD Thesis, St Andrews University, 1997, pp. 26-34.

preparing his lectures and in managing his correspondence, an occupation that allowed him ample time to return to his studies in moral philosophy at Edinburgh University. In Edinburgh it was then against the spirit of the times and the contemporary belief in the unity of knowledge to confine one's interests to one academic discipline. (Dugald Stewart had at one time thought that Alison might succeed him as Professor of Moral Philosophy but the chair had gone to another physician, Thomas Brown.[3]) Throughout his long career Alison continued to be both a physician and a philosopher.

During his first years as a Fellow of the College, Alison made a number of journeys through France, Italy and Switzerland (including a failed attempt to climb Mont Blanc[4]). His European expeditions had some elements of the Grand Tour, then regarded as an essential part of a young gentleman's education; he studied historic sites, visited art galleries and attended theatres in the great cities. But his chief purpose was to observe the living conditions of the people, their physical well-being and the provisions made for the care of the sick poor. In the peasant communities he looked for evidence that might substantiate the theory that Malthus had famously proposed in his *Essay on the Principle of Population* in 1798. (That is, that the population increases geometrically while the food supply increases, at best, arithmetically. Consequently, the population is kept in balance with its food supply only by the 'misery' of famines, plagues or wars, unless it is checked by other unnatural means.)

ALISON AND THE POOR

In June 1815, Alison, with three other recently elected Fellows of the College, founded a public dispensary in the Edinburgh's New Town. There was some opposition from the staff of the Royal Public Dispensary that had been operating in the Old Town since 1776. But Alison held that a second public Dispensary was justified by the increase in Edinburgh's population; the new Dispensary would also offer additional services that were not provided by the Royal Dispensary. The Royal Dispensary was open only two days a week and had no set system of home visiting. The New Town Dispensary was to be open to the sick and disabled poor every day except Sundays; patients unable to attend the dispensary were to be seen in their homes and physician-accoucheurs would visit pregnant women in their homes at any time. Children would be vaccinated against smallpox free of charge and in general there was to be greater emphasis on prevention. With the help of the Destitute Sick and Clothing Societies, the New Town Dispensary would make some contribution to the patients' material needs.

Within the first months the number of patients 'far exceeded what was ever contemplated'. Every year, for the next twenty years, some 7,000 patients were treated at the Dispensary; 3,000 sick and disabled were visited at home; 150 women were attended by the physician-accoucheurs; 450 children were vaccinated.[5] During these years Alison not only gained experience of the ailments of the urban poor in Scotland, he also made his own unfashionable assessment of the causes of poverty itself.

3. W.T. Gairdner, *The Physician as Naturalist* (Glasgow, 1889), p. 391.
4. A.H. Douglas, *The Life and Character of Dr. Alison* (Edinburgh, 1866), p. 5.
5. *Annual Reports of the Edinburgh New Town Dispensary, 1815-1841.*

Alison did not publish his *Observations on the Management of the Poor in Scotland* until 1840 but the principles on which his observations were based were already becoming clear in his mind when he was still a young man. In his sermons his father, the Rev Archibald Alison, had instructed his congregation – and his children – that it was their Christian duty to be charitable, to minister to the needs of the poor and to work towards the prevention of poverty by educating the poor and encouraging in them in habits of industry and independence. W.P. Alison was a very charitable man; to his friends it often seemed that his generosity was likely to cause his own financial embarrassment. But to Alison, it was not enough to be charitable and to encourage the poor to rescue themselves from poverty. Alison had studied under Andrew Duncan and had absorbed his ideas on medical police. But while Duncan had defined medical police as 'the application of the principles deduced from the different branches of medical knowledge for the promotion, preservation and improving the public health', Alison redefined it as 'the consideration of the means of improving health *adopted by the legislature and magistrates and the consideration of the principles of the enactments themselves*'.

Duncan had taught his students that the health of the people should be promoted not 'by rigid laws' but by 'recommendation and example' and that such regulations as were required should be drawn up by local magistrates acting on the advice of local doctors. Alison agreed that it was 'an established maxim of political economy that legislative interference whenever it is unnecessary is hurtful', but he believed that when persuasion, voluntary effort and locally agreed regulation failed, legislation by central government was not only justifiable but also essential. Alison's views followed from the political economy he had been taught by Dugald Stewart. Traditionally, political economy had been concerned with the material resources – that is the wealth and population – of the state; Dugald Stewart had argued that since the ultimate objective of political economy was the promotion of 'the happiness and improvement of society, the management of wealth and population were only 'subordinate and instrumental'. Those who wielded political power must be responsible for ensuring the well-being of everyone in society and when charity and voluntary efforts failed 'the question no longer admits of discussion, a compulsory law is the only expedient which can supply an effective remedy'.

In time Alison was to acquire a large and fashionable private practice and was appointed first physician to Queen Victoria in Scotland. At Edinburgh University he became successively Professor of Medical Jurisprudence and Medical Police, Professor of the Theory of Medicine and Professor of the Practice of Medicine. But in a long career his chief energies were devoted to the shaping of the laws relating to public health and the welfare of the poor in Scotland. The platform from which he was able to bring his influence to bear was the Royal College of Physicians of Edinburgh. From 1817, he was a member of every College committee appointed to advise on problems of public health, poverty and the diseases that afflicted the poor.

ALISON AND THE CAUSES OF CONTAGIOUS FEVER
On 6 May 1817 the College appointed a committee to report 'on the contagious fever said to be prevalent in Edinburgh, to enquire into the truth of the report and to draw such regulations

as the case may require'. Within a few days the Committee (the President, Thomas Hope, James Hamilton, James Home, Thomas Spens, Andrew Duncan jun. and W.P. Alison) reported that a continuing fever was indeed 'more frequent than usual in Edinburgh, that it was in general of a mild description and that it did not seem necessary or expedient for the Royal College to pursue any measures respecting it'. Alison dissented from this decision, commenting that 'some people are averse to taking any active measures of prevention because the first cases of fever they see are mild and not alarming; they might as well refuse to make use of vaccination in an unprotected place because one case of smallpox first appearing may happen to be mild and distinct'.

In 1810, Andrew Duncan had published a pamphlet in which he argued that since the common febrile illnesses, mumps measles and scarletina, were discrete clinical entities they must have distinct specific causes. By 1817, Alison had gained extensive experience of 'contagious fever' from his dispensary practice and in the *New Town Dispensary Disease Reports* for the early months of 1818, he had published his conclusion that 'contagious fever' also had a specific or 'exciting cause' but that its severity and its rapid spread among the poor was due to the operation of predisposing causes. These predisposing causes were:

> that the habits of the lower orders are in general very uncleanly, that many parts of the town, inhabited by them are very close and dirty, the whole families or even more families than one (particularly in hard times) are often crowded into single rooms that a great number of the inhabitants of such places have suffered severely during the winter both from want of the necessities of life and likewise from the depression of spirits that attends the want of employment.

In his *Reports of the Diseases Treated at the New Town Dispensary*, Alison proposed a number of measures that could be put in place immediately to prevent the spread of contagious fever. These were limited to the isolation of cases, fumigation of houses and the amelioration of poverty. As they pointed out, the removal of dirt, refuse and waste from public places was the province of the city magistrates and required government legislation. Alison's *Reports of the Diseases Treated at the New Town Dispensary* were published in *The Edinburgh Medical and Surgical Journal*. It may have been the publication of these reports that prompted a letter to the College from the Lord Advocate on 14 May 1817:

> Having learned from the public prints as well as from common reports that a typhus fever has for some time prevailed in the city and suburbs I consider it my duty to request of you to ascertain for my information whether in the opinion of the Royal College of Physicians there is any particular cause assignable for the unusual extent of this disease for which it is in the power of the police to provide a remedy. In particular I am desirous of learning whether it is the opinion of the College that the prevalence of this disorder may have been occasioned by masses of putrescent matter which have been collected in the vicinity over which the winds must pass before it enters the city.

The College's Committee on Contagious Fever (which now included Andrew Duncan sen.) replied that 'the fever of a typhoid charter' present in Edinburgh was a disease rarely absent from populous towns and that its prevalence could be attributed to a number of causes including ill ventilated crowded houses, to fatigue and intemperance, to bad or too little food. As to the masses of putrescent matter, the Committee 'could not presume to assert that the exhalations from them have actually given rise to the fever prevailing at present'. Nevertheless, the College advised that such putrescent matter should not be allowed to accumulate in the city or its immediate vicinity.

In the following months there were many in Edinburgh who believed that the limited measures to control the contagion advocated by the College and put in place by the city authorities were causing unnecessary alarm.[6] On 23 October, the Lord Provost referred the problem once again to the College. The College's Committee on Contagious Fever replied that although the fever was now in a mild form it was nevertheless advisable to take measures to prevent its becoming more severe and more widely dispersed. Much could be done by 'inculcating among the ranks of the lower classes due attention to the various means such as ventilation, cleanliness, separation of sick from the healthy, purification of apartments' bedding and clothes so often recommended'. [The purification recommended was fumigation with nitrous gas or chlorine gas from muriatic acid.] In the last weeks of 1817, a Fever Board, financed by the Town Council, the College and other public bodies in Edinburgh, was established to ensure that these preventive measures were introduced and to oversee their operation.[7] Thereafter the Fever Board continued to coordinate the activities of Edinburgh's hospitals and dispensaries and its Destitute and Clothing Societies during all forms of health crisis in the city.

The *Report* of the College Committee that led to the establishment of the Fever Board was written by Alison. In it he had commented that it was '*a matter of much difficulty to ascertain with any degree of accuracy the precise proportion which cases of fever occurring in Edinburgh at any one period bear to those prevailing at another*'. He later persuaded the new Edinburgh Fever Board to support a study to establish the true incidence of urban fever and to assess the factors that might contribute to its onset. The result of this study was the rejection of the popular theory that urban fever was caused by 'miasma', a toxic and potentially lethal vapour that was supposed to rise from accumulations of the town's putrescent waste. In 1818, Alison wrote in the *Edinburgh Medical and Surgical Journal*:

> It is quite impossible to ascertain whether every case of the fever now existing in this city be the offspring of a specific contagion or not. But we have no doubt that contagion is the exciting cause of by far the greater number of them. We conclude this, not merely from observing that about five-sixths of our fever patients are certainly exposed to the contagion before they fall sick but likewise from remarking the frequency of the disease in certain districts of the town and the comparative exemption of other districts.

6. College Minute, 23 October, 1817.
7. Martin, William Pultney, p. 75.

Now if we suppose that a specific contagion is the principal, or even the sole cause of continued fever we can easily explain its breaking out occasionally where the application of this cause is not suspected. But if we are to suppose that it is excited by dirt, bad air, foul air and accumulated human effluvia it is exceedingly difficult to understand its great prevalence in one place or in one district of a town and its extreme rarity or total absence from another for a considerable time during which those causes are undeniably present in both. When we add the well known fact that, in the ill-aired and dirty districts where it does prevail among the poor, the disease extends itself from individual to individual, from family to family and from house to house … and the almost total exemption from fever which is occasionally enjoyed by very large towns in which poverty, dirt foul air and accumulated human effluvia must exist in great abundance, it seems impossible to resist the inference that the number of cases in which fever proceeds from these causes alone must be trifling in comparison with the number of those on which it is excited by contagion.

The practical conclusion is not that cleanliness, fresh air and nourishing diet are not of the utmost importance in checking the progress of continued fever but that where it is unfortunately impossible to apply those modes of prevention we may nevertheless hope to preserve the population in a great measure or entirely if we can preserve them from the application of the specific contagion.[8]

A century before, in 1721, the College, in a long and detailed report, had advised Edinburgh's Town Council that 'to guard against any pestilential infection' all refuse and human waste should be collected and removed some distance from the town; all putrescent matter should be buried and not left to rot; and the town's streets should be cleaned 'frequently with water'. That advice had been repeated by the College during the eighteenth century and, in 1816, when a new Police Bill was being drafted for Edinburgh, the same advice had been given yet again. Following Allison's report the College continued to give due emphasis to the importance of waste disposal, sewerage and water supply. But in advising on measures to protect the health of the public the College now gave new prominence to the need to overcome poverty and its attendant problems of overcrowding, malnutrition, unemployment and depression which together predisposed Scotland's ever-growing urban population to disease and early death.

CHOLERA: THE EPIDEMIC OF 1832

By the spring of 1831 the epidemic of cholera spreading from Asia into Europe had reached the coastal cities of the Baltic and north Germany. Since these were the entry ports of much of the country's trade with Europe, it seemed almost inevitable that the disease would soon spread to Britain. On 2 August 1831 a special meeting of the College expressed surprise that no communication had been received from central government in London; it was proposed

8. *Edinburgh Medical and Surgical Journal*, 1818, Vol., 14, p.123.

that the College should take the initiative and immediately issue its own 'assistance and advice as to the best measures to be adopted for preventing its being introduced in this country'. However, Alison persuaded the meeting to appoint a Cholera Committee to consider what measures would be appropriate for Edinburgh but thereafter to take no further action until the College received a clear statement of government policy for the United Kingdom. By the end of August, since there had still been no statement of policy from central government in London, the College's Cholera Committee and the Town Council proceeded to set up a Cholera Board of Health in Edinburgh on the model of the Boards of Health that had been established during previous epidemics of disease.[9]

DELAYS IN LONDON

The government body responsible for the prevention of epidemics was the Privy Council; in practice, its responsibility was delegated to its Clerk, Charles Grenville, and the civil servants of the Privy Council Office. When cholera reached Riga in the spring of 1831, Grenville, had ordered that all ships from Russia, the Baltic, the Cattegat and the Elbe should be detained for 14 days at one of the designated quarantine stations round the coast of the country from the Medway, to Milford Haven, the Forth and Cromarty Bay. On 9 June, Grenville passed all the information on the epidemic that the Privy Council had received from its agents in Eastern Europe to Sir Henry Halford, the President of the Royal College of Physicians of London.[10] Halford reassured Grenville that since cholera was contagious and could be carried in the hemp, flax and other materials that made up the cargoes in ships arriving from the Baltic, the strict quarantine measures that Grenville had been put in place were fully justified and necessary.

On 18 June, Grenville asked Halford for names of Fellows of the London College to serve on a Central Board of Health to advise on what further measures were required as defences against cholera. The seven Fellows nominated were the elite of the College, all successful physicians and all able to number members of the royal family and members of the highest ranks of London society among their patients.[11] (The *Lancet* later dismissed them as drones, sycophants and courtiers who had never had any experience of treating cholera. When the treatment regime they advocated was made public, it was seen to be perhaps appropriate for their wealthy patients but not for the poor who made up the vast majority of the victims of cholera.) They were divided among themselves. They could not agree on whether the disease was contagious or likely to be carried in ships' cargoes. They were therefore unable to give Grenville the authoritative support that Halford had led him to expect. This was a serious failing since Grenville was under pressure from a powerful lobby that maintained that his quarantine policy that left ships idle for weeks at time was unjustified and was seriously damaging to the country's economy. Grenville's policy was further undermined in July 1831 when the Central Board of Health interviewed seven army and civilian surgeons who had

9. Martin, William Pulteney, p. 86.
10. Sir George Clarke, *A History of the Royal College of Physicians of London*, Vol. 2 (London, 1966), p. 670.
11. R.J. Morris, *Cholera 1832: The Social Response to an Epidemic* (London, 1976), p. 26.

treated cholera in India; not one of these supposed experts supported the idea that cholera was contagious and could be carried in ship's cargoes. Three months later, on 23 October 1831, cholera was reported in Sunderland, making it evident that Grenville's strict quarantine policy had indeed been ineffective and that the advice he, and through him the Privy Council, had received from the representatives of the London College of Physicians on the Board of Health had been less than helpful.[12] On 22 November, the Privy Council announced the appointment of a new Cholera Board of Health. The *Lancet* was scathing:

> How are the mighty fallen! The Physician General to the Court of St James, poor Sir Henry Halford, has at last dropped down to his legitimate level. This good old gentleman all at once has sunk, quite destitute of Sovereign ballast, from the Council Chamber of the Monarch to the dirty Hall in Pall Mall East.
>
> What a job – what a scandalous job – over which this titled courtier was appointed to preside; A Board of Health founded for the protection of England from the ravages, made to consist of men, not one of whom had ever been an eyewitness of the disease. As well might the Government seek information on the subject of Asian cholera from the old women of Wapping.[13]

The *Lancet* was equally scornful of the *Public Notification Respecting the Cholera Morbus* that had been published by Halford's Board of Health on 20 October. The measures it advised for control of cholera were said by the *Lancet* to be no different from those that had been adopted during outbreaks of plague in previous centuries; Halford's Board had advised the public that it was of the utmost importance that:

> to separate the sick from the healthy, one or more houses should be kept in each town or its neighbourhood to which every case of the disease might be removed, provided the family of the affected person consented to such removal, and in case of refusal a conspicuous mark ('Sick') should be placed in front of the house to inform persons that it is in quarantine and even when persons with the disease shall, have been removed the word 'Caution' should be substituted.

The houses from which the sick had been removed were to be cleaned, the 'walls from cellar to garret lime washed' and all 'papers, cordage, old clothes and hangings burnt'. As treatment the board advocated:

> White wine, whey with spice, hot brandy and water or sal volatile in the dose of a teaspoonful in hot water frequently repeated or from five to twenty drops of some of the essential oils as peppermint, cloves or cajeput in a wine-glass of water may be administered; where the stomach will bear it, warm broth with spice may be employed.

12. Clarke, *A History*, p. 673.
13. *Lancet,* 1831-32, Vol. I, p. 304.

The *Lancet* commented:

> Singular comicality! In the name of wonder who is to refer to them? The old dowagers and duchesses, we presume …Verily, Sir Henry's Board is already the target which is destined to receive the most piercing shafts of ridicule from all branches of the medical profession.

In place of the representatives of the London College of Physicians, the Privy Council appointed the Hon Edward Stewart, as chairman, William MacLean as secretary with William Pym seconded from the quarantine department and two half-pay officers of the British army (Lt.-Colonel John Marshall and Major R. McDonald) and two from the East India service (J. Russell and David Barry); the representatives of the London College of Physicians were retained only as advisors to the board. This distancing of the London College of Physicians caused a tension between the London College and key officials of central government that soon led to a more general souring of the relationship between the medical profession and government administrative bodies. It was a souring that was made worse by the tactless behaviour of Edwin Chadwick (Chapter 9) and it was to bedevil the development of public health services for half a century.[14]

PREPARATIONS IN EDINBURGH

In Edinburgh planning had continued during August and September 1831. When, in October, the long-awaited guidance was at last received from Halford's board in London it was greeted with the ridicule predicted by the *Lancet*. Edinburgh's Cholera Health Board was already in place. It consisted of 27 members appointed by the City Council with a medical committee of 15 made up of 6 Fellows of the College of Physicians, 6 Fellows of the College of Surgeons and 3 doctors who had practised in India and had experience of treating cholera. The services put in place by the board were modelled on those introduced to combat 'contagious fever' by Alison's Fever Board in 1817. Nine soup kitchens were opened to feed the poor with a store to provide them with free clothing. Restrictions were placed on the movement of vagrants and beggars into and within the city. Four hospitals to accommodate a total of 270 cholera patients were set up in the city, the largest at Castlehill, Queensbury House and Surgeons' Square. Arrangements were made for the fumigation of houses following the removal of cholera victims to hospital. Ten quarantine houses were designated to hold family members and others who had been in contact with the disease. The city was divided into 30 districts in each one of which a station for the supply of medicines was set up. A team of doctors was assigned to make daily visitations within each of these districts; in all some 150 physicians and surgeons were enlisted as an 'Association' under the direction of John Abercrombie, a Fellow of the College. Posters were displayed throughout the city explaining the measures being put in place and justifying the restrictions that were to be imposed on the freedom of the individual citizen. These measures, taken independently in Edinburgh, were later endorsed by the Central

14. Morris, *Cholera*, p. 34.

Cholera Board of Health in London and Edinburgh's Cholera Board of Health was formally established by warrant of the Privy Council on 14 January 1832, two weeks before cholera arrived in the city.

THE CHOLERA EPIDEMIC IN SCOTLAND

The first cases of cholera in Scotland were diagnosed at Haddington on 17 December 1831; it was thought that disease had been carried by three cobblers who had 'lodged in a low filthy part of the town' after walking there along the Great North Road from Newcastle. An explosive outbreak followed a few days later among the collier families at Tranent. The disease then travelled through the colliery and fishing communities along the south shore of the Firth of Forth to Leith. From there the disease passed to Edinburgh where the first cases of cholera were reported on 27 January 1832.

In the city the disease rumbled on for over nine months, twice seeming to die out before breaking out once again. The measures devised by Edinburgh's Health Board were carried out as planned and on 20 February 1832 the government passed a Cholera Act for Scotland which allowed the board to raise funds through the city's police rates to finance its activities. The standard treatment used was the administration of large doses of calomel and opium. Patients went very quickly into a state of circulatory collapse; the venesection and bleeding that was commonly practised in cases of fever therefore seemed unwise and, in any case, would often have been almost impossible. Since, after the onset of symptoms, the patients very quickly became cold to the touch and it was generally recommended that they should be put in a hot bath. This could seldom be done as the patients were collapsed, semi-conscious and suffering muscle spasms. For the Edinburgh Board, Dr Bell (one of the members of the Board's Medical Committee who had treated cholera in India) devised a hot air bath. A wickerwork canopy was placed over the patient and under the bedclothes and hot air was introduced through a wide copper pipe heated at the foot of the bed by a spirit lamp; for sixpence worth of alcohol the patient could be nursed for an hour at a temperature of 120–160 F. However, this was so expensive and cumbersome that it was seldom used.

In spite of the best efforts of the medical attendants, the treatments they offered seemed to have little effect. Alison's long experience of the 'contagious fevers' that had afflicted Edinburgh for so many years had led him to conclude that none of the accepted forms of treatments were of any curative value. He was equally sceptical of the effectiveness of treatments being offered during the epidemic of cholera and was at first dismissive of a promising form of treatment introduced in the last weeks of the epidemic.

In 1831, the Royal College of Surgeons in London commissioned W.B. O'Shaughnessy, an Edinburgh medical graduate, to investigate the changes in the blood of the victims of the outbreak of cholera at Newcastle. He reported his preliminary results in the Lancet on 31 March 1831 (later published in full in his book, *Report on the Chemical Pathology of Malignant Cholera*). His analyses revealed 'a great but variable deficiency of water in the blood in four malignant cholera cases; a total absence of carbonate of soda in two and a remarkable diminution of other saline ingredients'.[15] He concluded that in treating cholera it was necessary '1st to restore the blood to its natural specific gravity; 2nd to restore its deficient saline matters'. O'Shaughnessy's report in the *Lancet* was read by Thomas Latta, an Edinburgh graduate practising in Leith, a town in which the outbreak of cholera had claimed a very large number of victims. Latta at first attempted to follow O'Shaughnessy's recommendations by administering fluids by mouth or per rectum. When these efforts failed he gave fluid intravenously; the fluid he used was made up of 'two or three drachms of muriate of soda and two scruples of the subcarbonate of soda in six pints of water'. All six pints were injected through the basilic vein in thirty minutes. Of the first five patients treated, three survived. On 22 May when Latta described his procedure in the Lancet, he concluded:

> I have no doubt that it will be found, if judiciously applied, to be one of the most powerful and one of the safest remedies yet used in the second stage of cholera or that hopeless state of collapse to which the system is reduced.[16]

Latta's procedure was used in the treatment of patients at the Drummond Street Cholera Hospital who had 'reached the last moment of earthly existence;'[17] nineteen survived while 'no such miracle' had been seen before. Robert Christison (later President of the College) reported a series of thirty-seven patients of whom twelve survived. Alison's initial scepticism was overcome and but not every member of Edinburgh's Board of Health was convinced; James Gregory continued to insist that cholera was 'an obvious affection of the nervous system' to be treated with opium. Elsewhere in Britain opinion was similarly mixed. In the autumn of 1832 the epidemic of cholera came to an end; a year later Latta died and O'Shaughnessy departed to India. Interest in intravenous treatment faded away.

In Edinburgh 1,159 people died of cholera during the cholera epidemic. Its management of the epidemic had been devised on the assumption that cholera was a contagious disease. But the experience of 1832 cast doubt on that assumption. Those who died were not the very young and the very old as was the case in outbreaks of contagious fevers but the middle-aged poor, especially the badly fed, badly clothed, badly housed and intemperate poor. The disease had spread across the country in fits and starts, causing explosive outbreaks in some towns and villages while missing others apparently at random. At Symington those who lived on one side of the village street had died of cholera but not those who lived on the other side in houses which had their own wells. The superintendents of the Edinburgh's cholera hospitals noticed that it had been common for one member of a family to be admitted *in extremis* while the others remained unaffected. Civic dignitaries visiting the cholera hospitals had never contracted the disease and the same was generally true of the medical and nursing staff who, over long periods, had been in frequent and close contact with the patients. As the epidemic

---

15. W. B. O'Shaughnessy, *Lancet* 1831–32, Vol. 1, p. 401; W. B. O'Shaughnessy, *Report on the Chemical Pathology of Malignant Cholera* (London, 1832).

16. *Lancet*, 1831–32, Vol. 2, p. 274.

17. N. MacGillivray, Dr Latta of Leith: Pioneer in the Treatment of Cholera by Intravenous Saline Infusion, *Journal of the Royal College of Physicians of Edinburgh*, 2006, Vol. 36, p. 82.

came to an end it seemed to many that cholera was no ordinary contagious disease and that measures that had been adopted for its management had been based on a false premise.

PUBLIC REACTION

The conspicuous failure of the measures imposed by the Board of Health to treat and to control the spread of cholera provoked the resentment and hostility of many, perhaps even a majority, of the people of Edinburgh. The resentment and anger was greatest among the poor. While the epidemic continued, a great many of their number were put in quarantine or confined to hospital against their will and, separated from their families, hundreds died. It seemed to the poorer sections of society that their freedoms and even their lives were being sacrificed to no effect other than to increase their misery. In Edinburgh, there were violent protests when families said to have been in contact with cholera were forcibly removed from their homes. In the industrial towns elsewhere in Scotland, where the incidence of the disease was much greater, the protests were more frequent and even more violent; in Glasgow a mob of 2,000 was, with great difficulty, brought under control by the police; in Paisley a riot was dispersed only after the intervention of the 4th Dragoons.

The resentment and hostility of the poor were aimed principally at the medical profession; there were cries of 'murderers' and 'Burkers' and 'humbug'. Doctors had been regarded with growing suspicion for some time. In January 1829, William Burke had been hanged in Edinburgh for 'secretly killing by suffocation or by strangulation in order to sell the victims' bodies for dissection'; many believed that the outbreak of 'cholera' was a humbug and that the real purpose of the measures introduced by the medical profession 'to control the disease' was to procure more bodies for dissection. Others believed that the deaths of these large numbers of the poor had been ordered by the government to reduce the burden of an unwanted surplus in the population. Their experience of the cholera epidemic of 1832 left the poor even more distrustful of the intentions of the medical profession at a time when the leaders of the profession in Scotland were intent on improving the provisions of the country's Poor Laws and in framing new Public Health legislation from which it was the poor who had most to gain.

THE LEGACY

The epidemic of cholera had been spreading westwards from Asia since 1829 and had reached across northern Europe in the summer of 1830.[18] But in the spring of 1831, the Privy Council in London, the body responsible for the protection of the people of the United Kingdom, was still uncertain about what action should be taken to prevent its arrival in Britain; an effective Central Cholera Board was not appointed in London until 22 November 1831,[19] three months after the first cases of cholera were diagnosed in Britain.

By then, in August, the Edinburgh College of Physicians had already appointed a Cholera Committee. On 26 September its secretary, James Gregory, wrote to London asking for a

18. Morris, *Cholera*.
19. Ibid., p. 32.

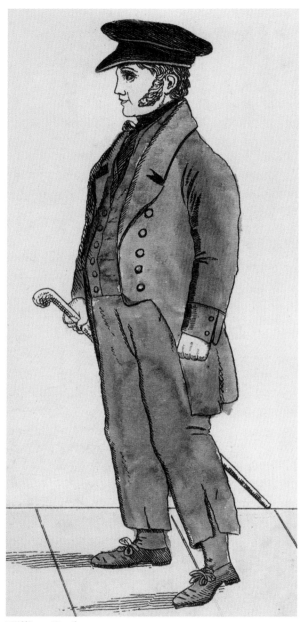

William Burke

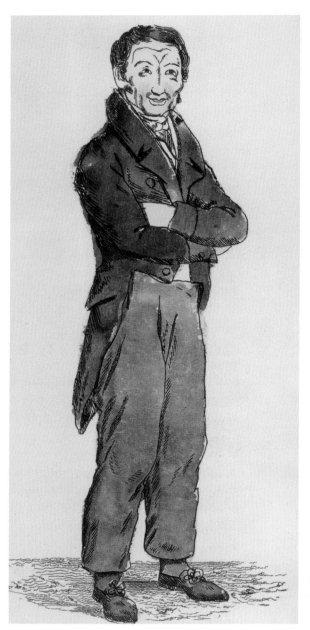

William Hare

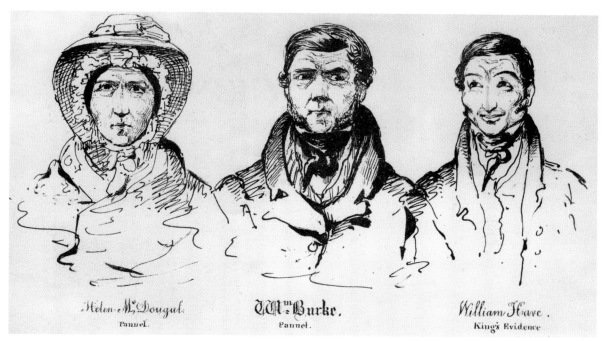

Helen McDougal.
Pannel.

Wm Burke.
Pannel.

William Hare.
King's Evidence

Cartoon of Burke, Hare and Helen McDougal

statement of government policy but the reply, received on 30th September, was unhelpful. Edinburgh then took the initiative and established a local Cholera Health Board; the Board's arrangements for the containment of the epidemic were in place two weeks before the disease reached the city.

The difference in the readiness of the response in London and in Edinburgh was a reflection of the importance given to the teaching on public health ('medical police') at Scotland's medical schools and the relative neglect of the subject in England.[20] It also reflected the greater experience of Royal College of Physicians of Edinburgh than that of its sister College in London in the devising and enforcement of public health measures; in 1817, the Edinburgh College of Physicians had established a Fever Board which served as a model when a new Health Board was called for on the approach of cholera in 1831.

In the absence of useful guidance from London during the anxious weeks of the summer and early autumn of 1831, local authorities across Scotland had turned to Edinburgh – to the Cholera Committee of the College of Physicians and Edinburgh's Cholera Board of Health – for advice and assistance. This experience was remembered when, in the aftermath of the cholera epidemic, poor law and public health reforms were being planned for the United Kingdom. The College, with the universal support of the country's local authorities, was able to insist that central control of the new services for Scotland was vested, not in London, but in Edinburgh.[21]

20. Martin, William Pulteney, p. 97.
21. Ibid., p. 350.

10

ALISON AND CHADWICK
Health Care for the Poor

Over nine thousand five hundred people in Scotland died in the cholera epidemic of 1832.[1] When the 'infective fever' that had long been endemic in Scotland's great cities became epidemic, as it did again in 1843, the death rate was almost as high.[2] As in the epidemic of cholera, the greatest mortality was among the poor. In 1843 Alison wrote:

> I have stated, and still maintain ... that the rapid extension of fever in any community may always excite suspicion of the provisions against destitution there being imperfect; and that where such extension of the disease is found chiefly to affect the poorest classes of the community it may held as a test of the inadequacy and inefficacy of the measures there adopted for the relief of poverty.[3]

In Britain poverty had increased dramatically since the end of the Napoleonic Wars in 1815. The wars had been long and costly.[4] For more than twenty years the British economy had been geared to war and the country's manufacturing industries struggled to find new markets. After a brief period of success, industry suffered economic depressions in 1819–20, 1826–27, 1829–31 and again in 1837 causing long periods of unemployment for much of the industrial workforce. Competition for what little employment was available was made more intense by the discharge of large numbers of men from the armed forces first at the end of the war and again when Britain's army of occupation was withdrawn from France. The high level of unemployment added to the social pressures caused by an unprecedented rate of increase in the population; in the thirty years from 1801 the population of Britain increased from 10.5 million to 16.3 million.

In these first decades of the nineteenth century, agriculture was still the dominant industry in Britain. In 1815, it was given special protection from competition by the passing of 'Corn Laws' that effectively excluded the importation of foreign wheat if the domestic price per quarter should fall below eighty shillings. The country's most important industry was secured and landowners who had over-extended their holdings during the war were saved from bankruptcy. But all this was achieved at the cost of high food prices for everyone, in town and country alike, and in the country the wages of those working the land remained as low as they

1. R.J. Morris, *Cholera 1832* (London, 1976), p. 12.
2. Ibid.
3. W.P. Alison, *Observations on the Epidemic Fever of 1843 in Scotland and its Connection with the Destitute Condition of the Poor* (Edinburgh, 1843), p. 2.
4. Inflation during the war years had seriously devalued Britain's currency.

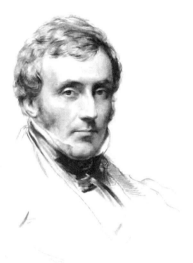

W. P. Alison

had always been. Many in the rural workforce, finding they could now barely afford to eat, moved away, hoping to find better paid employment in the towns. Their migration from the countryside served only to increase still further the problem of urban poverty.

In towns throughout the United Kingdom, charity organisations made great efforts to relieve the growing distress. In Edinburgh, local charities provided the needy with food and clothing. The College increased its commitment to the charitable institutions that its Fellows had served since they were founded. The Charity Workhouse was extended to accommodate 700 poor, 4 out of 5 of them women and children. At the Dispensaries founded by Andrew Duncan in the Old Town and later by W.P. Alison in the New Town, the number of indigent patients receiving outpatient medical assistance increased from 3,223 in 1815 to 10,570 in 1838. Over the same period, admissions to the Royal Infirmary more than doubled from 2,200 to 4,903;[5] the College responded by adding to the number of attending physicians. In 1832 Alison, President of the College during some of the worst years, had established a House of Refuge for the Destitute to give short term shelter for families in distress; it was soon admitting over 1,600 refugees from destitution each year. The city was divided into 18 districts and medical officers (9 from the College of Physicians and 9 from the College of Surgeons) were appointed to provide free medical aid in each of these districts.

Great as it was, the suffering in Edinburgh was less than in the industrial towns of the west of Scotland. There the distress was greater than anywhere in Britain. Scotland's new industries

---

5. W.P. Alison, *Observations on the Management of the Poor in Scotland and its Effect on the Health of the Great Towns* (Edinburgh, 1840), p. 3.

were of more recent origin, had grown more rapidly and were therefore more vulnerable to failure than those in England. Periods of unemployment and poverty were more frequent and more severe and Scotland's industrial towns were further burdened by a steady influx of the rural poor from both the Lowlands and the Highlands and a flood of the totally destitute from Ireland, that caused Alison to comment that 'if we are to cut off mendicancy in Scotland we must first cut off Ireland'.

In every part of the United Kingdom, where the combination of unemployment, poverty, overcrowding, high food prices and starvation had afflicted the industrial towns, there were public protests, disturbances and riots. The Government was less than sympathetic. Within the Cabinet the disturbances were talked of as 'mischief';[6] the Duke of Wellington was certain that the rioters 'won't be quiet until a number of them bite the dust or till some of their leaders are hanged'. As temporary measures, six Acts were passed by Parliament, one banning 'seditious' meetings, two against drilling with arms and three limiting the freedom of the press. In these troubled times Parliament voted to retain the death penalty for the stealing of even five shillings worth of food.

As economic depression and unemployment continued, the Government found the ever increasing amount of money being paid to support the poor an 'embarrassment'.[7] Before the war the annual amount being paid out under the Poor Law had been £2 million; by 1818 that sum had increased to £9.3 million.[8] There were imputations of corruption but even more complaints of waste and extravagance. In 1817 a select committee of the House of Lords had been appointed to review the working of the Poor Law but without any notable outcome. In 1832, in the aftermath of the cholera epidemic, a new and more interventionist government appointed a Royal Commission of Inquiry on the Poor Laws; Edwin Chadwick (a former journalist and lawyer who, as the secretary of Jeremy Bentham, had become an enthusiastic convert to Utilitarianism) was made an Assistant Commissioner responsible for collecting the relevant information.

SCOTLAND AND THE ROYAL COMMISSION OF INQUIRY ON THE POOR LAWS

When the Select Committee of the House of Lords was appointed in 1817, the Government intended that it should review the working of the Poor Laws both north and south of the border. The administration of the Poor Law in Scotland was then the province of the Church of Scotland; the committee therefore wrote to the General Assembly that 'as it is evident that the management of the poor in Scotland must have been conducted upon a different principle [from England] whatever information can be furnished will be extremely useful'.[9]

The Poor Law in Scotland had been established in 1574 by an Act of the Scottish Parliament modelled on the Act that had established the Poor Law in England in 1572. The

6. E. Longford, *Wellington: Pillar of State* (London, 1972), p. 58.
7. Ibid.
8. Taking into account the fall in the value of the pound the real increase was considerably less.
9. General Assembly Papers. SRO CH1/78-9.

English and Scottish Acts both laid down that the poor, aged and 'impotent'[10] of the country's parishes were to be supported by a local tax or stent set in proportion to the local property owners' resources. In these early years the only material difference was that, in England, parishes were ordered to provide work and work materials for those needing employment while Scottish parishes were not.[11] But later, in 1592, an Act of the Scottish Parliament made the church, through its kirk sessions in every parish, the supervising authorities of the Poor Law and a further Act in 1597 gave the kirk sessions full overall responsibility for its administration.

In time, it became unusual for the stent (more generally known as the 'assessment') to be legally enforced and the Poor Law fund in each parish was supplied by collections at church services, by legacies and by voluntary assessments. More radical ideological change came about in the early years of the nineteenth century. The General Assembly of the Church had become dominated by its evangelical members who abandoned the traditional Calvinist emphasis on the congregation as the unit of the true church and stressed the personal responsibility of the individual.[12]

This was made clear in the General Assembly's reply to the House of Lords select committee in 1817: 'The Scotch have proceeded on the principle that every individual is bound to provide for himself by his own labour as long as he is able to do so and his parish is only bound to make up the proportion of the necessities of life which he cannot earn or obtain for himself by other lawful means'. However, in 1817, the Assembly had little direct knowledge of how the Poor Law was being conducted or how much was being spent on the relief of the poor in the widely scattered and very diverse parishes of Scotland. A hastily arranged survey by questionnaire provided only limited and somewhat uncertain evidence that seemed to show that the cost of the Poor Law in Scotland had not risen significantly since the end of the eighteenth century. What did become clear from the survey was that over the years the meaning of the words used in the Act of 1574 had changed. 'The poor' was now generally taken to refer to the whole of the labouring class. And it had now become understood that the Poor Law should provide, not for the poor, the aged and the impotent, as laid down in 1574, but only for the poor aged and the poor impotent. At the General Assembly the principle that the 'merely poor' should have no right to aid under the Poor Law was vigorously defended by the Rev. Thomas Chalmers, the Assembly's most charismatic and most powerful orator. Chalmers insisted that granting the poor a statutory right to maintenance by the state would 'encourage the poor to think more of their rights than of their responsibilities'; they would become 'morally degraded' conditioned to pauperism and made 'less industrious'.[13] State aid would create, within the population, a large redundant section, making no contribution to the economy but enabled to marry and multiply, placing an increasing burden on the state and eventually making unsustainable demands on the resources of the country. In the *Edinburgh*

10. The word was then used in the sense of weak, disabled or decrepit.
11. R. Mitchison, *The Old Poor Law in Scotland* (Edinburgh, 2000), p. 7.
12. Ibid., p. 135.
13. S.J. Brown, *Thomas Chalmers and the Godly Commonwealth in Scotland* (Oxford, 1982).

Review in 1817 (in a review of the current debates in Parliament on the Poor Laws of England) Chalmers wrote that 'it would have been better for the English poor if there had never been any legislation prescribing relief; a system such as the Poor Law destroys the natural notions which arise from human feelings and replaces them with artificial legal requirements. The English Poor Law should be abolished and the country allowed to revert to the practice of the least corrupted part of Scotland where the support of the poor was based on the simple distribution of alms voluntary giving between people who knew each other'.[14] These same assertions were repeated in the House of Commons by a number of young Whig members from Scotland. In was in consequence of these very confident protestations by the General Assembly, by Chalmers in the *Edinburgh Review* and by Scottish MPs that Parliament concluded that legislation to amend the existing Poor Laws should apply only to England and Wales.

A POOR LAW FOR ENGLAND AND WALES

The Select Committee of the House of Lords appointed in 1817 to review the Poor Laws reached no firm conclusion. A second Select Committee appointed in 1824 was no more successful. In 1832, in the aftermath of the cholera epidemic, a new and more actively interventionist government appointed a *Royal Commission for Inquiring into the Administration and Practical Operation of the Poor Laws*. The cost of the Poor Law was continuing to increase 'by leaps and bounds' so that 'the poor rate threatened to engulf the whole landed property of the country'.[15] The controversy on how problems should be solved had now raged for years. Some thought that paupers should be put to work to earn their keep or even to make a profit for the community; others believed that the poor laws should be abolished and that the poor should have no right to relief of any kind. In 1832 a new scheme was proposed by Edwin Chadwick.

Chadwick was a lawyer who had been secretary to Jeremy Bentham and had become an enthusiastic disciple of Utilitarianism; when the Royal Commission was appointed he was made the Assistant Commissioner responsible for the investigation of the operation of the Poor Law in London. In his report to the Commission, Chadwick claimed that the essential 'evil' that had to be eliminated was the increase in able-bodied pauperism. Since 1795, local Poor Law authorities had been permitted to grant relief to able bodied but indigent poor in their own homes. This Poor Law allowance made it possible for able-bodied paupers either to withdraw from the labour market or, if they did not, to compete in that market with an advantage over workers who were entirely dependent on their own industry. Chadwick proposed that the poor should be forced to maintain themselves; if they did not they should be 'separated by a wide margin from the rewards of independent work' and removed from normal society by being confined in a 'well regulated workhouse'. Chadwick understood that such a harsh regime was most unlikely to be willingly enforced by the unpaid volunteers (nominated annually by the neighbouring Justices of the Peace) who had traditionally been responsible for the local administration of the Poor Law; the scheme was therefore to be

14. Mitchison, *The Old Poor Law*, p. 143.
15. S.E. Finer, *The Life and Times of Sir Edward Chadwick* (London, 1952), p. 42.

carried out by paid officials appointed by and acting under the supervision of a strong central agency.

In 1833, at the request of the Commissioners, Chadwick set out his proposals in detail and in legal form in a pamphlet, *Notes of Heads for a Bill*. When the pamphlet was published, it was well received by the public and much praised by the national press. It was then circulated to members of the Royal Commission as a draft for its Report. Thereafter Chadwick's proposals became the basis of the Poor Law (Amendment) Act of 1834.

The Act withdrew the right of the able bodied labourer to sustenance and withdrew the ratepayers' responsibility for him. The indigent and helpless retained their right to sustenance but only if their pauperism was judged to be no fault of their own and only if they had no immediate family who could support them. Out-door relief was abolished and sustenance was to be given only to those who, as registered paupers, gave up what civil right and property they had and became resident in a workhouse in conditions deliberately made unattractive to all but the most desperate. The workhouse was to be 'an uninviting place of wholesome restraint' and its manager 'the hardest taskmaster and the worst paymaster that the idle and the dissolute can apply to';[16] the paupers were to be forced to do hard manual labour (breaking stones for the men; oakum-picking for the women and children) on tasks chosen to be the more heartbreaking for the paupers since they were so clearly of no commercial or economic value; the food was deliberately made unpleasant; beer and tobacco were forbidden; husbands, wives and children were separated and no visitors were allowed.

Groups of parishes were brought together as 'Unions' large enough to afford to build workhouses that could accommodate all the different categories of pauper (males, females, children, the aged, the disabled, the sick and the insane). The magistrates, invariable drawn from the local squires and worthies, who had traditionally managed the Poor Law in their parishes were relieved of their responsibilities; under the new Poor Law each Union was presided over by a Board of Guardians elected by the ratepayers and supervised centrally by three Poor Law Commissioners in London.

Although Chadwick recognised that disease was a major cause of poverty he made no provision for medical aid in his Poor Law (Amendment) Act. He believed that the diseases that caused poverty could be prevented by removing the miasma that caused them and that this could be done by improved sanitation. Following his experience with leaders of the medical profession in London during the cholera epidemic (Chapter 8) he had little respect for doctors in general and regarded them as 'necessary evils' that were 'not likely to last' since they would be made redundant by improvements in sanitation and public hygiene.[17] However, a provision in the Act allowed Boards of Guardians to appoint 'officers' to assist them and a number of Boards used this loophole to appoint 'medical officers'. Unfortunately their selection of candidates was often arbitrary and made with little regard for training or qualifications; many of the 'medical officers' appointed in the 1830s and early 1840s were unlicensed. It was only the ensuing scandal that led the Poor Law Commissioners in 1842, to make formal provision

16. Quoted in J. Ridley, *Lord Palmerston* (London, 1970), p. 278.
17. R. Hodgekinson, *The Origins of the National Health Service* (London, 1967), p. 639.

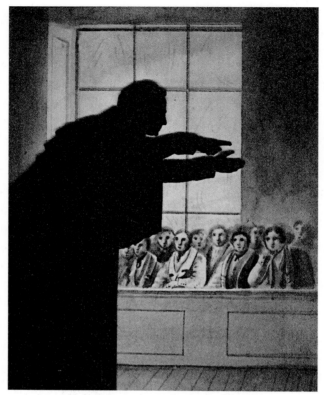

Thomas Chalmers (National Portrait Gallery)

for the appointment of medical officers and issue regulations to ensure that those appointed were licensed to practise in England.[18]

The amendment of the Poor Law in England achieved its primary aim; when the Chancellor of the Exchequer presented his budget in December 1852, he was able to inform the House of Commons that the cost of poor relief in England and Wales had fallen by 20 per cent. However, the new Poor Law had already proved unpopular with the public at large. The brutality of its Poor House system had made its author, Edwin Chadwick, 'the most unpopular single individual in the whole kingdom'[19]

ALISON AND THE CARE OF THE POOR IN SCOTLAND

Edwin Chadwick confidently expected that when Poor Law (Amendment) Bill became law in 1834 he would be made a Poor Law Commissioner and invited to take charge of the implementing of the scheme of which he was the author. However, the three Commissioners appointed were to be paid salaries of £2,000 a year and such lucrative posts were normally given to useful placemen to whom government ministers felt under some obligation. When

18. A Scottish medical degree was not accepted as a sufficient licence to practise in England.
19. Finer, *The Life and Times*, p. 187.

Chadwick was proposed as a Commissioner, the Cabinet decided that 'his station in society was not as would have made it fit that he should be a Commissioner'.[20] Chadwick felt humiliated and it was only with great difficulty that Lord Althrope the Leader of the House, who had managed the Bill through Parliament, persuaded him to accept appointment as the Secretary of the Poor Law Commission. He accepted office only on Althrop's assurance that in practice his authority would be at least that of a Commissioner.

This was an arrangement that the chairman of the Commission, Frankland Lewis, refused to accept. When Chadwick attempted to act independently Frankland Lewis attempted to have him dismissed but for a time Chadwick continued to have the support of government ministers. Then, in the general election of 1837 the government's majority in the House of Commons was reduced to thirty and the loss of so many seats was blamed on Chadwick's new Poor Law. (When the Whigs were totally defeated in 1841, the unpopularity of Chadwick's Poor Law was blamed once again.) Chadwick's authority as Secretary of the Poor Law Commission became progressively eroded and, only some five years after it had been introduced, his interest in the development and management of the Poor Law system that he had devised for England had come to an end.

His attention had already turned to the great and growing deficiencies in the sanitation of the country's towns. In 1838, in a letter to the Home Secretary, he wrote:

> All epidemics and all infectious diseases are attended with charges, immediate and ultimate on the Poor Rates. Labourers are suddenly thrown by infectious disease into a state of destitution for which relief must be given. In case of death, the widow and children are thrown as paupers on the parish. The amount of the burdens thus produced is frequently so great as to render it good economy on the part of the administration of the Poor Laws to incur charges for preventing the evils where they are ascribable to physical causes.[21]

In a second letter he identified these 'physical causes':

> When acting as Secretary to the Commission it came under my observation that claims for relief on account of sickness came regularly in the greatest proportion from ill-drained places where ordure was retained in cesspools.

In 1839 Chadwick persuaded the Home Secretary to appoint his medical friends, Neil Arnott, Southwood Smith and James Kay-Shuttleworth (all medical graduates of Scottish universities) as a committee to investigate sanitary conditions in London. A few months later, after a change of government he contrived to have a motion introduced in the House of Lords that led the new Home Secretary to extend the inquiry into sanitary conditions of the labouring classes in all the large towns in the of England and Wales; Frankland Lewis was more than happy to give Chadwick leave from his secretarial duties with the Poor Law Commissioners to take charge of the new inquiry.

20. Ibid., p 109.
21. Ibid., p. 156.

In Edinburgh, the College immediately sent a petition to the Home Secretary. The petition:

> Humbly Sheweth
>
> That at present the Poor Law Commissioners have been directed to make inquiries as to the sanitary condition of the labouring classes both in England and Wales.
>
> That the sanitary condition of the labouring classes of her Majesty's subjects in Scotland equally demand investigation; and that in the cities of Edinburgh and Glasgow, it is known to your petitioners to be worse in several respects and particularly as regards the liability to contagious fever than that of the labouring classes in most if not all of the great towns in England.
>
> That your petitioners therefore humbly pray that the Poor Law Commissioners may be directed to extend their inquiries into Scotland.

In February 1840 the Home Secretary informed the College that 'the Poor Law Commissioners have undertaken to extend their labours to Scotland'.

The findings of Chadwick's inquiry were published as Blue Book by the House of Lords in July 1842. The *Report on the Sanitary Condition of the Labouring Population of Great Britain* became the most famous and most widely read government report of the nineteenth century. It formed the basis for new legislation extending government intervention to improve the protection of the health of the labouring poor in both England and Scotland.

By 1842, there had been a major shift in opinion in Scotland on the need for government intervention in the provision of care for the poor. In 1840, writing as 'Fellow and Late President of the Royal College of Physicians of Edinburgh', Alison had published his *Observations on the Management of the Poor in Scotland and its Effect on the Health of the Great Towns*. From his early studies in a number of counties in Europe (Chapter 4), Alison claimed that 'where indigence has been long admitted as having a legal claim to such an extent as to preserve all the inhabitants from the want of the first necessities' the 'evils' envisaged by Chalmers and his supporters in 1817 had not been the result. Alison admitted that it was perhaps possible that if aid to the poor were to be 'lavished with indiscriminate profusion' such evil consequences might follow but 'no one who knows the Scottish character can entertain the smallest apprehension of their being too liberally or incautiously expended here'.[22]

Alison claimed that the views that Chalmers had put forward since 1817 had not only been wrong but 'the general diffusion through Scotland of the opinion that all poor rates are evil has rendered the law [the Old Poor Law] of the country in many ways inoperative'. Assured that the provision of free aid to the poor was evil, the 'higher ranks in Scotland', who already contributed 'much less than those of any other country in Europe' had reduced their voluntary contributions to Poor Law funds still further.[23] Their withdrawal of support from the poor was

22. Alison, *Observations on Management*, p. 175.
23. Ibid., p. vi.

all the more understandable since they had been encouraged by the church to believe that poverty was the result of moral failure, drunkenness or idleness

Alison disputed Chalmers's understanding of idleness. Alison believed that it was impossible

> to suppose that all the persons who wander about this and other great towns in this country in a state of destitution, subsisting on alms and very precarious occasional employment can find regular work if they choose. In every long established and rich community there is a surplus population beyond what is required for any kind of employment of which the community stands in need.

Alison also believed that the depression that resulted from prolonged unemployment and extreme poverty made drunkenness 'almost unavoidable'.

> A certain duration of hopeless and extreme poverty will make any man, whatever his former character may have been, utterly reckless of the future.

Having discussed the nature of poverty and ideas on its management at some length Alison proposed:

> That the Poor Law should be financed by an assessment imposed uniformly throughout the country and that no parish nor any body of men should be allowed to avoid assessment.
>
> That the assessment should everywhere be very considerably more than before and that allowances to widows and orphans and to the aged, disabled and impotent persons should be much raised.
>
> That the Poor Law should be administered, not by a body elected by the ratepayers but by a body appointed by the state.
>
> That the workhouse system should be introduced into every considerable town in Scotland; elsewhere unions of parishes should be formed to support workhouses for the permanent reception of aged, disabled or incurable persons and of orphans who have no relations with whom they can be comfortably settled; for the reception of women and children left or deserted by their husbands and fathers; and also for the reception and confinement of all destitute persons entitled to legal relief who are judged to be improper objects for outdoor relief on account of intemperance or immorality.
>
> That relief should be regularly given to those of the poor who are proved to be destitute from want of employment. With a view to the maintenance of a desirable standard of comfort and discipline for them and with a view to the tranquilly of the community relief should normally be provided within the workhouse. This he justified by the observation that 'the younger generation, those on whom this evil has chiefly fallen, are far less educated and more prone to vice than the elder' and 'in the habit of spending their money as fast as they get it and often before'.

Alison also argued that the unemployed should be provided with aid under the Poor Law since long continued unemployment predisposed to disease, disablement and even death, condemning whole families to destitution.

> While there has been much disposition to relieve the sick poor there has been very general discouragement of institutions for the relief of [the] mere poverty of the unemployed poor … The kind of assistance to the poor which all medical men know to be of the utmost importance for the prevention of many of their most formidable diseases has as much as possible withheld.[24]

THE ROYAL COMMISSION ON THE POOR LAWS OF SCOTLAND.

Alison's *Observations on the Management of the Poor in Scotland and its Effect on the Health of the Great Towns* was widely read and was very favourably reviewed in the press *The Scotsman* was especially supportive. It acknowledged that Alison had 'studied poverty as it really existed over many years' and that his book had shown that it was 'that the allowances made to the impotents in this country are shamefully inadequate'. After reading Alison's work 'no sane person will be found to deliberately deny the right of every human creature when disabled by infirmity or want of employment to obtain the means of subsistence from the community in which he lives'.[25] The medical press – *Edinburgh Medical and Surgical Journal, London Medical Gazette, British and Foreign Medical Review* – was also supportive and agreed that the publication of Alison's Observations could not fail sooner or later to lead to a legislative enactment to cure the evils depicted in it'.[26]

Popular support for Alison's call for reform led, in March 1840, to the formation of an Association for Obtaining an Official Inquiry into the Pauperism of Scotland; its objective was 'to raise the condition of the poor in Scotland to the same standard as that already existing in the best regulated countries in Europe'. In April, a group of landowners who had 'doubts of the prudence of hastily interfering with or altering the present system of Poor Laws or superseding the means which the existing institutions afford of ascertaining the extent of destitution' formed a Local Inquiry Association. They immediately set out to pre-empt an official government inquiry by conducting one of their own; they asked that all burgh and county magistrates in Scotland should report to them on the extent of poverty and the workings of the poor laws in their parishes.

For three years these two Associations struggled in a flurry of pamphlets to corroborate or refute the claims made in his *Observations on the Management of the Poor*. The issues were also debated at length at the meeting of the British Association in Glasgow in September 1840 and at meetings of the General Assembly. Alison's opponents first attempted to show that the problem of poverty as described in *Observations* existed only in Glasgow and Edinburgh and that elsewhere poverty was not increasing and that the provisions of the Poor Law were entirely adequate for its relief. When these claims proved unconvincing, Alison's opponents

24. Ibid., p. 36.
25. Quoted by S.M.K. Martin, St Andrews University, PhD Thesis, 1997, p. 200.
26. *British and Foreign Medical Review*, 1840, Vol. 9, p. 544.

focused their objections on two particular issues. They objected to the proposed introduction to Scotland of the provisions of the English Poor Law, provisions that the Lord Chancellor, Lord Brougham, had described in the House of Lords as an 'evil of bad laws and worse administered'; they objected particularly to the English workhouse system which was disliked and disapproved by the general public in England and greatly feared by those facing poverty and the awful possibility of destitution. Alison's opponents also refused to accept his claim that destitution was so potent a factor in the aetiology of 'fever' that the prevalence of fever was a reliable indication of the 'utter inefficiency of the Scotch Poor Laws'. In denying that fever was caused by destitution they quoted the opinion of Arnott, Kay and Southwood-Smith, published in their *Report on the Sanitary Condition of the Labouring Population of Great Britain*, that appropriate sanitary measures alone would effectively eliminate the cause of fever; even Arnott agreed with Alison that destitution, while not its immediate cause, was an important predisposing factor in the aetiology of fever,[27] this was a concept that the great majority of Alison's opponents were either reluctant or unable to grasp.

In 1843, although many of the objections to Alison's scheme remained unresolved, the Association for Obtaining an Official Inquiry into the Pauperism of Scotland achieved its primary aim with the appointment of a Royal Commission for Inquiring into the Administration and Practical Operation of the Poor Laws of Scotland.

In his evidence to the Royal Commission, Alison made his case for the establishment of a state medical service that would provide free care, not only for the poor registered as paupers on their parish roles but also for the working poor who could not afford to pay for the services of a doctor.

> The medical aid to the poor I believe to be generally very deficient; and where it is sufficient for them, it is a heavy and unjust burden on the medical men who devote often, I believe, a larger portion of their time and money to the service of the poor than any other class in the community. I remember a very excellent man, a practitioner in the Grassmarket here, who told me that he had sometimes given away in a day among the poor in the Grassmarket more than he had earned in that day.
>
> In most towns there are dispensaries by which medical men are relieved of the great part of the expense of medicines for the sick poor and in some of them, I believe the duty of visiting the sick is very carefully performed; but being always on the voluntary principle there is no security for its being regularly or uniformly performed or for that early attention to cases on which the success of treatment, in most cases admitting of successful treatment depends. For example, in Edinburgh for thirty years before 1815, there was a public dispensary but it was opened only twice a week and it was no part of the duty of the medical officers to attend the sick poor at home. Any other medical aid which the sick poor had at home was private charity on the part of the medical

27. Martin, p. 221.

men. Since then the duty of attending the sick poor has been undertaken by several dispensaries; but the assistance given in this way is neither so regular nor effectual as it ought to be. During the present epidemic many of the young men, students, upon whom the duty of visiting chiefly devolves, have been deterred from attending the dispensaries by fear of having their studies interrupted.

Alison proposed that the town should be divided into a number of districts each with its own dispensary and its own medical officer. Each medical officer would come to know the people in his district and, with one or two assistants he would be able to carry out his duties quickly and efficiently. This arrangement had been proposed before but had not been adopted; it had been argued that there would inevitable be competition between the districts in finding subscribers, leading to a very unequal distribution of the charitable resources of the town.

> This illustrates the evil of leaving an object of such importance to the voluntary system of charity. I have no doubt that the system of medical relief to the poor by medical officers, appointed and paid by the managers or guardians of the poor in each district might easily be made much better for the interests of the poor and more uniformly efficient than the system of voluntary relief from dispensaries such as exists here. There can be no doubt that by a well regulated system of medical relief and by judicious measures of medical police, many of the working-classes who are now reduced to pauperism by diseases, by premature old age or by the death of relations might be enabled to maintain themselves in independence.[28]

The Royal Commission reported in 1844. It condemned the gross inadequacy of the financial relief provided in many parts of Scotland; the sums offered (to support perhaps a widow and a number of children) ranged from a shilling or two in assessed parishes to a few pence in rural parishes where there was no assessment. It also found that 'there is scarcely any provision made for medical relief to the poor out of the poor funds. This seems to be left systematically to charity'.[29] The evidence had also shown that if the poor were ever seen by a medical man it was owing to the benevolence of the doctor who frequently had to pay for any necessary medicines out of his own pocket. In the cities and some of the large towns dispensaries and infirmaries, financed by charity, went some way to supply the lack of any parochial care; otherwise the poor were left dependent on the charity of medical men, both for medicines and advice.[30]

The recommendations published in the report were an amalgam of ideas that had been put forward by both sides in the three years of debate. Alison commented that the Commissioners had 'gone just about half the length I had represented as necessary'.[31] Nevertheless, it was the

28. W.P. Alison, *Remarks on the Report of Her Majesty's Commissioners on the Poor-Law of Scotland* (Edinburgh, 1844), p. 67.
29. *Report of Her Majesty's Commissioners for Inquiring Into the Administration and Practical Operation of the Poor Laws of Scotland*, 1844, p. 13.
30. J.H.F. Brotherston, *Observations on the Early Public Health Movement in Scotland* (London, 1952), p. 71.
31. Alison, *Remarks*, p. vi.

recommendations of the Commissioners that shaped the Poor Law Amendment Act passed for Scotland in 1845.

The Act transferred to the state the responsibility for the administration of the Poor Law that had for three centuries been devolved to the Church. The parish remained the unit of administration but parochial boards were set up to 'have and exercise all the powers and authority hitherto exercised by the Heritors and the Kirk Session'. It was left to the parochial boards to decide whether or not assessment was necessary to fund the provision of relief to the poor in their parishes. Financial relief was still to be given only to the aged and the infirm poor. (In spite of the mass of evidence presented by Alison, the Royal Commission had recommended that it 'was neither necessary nor expedient' to give funds *raised by assessment* to the able bodied in times of depression.) The draconian workhouse system that was so feared by the poor in England was not imposed in Scotland. The traditional emphasis on 'outdoor' relief was to be maintained as far as possible although large parishes were encouraged to build poorhouses where they were thought necessary. A central Board of General Supervision was established but its responsibilities were limited to offering advice to the parochial boards and reporting on their work to the Home Secretary.

In most of its provisions, the new Poor Law Act was cautious and, in general, conservative. However, major innovations, secured later after continuing political pressure, came in its medical provisions. The Act stated that any new poor houses erected in Scotland were to have 'sufficient arrangements' for the care of the sick poor and that *'it would be lawful'* to appoint a properly qualified medical man to be in regular attendance. The Act also stated that in every parish the parochial board must provide all of its sick poor with nutritious diet, clothing, medicine and medical attendance but only *'to such an extent as may seem equitable and expedient'*.

In the House of Commons, Scottish members, successfully lobbied by Alison, Abercrombie and other Fellows of the College, objected that these medical provisions did not go far enough. They demanded that the Poor Law must ensure that every parish had the services of a resident medical officer and that to provide the necessary funds general assessment must be made obligatory. The Home Secretary, Sir James Graham, agreed that 'general assessment must be desirable but considering the difference of opinion he thought it infinitely more wise to leave the public of Scotland, by a voluntary act to adopt the assessment themselves rather than by an enactment to make it compulsory'.[32] The Prime Minister, Sir Robert Peel, considered that the provision of a paid medical officer was impractical and that the Scottish members were being over-ambitious. 'He entertained a strong objection to giving the people of Scotland a positive assurance that the poor should at all times be supplied with medical relief. He thought they should be cautious in how they excited expectation which could not be realised. Everything that was possible ought to be done but fallacious hopes should not be raised'.[33]

32. Hansard, lxxx1, HC 12 June 1845.
33. Ibid.

Nevertheless pressure continued and in 1848 the government offered a compromise. An annual grant of £10,000 (increased in 1882 to £20,000) was made to the board of supervision to provide a financial supplement for every parish willing to raise an equivalent sum to employ its own medical officer. Sir John McNeil, the chairman of the board was confident that, with this inducement, a full complement of medical officers would be recruited in every parish in Scotland.

A COLLEGE ASSESSMENT OF THE MEDICAL AID UNDER THE NEW POOR LAW

When introducing the Poor Law (Amendment) Bill to the House of Commons in 1845, the Lord Advocate had drawn the attention of the House of Commons to the great and increasing problem of poverty in the Highlands and Islands.

> In many districts a great change of circumstances has been occasioned by the alteration in the system of management of land. Small farms have been thrown together into large farms and the consequence is that there are fewer people able to contribute to the relief of the poor now than formerly... While the means of the contributors has decreased and the fund for relieving the poor has become lessened the poverty and misery of the labouring classes has naturally increased.

As the Lord Advocate was well aware, the long-standing poverty of the people of the Highlands and Islands had been increased even further since the end of the Napoleonic Wars. A sharp fall in cattle prices had made their few beasts almost worthless and the collapse of the kelp industry had closed their chief opportunity for local employment. The great majority lived in dire poverty, badly housed and poorly clad. 'Their domestic economy is frugal beyond conception. Their ordinary food consists of oat and barley meal and potatoes'.[34]

A year after the new Poor Law (Amendment) Act the Highlands and Islands were further 'blasted by providence'. The potato blight that had been devastating Ireland since 1845 had spread to Scotland and for almost a decade the people of the Highlands and Islands were unable to grow the crop on which they chiefly depended for their sustenance. Meal had to be brought in by relief organisations and paid for by the people in whatever cash they still possessed or, when that was exhausted, by their labour. Whereas in Ireland during these years the structure and functioning of society was undermined, 20,000 died of starvation and a further 193,000 died from typhus ('famine fever'),[35] in the Highlands and Islands social order was maintained and enough meal was shipped in to prevent deaths from starvation. Typhus never reached epidemic proportions in the Highlands and Islands;[36] the Great Highland Famine therefore caused few deaths but was the cause of greatly increased poverty and destitution.

Four years into this period of intense distress, John Coldstream, drew the attention of the College to the lack of medical aid in the Highlands and Islands. Coldstream was a friend of

34. Ibid.
35. K.F. Kiple, *Cambridge World History of Human Disease* (Cambridge, 1993), p. 161.
36. W. P. Alison, *Observations of the Famine of 1846–47* (Edinburgh, 1857).

Charles Darwin and after graduating at Edinburgh he too had made his early career in natural history.[37] Then in 1845, as a newly elected Fellow of the College, he had returned to Edinburgh to practise medicine and to take part in the missionary work of the new Free Church of Scotland.[38] The Free Church had been one of the principal agencies delivering relief to the Highlands and Islands during the potato famine and Coldstream was able to give an account of conditions there in a paper presented to College in July 1850. He claimed that because of the very small number of medical men practising in the region it was quite impossible for them to provide an adequate service for the sick.[39] Since he could give no exact figures, the College applied to the Board of Supervision 'for such information as it happened to be possessed of, regarding the supply of medical aid in the northern districts of Scotland'.[40] On being informed by the chairman of the board that the relevant information 'was not to be found', The College appointed a committee 'to determine the proportion which the Practitioners bear to the whole population and to ascertain whether there be much complaint on the part of the people of the difficulty in getting medical aid'.[41]

A questionnaire was sent to the 320 ministers in the 170 parishes of Argyll, Bute, Inverness, Ross, Sutherland, Caithness, Orkney and Shetland. The Ministers were asked to give the names and addresses of the doctors practising in their parishes, to state whether the number of doctors was increasing or decreasing and to assess the extent the inadequacy of medical aid in their districts. A similar questionnaire was also sent to all the doctors known by the College to be practising in the region at that time.[42]

There were then 370,000 people living in the 14,000 square miles of the Highlands and Islands. Only the aged and the infirm poor formally recognised and listed by their parishes as paupers (between 2 per cent and 4 per cent of the population[43]) were entitled to free medical care under the new Poor Law and that number had hardly changed since the famine began. But by the winter of 1850 there was little to distinguish the paupers from the general population and very few had access to medical aid. The College inquiry found that no fewer than 92 of the 170 parishes in the Highlands and Islands were without a resident doctor. In a number of these parishes, a doctor could be called from a neighbouring parish in cases of absolute necessity, but as many as 41 parishes were 'never visited by any regular practitioner and may therefore be regarded as destitute of medical aid'.[44]

The parish ministers of the Highlands and Islands were able to identify only 133 medical men in the whole region and not all were regarded as reliable. In many cases it was suspected, with some justification, that the practitioner had no proper training or qualification. The

37. Veronica Cecil, great-great-granddaughter of John Coldstream. Personal communication.
38. At the General Assembly in 1843, over a dispute that had little to do with the care of the poor, Thomas Chalmers had led the evangelical members in walking out to form the Free Church. In what became know as the Disruption the national church was almost broken in half; 454 of and some 40 per cent of the lay members left the established Church of Scotland.
39. College Minute, 16 July 1850.
40. Ibid., 5 November 1850.
41. Ibid., 2 July 1850.
42. There was no Medical Register until 1858.
43. I Levitt and T.C. Smout, *The State of the Working Class in Scotland in 1843* (Edinburgh, 1979), Table 8A.
44. Report of a Committee of the Royal College of Physicians of Edinburgh, 3 February 1852. College Archive.

distribution of the medical practitioners bore little relation to the parish structure of the region. Although many were receiving a 'salary' under the new Poor Law, medical practitioners did not necessarily base themselves on parishes which employed them. Those medical men who were wholly dependent for their livelihood on the fees they could earn in the practice of their profession based themselves in towns or villages which had a few shops, a post office and some promise of commercial activity. For the majority of the people of the more landward areas these 'commercial' doctors were remote and their services were neither immediately available nor affordable.[45] In the remote landward districts medical men could not make a living from private practice, the 'people being so much scattered' and 'being so poor and unable to pay either for attendance or medicine'.[46] Most doctors combined medical practice with 'small' farming and for some farming was their chief source of income. On some great estates the proprietor lent financial support. On his vast estates in the north the Duke of Sutherland employed a number of district surgeons on an annual salary of £40, which, with their other earnings made them among the most financially secure medical practitioners in the Highlands. However, few proprietors were so wealthy and able to spend such sums on medical aid for their tenants.

As poverty increased in the years after the Napoleonic Wars, even some of the medical practitioners who had seemed well established in the Highlands had begun to drift away. When, in 1846, the arrival of the potato blight in the Highland and Islands turned poverty into destitution, that drift increased. The measures introduced in 1845 by the Poor Law (Amendment) Act, even when strengthened by the subsidy added in 1848, did nothing to halt that trend; in response to the College's inquiry, ministers in the Highlands and Islands reported the loss of 35 medical practitioners from the region. Of the 200 ministers (Free Church and Church of Scotland) who replied to the College's inquiry, the great majority (141) reported that the new Poor Law had brought no improvement in medical services in their parishes and 32 reported that medical help had become even more difficult to find.

By 1850 it had also become clear that the medical provisions of the Poor Law (Amendment) Act, and in particular the Treasury grant, had, in many cases not been implemented and in others that had been mismanaged. Parochial boards had often found it impossible to appoint a medical officer since the Treasury grant had to be matched by an equal contribution from parish funds that did not exist. In parishes where the subsidy was taken up, it was often used arbitrarily and unfairly. Some parishes allocated the grant to favoured practitioners who did not live or practise in the parish. Others subsidized practitioners with no formal training or any recognised qualification. But even where the grant was used to the best effect, it often proved insufficient to relieve the almost overwhelming financial pressure on the local medical practitioner.

> Although the medical practitioners of this place are allowed thirty pounds and some odd shillings for attending the paupers on the roll, some of us have to

45. A single visit at a distance of a little over ten miles might command a fee of 30 shillings.
46. John Ferguson, surgeon, Dunvegan. College Archive CI/535.

expend a large proportion of that sum on medicine for the people in indigent circumstances who, though not in receipt of parochial relief, cannot pay for medical attention.[47]

By 1850 it was apparent that the Poor Law (Amendment) Act, even with the addition of the annual Treasury grant, had not succeeded in ensuring the provision of adequate medical care in a poor community. The fundamental problem was the overwhelming extent and severity of the poverty. The few paupers whose care was directly financed by the state, formed only a very small proportion of the number of those who were too poor to pay for medicines and medical attention. In many prosperous regions in Scotland, medical practitioners could earn enough in fees from those who could afford to pay to allow them to provide services gratis to that manageable proportion of their patients who could not. In the majority of parishes in the Highlands and Islands, those who could pay were too few to provide more than a very modest income for a medical practitioner; by providing medicines and service freely to all those who required it, he faced financial ruin. In many cases the practitioner was only saved from being overwhelmed by the restraint of the great majority of poor. 'The people seldom think of calling a medical man until there is manifest danger and often cases are too far gone before advice is had'.[48] Fortunately, throughout the Highland Famine the population remained 'generally healthy'.[49]

In 1850, the poverty that was at the root of the problem in the Highlands and Islands was not related specifically to the failure of the potato crops. Indeed in the 232 reports received by John Coldstream, the parish ministers and medical practitioners seldom mentioned the potato famine. Without exception they saw the problem of poverty as endemic and set to continue indefinitely and many described the situation as hopeless. There was also general agreement that, while the level of poverty in the Highlands and Islands continued, it would be impossible to maintain adequate medical services without government intervention. Some suggested that government 'should oblige parishes to combine in small groups and be required, with Treasury support, to employ salaried medical officers to provide free medical aid for all those in need'. Others agreed that:

> The simplest and cheapest plan to give medicines and medical aid to tens of thousands in the Hebrides would be for the government to employ a few sober men of good character and energy, provided with medicines and instruments and a small steamboat (as the Marquis of Salisbury has done for Rum) to move constantly about among the people where they could conveniently assemble to be cured of their diseases. By this plan medical men would more economically and efficiently be brought into contact with the sick and the maimed than by the establishment of stationary practitioners

47. Colin MacTavish, Collge Archive CI/477.
48. Rev. Allan Gunn, Watten. College Archive CI/275.
49. Ibid.

Yet other doctors proposed that a government service should be established in every district and staffed by 'many of our own Army and Navy surgeons, unemployed and inadequately provided for'.

> Already in 1850, the College inquiry had shown that the Poor Law (Amendment) Act of 1845 had done almost nothing to improve medical services in the poorest and most sparsely populated parts of Scotland.

MEDICAL SERVICES FOR THE WORKING POOR IN THE HIGHLANDS AND ISLANDS

In his *Observations of the Famine*,[50] Alison asserted that the plight of the working poor in the Highlands was essentially no different from that of the working poor elsewhere in Scotland. This was a view that was shared by the Fellows of the College. At a meeting of the College in February 1852 it was also agreed that the government must intervene to prevent 'the evils of deficiency of medical aid' and particularly to correct the 'anomaly of the very poor, who are recipients of parish aid, receiving more attention than those who are in comparatively independent circumstances, although unable to pay for medical aid'.[51]

However, in August 1852, when the College published its *Statement Regarding the Existing Deficiency of Medical Practitioners in the Highlands and Islands*, it did not lend its support to any of the proposals that practitioners in the Highlands had put forward for the creation of some form of state medical service. The President ruled that 'keeping in mind that the College should never aim at any object which they are unlikely to obtain'[52] However, the College provided Sir John McNeil, the Chairman of the Board of Supervision in Scotland, with a full account of the deficiencies that had been revealed in the medical services in the Highlands and Islands and made clear its view that the lack of affordable medical aid for the able-bodied working poor documented by its Inquiry in the Highlands and Islands, illustrated a problem that was general throughout Scotland. In his reply, Sir John reassured the College that he was confident that, in time, the subsidies offered to doctors willing to provide services under the Poor Law would attract a sufficient number of medical men to those parts of the country that were as yet poorly served.

Sir John's confidence was not justified by events. By 1894, when the responsibilities of the Board of Supervision passed to a new Local Government Board, the number of doctors practising in Scotland had more than doubled, reaching a total of 3,696. However, there was no evidence that the subsidies paid to doctors for their services to the poor had played any part in this increase.[53] Nor had the these subsidies attracted doctors to sparsely populated areas such as the Highlands and Islands; the medical directories of the time show that doctors continued to become concentrated in the well populated areas of central Scotland, particularly in Lanarkshire and Midlothian.

50. W. P. Alison, *Observations on the Famine of 1846-47* (Edinburgh, 1857).
51. Report of a Committee of the Royal College of Physicians, 3 February 1852.
52. College Minute.
53. A. Digby, *The Evolution of British General Practice, 1850–1948* (Oxford, 1999), p. 23.

Even where a Poor Law medical officer had been appointed the Poor Law bureaucracy was deliberately arranged to prevent even those entitled to free medical aid from having direct and ready access to his services.[54] The patient or his relatives were obliged to apply first to the parish Relieving Officer for authority to call for the attention of the Poor Law medical officer and in a large and scattered parish both the Relieving Officer and the doctor might be several miles away and difficult to contact.

MEDICAL SERVICES FOR THE WORKING POOR IN URBANISED SCOTLAND

In the years after 1845, medical services under the Poor Law became increasingly centred on Scotland's new Poor Houses. The Poor Law (Amendment) Act had laid down that 'in cases in which Poor Houses shall be erected there shall be proper and sufficient arrangements for dispensing and supplying medicines to the sick poor and there shall be provided by the Parochial Board proper medical attendance for the inmates of every such poor house'. Within a few years the board of the supervision had sanctioned the building of sixty-six Poor Houses with accommodation for paupers of all ages. By 1868, one person in twenty-four in Scotland was receiving poor relief and of these only one in fourteen was in a poor house.[55] In the hospital wards of these poor houses the accommodation was primitive and medical equipment negligible. The beds were low so that should an inadequately attended patient fall out of bed there was less risk of serious injury. There was no trained nursing staff; the sick and bed ridden were cared for by other pauper inmates for whom 'nursing' was a welcome source of income. The respectable poor, who 'had a horror of being sent to such institutions'[56] made every possible effort to be admitted for hospital care at one of Scotland's many voluntary infirmaries.

The regime in Scotland's poor houses was never as harsh as in England's workhouses; in Scotland the inmates were not made to do hard labour. Nevertheless the poor houses became, like the workhouses in England, increasingly used as a test of poverty that ensured that only the desperate sought help under the Poor Law. By 1894 the incidence of pauperism had been reduced to one in forty-four of the population and, for the poor, the Poor Law medical services were only a last resort.

The medical service that followed from the Poor Law (Amendment) Act of 1845 fell far short of that envisaged by W. P. Alison and the College in 1840. Nevertheless, it represented the first step towards the creation of a state medical service in Scotland. And, in the Board of Supervision, Scotland at last had a government body in Scotland with responsibility for health.

54. D. Hamilton, *The Healers* (Edinburgh, 1981), p. 229.
55. Ibid, p. 228.
56. J.G.M. Main, Nursing, in G. McLachlan, *Improving the Common Weal* (Edinburgh, 1987), p. 461.

11

POVERTY OR MIASMA
Public Health

The Report on the Sanitary Condition of the Labouring Population of Great Britain was essentially the work of Edwin Chadwick, although its final version was re-drafted by the great exponent of Utilitarianism, John Stuart Mill. When it was published in July 1842, the three Poor Law Commissioners, under whose authority it had been carried out, refused to accept responsibility for so radical a document and it was issued in Chadwick's name alone.

In conducting his survey Chadwick had made full use of the staff and the administrative machinery of the Poor Law. The Assistant Commission in each region was given detailed instructions on the information required and asked to provide a full report of their observations. All Poor Law medical officers, relieving officers and clerks to the Boards of Guardians (and in some cases the Guardians themselves) were asked to visit schools where sickly or stunted children were to be identified and the houses in which they lived located; they were also asked to discover from hospitals, dispensaries or friendly societies the houses in which 'deaths occur from fever'; all these unfortunate houses were to be visited and full details of local drainage and sewers street cleaning were to be recorded in a questionnaire designed and supplied by Chadwick.

His Report on the Sanitary Conditions of the Labouring Classes of Great Britain was completed in 1842. It was a 'masterpiece of protest literature'.[1] In 372 pages of text and 85 pages of appendices Chadwick documented the inadequacies of the systems of sewerage, drainage and water supply in towns of all types and sizes, in country villages, in rural labourers' cottages and miners' lodgings. He offered statistics designed to show a direct causal relationship between these inadequacies and the diseases prevalent among the poor. He claimed that his investigations had shown that these 'various forms of epidemic, endemic and other diseases caused or aggravated or propagated amongst the labouring classes by atmospheric impurities produced by decomposing animal and vegetable substances, by damp and filth and close and overcrowded dwellings prevail amongst the population in every part of the Kingdom'. He concluded that to safeguard the health of the labouring classes of Britain:

> the primary and most important measures, and at the same time the most practical, and within the province of public administration, are drainage, the removal of all refuse of habitations, streets and roads and the improvement of the water supply.

---

1. A.S. Wohl, *Endangered Lives* (London, 1983), p. 147.

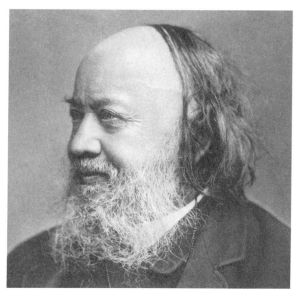

Edwin Chadwick

THE SANITARY CONDITION OF THE LABOURING POPULATION OF SCOTLAND

Chadwick's *Report on the Sanitary Condition of the Labouring Population of Great Britain* contained detailed information from almost every part of England and Wales but relatively little from Scotland. The Poor Law administrative network that had supplied Chadwick with the great mass of his information did not extend to Scotland. And although Glasgow in particular had reliable records, the civil registration of births, marriages and deaths had not yet become general throughout Scotland (and would not until 1855). Nevertheless, Chadwick was able to collect material for a Scottish supplement to his main report. The provosts of all Scottish burghs were circularised for information concerning the health of their citizens, the state of the streets, sewers and working-class housing. Doctors, ministers, lawyers and other 'knowledgeable individuals' were sent substantial questionnaires and encouraged to send more extensive personal accounts. Selected material from these many reports was published in July 1842 as *Reports on the Sanitary Condition of the Labouring Population of Scotland*.

This volume contained reports from thirteen towns in very different parts of Scotland and varying in size from major cities to mining villages. Only the Report on the Sanitary Conditions of the Working Classes in City of Glasgow was fully supported by tables of all relevant statistics. However, other reports which offered few or no statistics were no less persuasive. From Greenock Dr W. L. Laurie wrote:

> Like other towns in Scotland, Greenock has a large pauper population; the great bulk of these (I would say three-fourths) are natives of other places having come here in search of employment and from destitution, disease and other causes

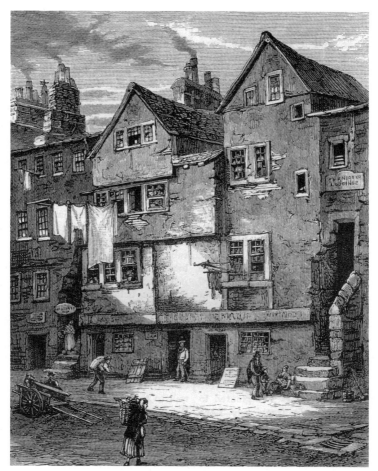

Cowgate in the nineteenth century

have been thrown a burden on the community. A great number come from Ireland and the Highlands with the express purpose of making a settlement, that is, supporting themselves in the best way they can for three years when they have a legal claim for relief from the parish. There are many who suffer much, especially during the winter, from want of food and fuel. Many are induced by their destitution to commit crime or fall a prey to disease in its most malignant form.

Last winter when visiting my district, I was informed of two sisters in a garret in great want. At one time they had been in good circumstances but had gradually reduced; they generally supported themselves by sewing but owing to want of work they had tasted almost nothing for three days; a neighbour had given them a few potatoes. Such cases are to be found in every close in the poor localities.

Typhus fever last winter carried off many heads of families and left their children destitute. As I was passing one of the poorest districts, a little girl ran after me and requested me to come and see her mother. I found the mother lying in a miserable straw bed with a piece of carpet for a covering, delirious from fever; the husband had died in the hospital of the same disease. There was no fire in the grate; some of the children were out begging and the two youngest were crawling on the wet floor. Every saleable piece of furniture had been pawned during the father's illness. None of the neighbours would enter the house; the children were actually starving and the mother was dying without any attendance whatever ...

The greater proportion of the dwellings of the poor are situated in very narrow and confined closes or alleys leading from the main streets; these closes end generally in a cul-de-sac and have little ventilation, the space between the houses being so narrow as to exclude the action of the sun on the ground. I might almost say there are no drains in any of these closes for where I have noticed sewers they are in such a filthy and obstructed state that they create more nuisance than if they never existed. In those closes where there is no dunghill, the excrement and other offensive matter is thrown into the gutter before the door or carried out and put in the street. There are no back courts to the houses but in nearly every close there is a dunghill, seldom or never covered in; few of these are cleaned out above once or twice a year; most are only empted when they can hold no more: to some of these privies are attached and one privy serves a whole neighbourhood. The people seem so familiarised with this unseemly state of things and so lost to all sense of propriety, that it is a matter of no small difficulty, in some of the backstreets, to make your way through them without being polluted with filth.

Behind my consulting rooms, where I am now sitting, there is a large dunghill with privy attached; to my certain knowledge that dunghill has not been empted for six months and the effluvium is so offensive that I cannot open the window. The land [tenement] is three stories high and the people, to save themselves the trouble, throw all their filth out of the stair window consequently a great part of it goes on the close and the close is not cleaned out until the dunghill is full. The filth reaches nearly to the sill of the back window of a shop in front and the malodorous moisture oozes through the wall on to the floor ...

When I come to speak of the cause and extension of fever I shall mention nuisances which, though not the sole origin of fever, yet contribute to its extension. The lands which the poor inhabit are divided into flats there being four or five families on each flat according as they possess one or two rooms each. The rent of these rooms varies from two pounds and ten shillings to seven pounds; the average size of each room would be from eight to nine feet square and about the same measure in height. The demand for this class of house is very great which induces the landlords to take such high rents.

Two articles by lawyers in Edinburgh and Glasgow discussed the difficulties that would have to be overcome in implementing in Scotland any legislation that might be drawn up primarily to improve sanitary conditions in England. Scotland had established bodies of law on the elimination of 'nuisance' and on the regulation of housing that was quite different from those in England. In Scotland the cleansing, lighting and paving of streets was not the province of the Town Council as in England but in a parallel administration of Commissioners of Police. The concept of 'medical police', the recruitment of the medical profession to assist in the control of public hygiene was familiar in Scotland and had been taught in Scottish medical schools for many years; in England the concept was still almost unknown.[2]

Almost the longest chapter in the Scottish Report was 'Observations on the Generation of Fever' in which W. P. Alison challenged the assumptions that had shaped Chadwick's inquiry and his subsequent Report:

> I take the liberty of observing that the queries of the Poor Law Commissioners appear to have been framed very much in accordance with the belief that the original cause of typhus or contagious fever is a malaria arising from putrescent animal and vegetable matters and from excretions of the human body, accumulating and corrupting; and that this malaria is developed wherever men congregate and bring together corrupting matters. This belief is distinctly avowed both in the Report of Drs Arnott and Kay and in that of Dr Southwood Smith and the recommendation of these gentlemen are accordingly founded on the supposition that by removing all such causes of vitiation of the Atmosphere contagious fever may be arrested at its source and thus the evils resulting from it prevented.
>
> Now, although I highly respect all these gentlemen, I think it my duty to state to the Poor Law Commissioners (and in doing so I am confident that I express the opinion of the great majority of the medical men in Scotland who have seen much of the diffusion of typhus fever among the lower orders) that this opinion is not merely a speculative one but one which ample experience entitles us to regard as erroneous; and at all, events, that there is no reason whatever for believing that the contagious fever which has prevailed more or less extensively in Edinburgh for the last 25 years has any such origin or can be suppressed by any such measures.

In elaborating on this theme at length, Alison made no claim to any insight into the originating exciting cause of typhus but wrote:

> I think I am justified in concluding that the want and misery of a certain portion

2. V. Berridge, Health and Medicine, in F.M.L. Thomson, *The Cambridge Social History of Britain 1750–1950* (Cambridge 1990), Vol. 3, p. 175.

of the inhabitants and the filth within the houses, the crowding, the negligent and reckless habits and the occasional intemperance which are the usual concomitants, and I believe the natural results, of this want and misery are the great predisposing causes of fever to which its frequent and general diffusion in this and other large towns is chiefly to be ascribed.

Alison believed that Chadwick was unrealistic in claiming that the typhus that afflicted the poor of Britain's towns and cities could be prevented merely by implementing new systems of drainage and sewerage designed to eliminate urban 'miasma'. However, he did not dispute that there was an urgent need for improvement in public sanitation. In 1840 he had drawn up the petition in which the College asked for Chadwick's Sanitary Inquiry to be extended to Scotland. In 1845, he founded the Edinburgh Sanitary Society to rally support for the measures advocated in the Report that resulted from that inquiry.

THE GOVERNMENT'S RESPONSE TO CHADWICK

Chadwick's Report was first issued as a House of Lords document in the official folio form used for all parliamentary papers and it had a very small and very limited circulation. Chadwick therefore arranged for it to be re-published in a more convenient and popular form. As many as 100,000 copies may have been printed but, although Chadwick was to claim that the number sold was 'much higher than anything the King's Printers have yet sold', it is unlikely that more than 20,000 were sold or given away.[3]

There was no immediate response from the government or in Parliament. The explanation for the government delay may be that, in his report, Chadwick had suggested the broad direction that reform should take but had made no specific proposals that could be immediately incorporated in new legislation. In 1844, the government decided to appoint a Royal Commission on the Health of Towns to review Chadwick's findings and to advise on whatever legislation seemed to be indicated. Chadwick was not a member of the Commission but he was very active in assuring that the Commission was provided with an ample flow of suitably prepared witnesses. And in London, Southwood Smith founded the Metropolitan Health of Towns Association 'to diffuse among the people the valuable information elicited by recent inquiries as to the physical and moral evils that result from the present defective sewerage, drainage supply of water, air and light and construction of dwelling houses'. The Association included leading politicians of both the Tory and Whig parties and the social and medical reformers, Lord Ashley and John Simon. Branches of the Association were formed in Manchester, Liverpool, York and several other towns in England; the Edinburgh Sanitary Society, founded by W. P. Alison in 1845, was the only branch or corresponding society formed in Scotland.

The Royal Commission issued its second and final report in 1845, confirming the findings of Chadwick's inquiry and making specific proposals for new legislation. However, in 1845

3. M.W. Finn (ed.), *Report on the Sanitary Condition of the Labouring Population of Great Britain by Edwin Chadwick* (Edinburgh, 1964), p. 55.

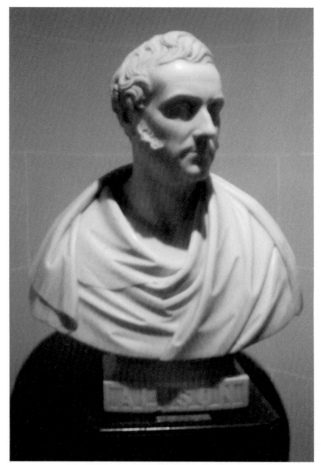

W. P. Alison

and 1846 Parliament was preoccupied by the great problem of the Irish Famine and the question of the Corn Laws. While the government delayed, campaigning by Chadwick, the Health of Towns Associations and the Sanitary Society in Edinburgh continued.

On 2 February 1847, Alison was able to inform the College that legislation was about to be introduced in the House of Commons 'regarding the sanitation of towns' in England and Wales. A committee of the College, chaired by Alison, was immediately appointed to 'to prepare a representation as to the application of a similar Bill to Scotland to be submitted to the College and afterwards laid to the government'.

On 14 May 1847, Alison's committee reported to the College that it had 'carefully examined the drafts of two Bills'. One was the Town Improvement Clauses Bill which brought together a number of private member's Bills that had already been submitted for the improvement of lighting, draining, cleaning and naming of streets in towns in England and Wales; the other, 'entitled a Bill for the Improvement of the Health of Towns in England', had been submitted to Parliament by Lord Morpeth, the Leader of the House, on behalf of the

Government. Morpeth's was a radical Bill drawn up in line with the general directions of Chadwick's report but more closely based on the recommendations of the subsequent Royal Commission. Alison and his committee reported that they were not yet ready to comment in detail on the possible …

> applicability of such measures to Scotland but desire to express their conviction that these measures are of great and general importance; and of a highly beneficial tendency; and further that such measures are even more demanded by the present sanitary condition of the towns of Scotland than those of England.

In Parliament, the Town Improvement Clauses Bill was passed without difficulty. Lord Morpeth's Bill, however, met with such effective opposition that it had to be withdrawn. A year later, the Government submitted a much less radical Bill. This Public Health Bill made provision for the establishment of local boards of health with extensive powers to introduce or improve local sanitation schemes. In town or districts in which the death rate was above 23 per thousand a General Board of Health in London would have the power to enforce the establishment of a local Board of Health. For towns or districts in which the death rate was lower than 23 per thousand, a petition to the General Board of Health by at least 10 per cent of the population would lead to an inspection of the town; when the findings of the inspectors became public, the local authority could, if it so wished, apply for permission to establish a local Board of Health. These provisions of the Bill were not to apply to London or any other large town in which health commissions or other relevant health bodies had already been established by Act of Parliament.

On 19 February 1848, Alison's committee presented its second report to the College. This presented two main objections to the Public Health Bill being made to apply to Scotland. First, the committee was sceptical of the advantage to Scotland in having its health authorities subject to the jurisdiction of a General Board of Health in London. This view had its origins in the College's experience during the cholera epidemic of 1832; the Board of Health in London had been unduly slow to issue its official guidance on the measures that should be taken in Scotland to control the epidemic; local authorities had made their own arrangements and when that guidance was finally received it proved to be unhelpful. Second, Alison and his committees pointed out that 'although they had the highest respect for the individuals who were to be members of the General Board of Health in London [Chadwick, Southwood Smith and Lord Ashley] yet the confident expression of opinion which these gentlemen have officially made on several important questions touching the diffusion of epidemic diseases, on which they know that some of the most experienced practitioners in Scotland hold a very different opinion, have by no means tended to increase their expectation of the efficiency of measures, applicable to Scotland for restraining the diffusion of epidemics which may proceed from that source'.[4]

4. College Minute; *First and Second Report by a Committee of the Royal College of Physicians appointed to consider any bills that may be brought into Parliament for the improvement of the Health of Towns and the applicability of such measures to Scotland* (Edinburgh, 1849), p. 18.

At the second reading of the Bill in the House of Lords on 30 June the Duke of Buccleuch, who had been chairman of the Royal Commission in 1845, expressed 'his anxious and earnest hope that the attention of the government would be directed to extending the benefits of the measure to the country with which he was more immediately connected. He would venture to say that the great cities of Glasgow and Edinburgh were perhaps in a worse condition with regard to sanitation than any city in England. For the government Lord Campbell replied that:

> there are at present difficulties in applying a measure of this kind to Scotland but
> he hoped that perhaps in the next session that country might enjoy the benefits
> of sanitary reform.[5]

On 31 August, the Bill became law as the Public Health Act (1848) 'for improving the sanitary conditions of towns and populous places in England and Wales'. In 1849, as Lord Campbell had indicated, a Public Health (Scotland) Bill was presented to Parliament by the government but it was rejected by the House of Commons.

CHADWICK AND THE IMPLEMENTATION OF THE PUBLIC HEALTH ACT (1848)

For Chadwick the Public Health Act was a disappointment. Its provisions made only limited and uneven progress in the direction he had pointed in the closing pages of his Sanitary Report in 1842. There he had advocated the establishment of a uniform national system of sanitation under strong central control:

> The advantages of uniformity in legislation and in the executive machinery and
> in doing the same thing in the same way (choosing the best) and calling them
> by the same names will only be appreciated by those who have observed the
> extensive public loss occasioned by legislation for towns which makes them
> independent of beneficent, as of what perhaps might have been deemed
> formerly aggressive legislation. Independence and separation in the form of
> legislation [has] separated the people from their share of the greatest amount of
> legislative attention or excluded them from the common interest or from the
> common advantages of protective measures.

As chairman of the new General Board of Health, Chadwick went as far as the provisions of the Public Health Act would allow in establishing strong central control and enforcing uniformity in sanitary practice. His efforts provoked widespread hostility. His policy of forcing towns with higher than average mortality rates (in many cases, towns in which the populace refused to accept the view of the General Board's inspectors that the existing sanitary arrangements were unsatisfactory) to establish local Health Boards was seen as intolerable state interference.[6] There was growing popular resentment at Chadwick's 'papal form of government',[7] a style of 'government' that was not only unpopular but often ineffective since

5. *Hansard*, 30 June 1848.
6. Wohl, *Endangered Lives*, p. 149.
7. Sir John Simon quoted in Wohl, *Endangered Lives*, p. 149.

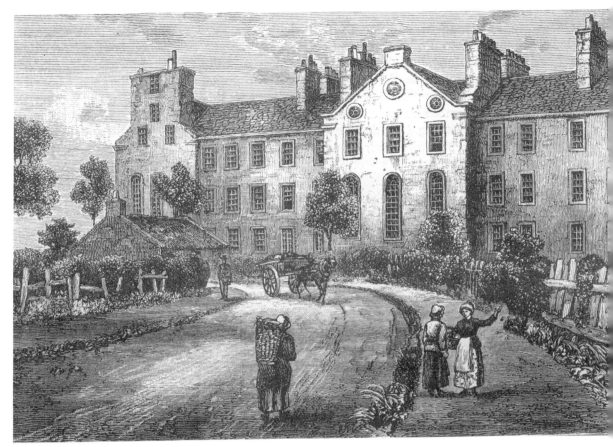

Charity Workhouse

Local Boards, unwillingly established, could choose to ignore the directives of Chadwick's General Board in London. Within a very few years Chadwick had lost the support of the country's Sanitary Associations and they gradually crumbled away.

He also lost the support of the country's engineers. In his drive for uniformity he insisted that all new sewage systems should be constructed using narrow bore glazed pipes rather than brick-lined tunnels favoured by professional engineers. His edicts provoked the opposition of the Institute of Civil Engineers.[8] Chadwick had always insisted that 'sanitary science is a subsidiary department of engineering, a science with which medical practitioners can have little or nothing to do'.[9] He was therefore unable to brush aside the Institute of Engineers as he had the London Royal College of Physicians in 1831. The Institute's well orchestrated lobbying found a ready audience in Parliament. The were a great many Members of Parliament who saw the General Board of Health as a new and dangerous bureaucracy answerable neither directly to Parliament or to any government minister and Chadwick himself was seen as a 'tactless bore'[10] already unpopular as the author of the unpopular Poor Law Act of 1834 and its notorious workhouse system.

8. S.E. Finer, *Life and Times of Sir Edwin Chadwick* (London, 1952), p. 440.
9. R. Lambert, *Sir John Simon 1816–1904* (London, 1963), p. 226.
10. J. Pollock, *Shaftesbury; The Poor Man's Earl* (London, 1985), p. 91.

In spite of growing opposition Chadwick survived until 1853 when an outbreak of a virulent fever in Croydon brought his career as a sanitary reformer to an abrupt end. Croydon's new sewage and drainage had been hailed as a model of Chadwick's system; the town's inhabitants demanded an independent inquiry and a government Commission was immediately appointed. The Croydon Report was devastating. It found that the outbreak of fever had been caused by a failure of the sewage system and that the reason for that failure was the use of narrow pipe drains. Lord Palmerston, the Home Secretary, persuaded Chadwick to retire with a generous pension of £1000; the other two members of the Board, Southwood Smith and Lord Ashley, resigned. After a period of debate on whether the Board should be abolished, a new Act of Parliament in 1855 continued the Board but now only on an annual basis. Three politicians, less interventionist and more diplomatic than Chadwick were appointed as the new Board and the 'judicious and conciliatory'[11] John Simon became the Board's first Medical Officer. But opposition to the continuation of the General Board of Health did not weaken and in 1858 it was abolished; through the intervention of the Prince Consort its Medical Department was transferred to the Privy Council and John Simon became its Central Medical Officer.[12]

PUBLIC HEALTH IN SCOTLAND

The creation of the General Board of Health in London in 1848 had led to confusion in Scotland. This was made evident when Britain prepared to face a second epidemic of cholera. An outbreak of the disease was reported on the Continent in the summer of 1847. In January 1848, representatives of the College, the College of Surgeons, the Town Council and Edinburgh's three parochial boards met to discuss the measures that could to be taken should the epidemic show signs of spreading to Britain. On 1 August 1848, the President, Sir Robert Christison, informed the College that 'it was probable that the epidemic could not be now far distant'; planning now began in earnest. Representatives of the two College and the Parochial Boards met frequently during August and September but on 5 October, when 'all parties were most anxious to proceed to carry into effect the necessary measures' the meeting was informed that 'by the recent Act passed on 4 September last [Nuisance Removal and Disease Prevention Act] the initiative had been taken out of the hands of the local authorities and placed in the hands of the General Board of Health in London. Christison, who had chaired the planning meetings in Edinburgh, immediately (5 October) wrote to Edwin Chadwick in London:

> I take the liberty of addressing the following statement to you as the only member of the Board with whom I am acquainted, leaving it to you to make what use you may think fit of my communication …
>
> From the concurrent testimony of several medical men there is no reason to doubt that cholera has broken out since Saturday last, the 30th September. If this be the advent of the epidemic we are taken quite unprepared. It is more

11. H. Williams, *A Century of Public Health in Britain* (London, 1932), p. 274.
12. Ibid., p. 275.

than a month since, as president of the College of Physicians, I was empowered by the College to put myself in communication with the city authorities on the subject of making preparations for the disease which I accordingly did. But its slow progress on the Continent led us here, as it seems also to have led you all in London, to be slow to believe that any great preparation would be necessary. We are all of a different opinion now, however … My opinion therefore is that preparations must be begun instantly and with energy. But it appeared that as all were in a mood to act that nothing farther can be done without authority first given by the General Board. The initiative rests with your Board. If we are wrong in thus interpreting the Act, you should get the necessary corrections sent as soon as possible. But if we are right, as I think is the case, it is most important that no time be lost by the General Board in determining and announcing them. (italic in original)

The President then set out in detail the measures that his planning committee had drawn up for Edinburgh. These measures were essentially those that been developed during the epidemic of 1832 but now including the appointment of a Local Board of Health. It had been agreed in Edinburgh that 'the General Board of Health should act, not with the parochial boards in detail but through the medium of a Local Board superintending the whole'. In his letter to Chadwick, Christison insisted unless a Local Board was appointed 'you will have great difficultly in getting the three Parochial Boards [in Edinburgh] to act in concert'.

On receipt of Christison's letter, Chadwick had the General Board of Health appoint the Lord Advocate, the Dean of Guild, the Sheriff of Edinburgh, the Chairman of the Board of Supervision, the President of the College of Physicians and the President of the College of Surgeons as a Local Board of Health for Edinburgh. This Local Board immediately ordered the publication of the measures that had already been drawn up for Edinburgh by Christison's committee and communicated to Chadwick. However, on 12 October, the College was informed that there had been 'unavoidable delay in authorising them to be put in force on account of doubt being entertained as to the extent of the powers conferred on General Board of Health upon the Local Board'.

On the 13 October, Christison, now as president of the College, wrote to the General Health Board in London to state once again the case he had already made on behalf of Edinburgh's cholera planning group to Chadwick in his letter of 5 October. On the 16th the Secretary of the General Board of Health replied unhelpfully that the members of his board:

have not at the moment time to enter into a statement of their views on the points brought under their notice by the College. On this subject the Board will again have to communicate with the College with which they will at all time be happy to take council on all matters relating to proposed measures for improving the public health in Scotland.[13]

13. College Minute, 7 Nov 1848.

The College received no further communication from the General Board of Health until 7 November when the College was informed that 'the Local Health Board in Edinburgh had been dissolved it having been found that the General Board of Health had no power to delegate its functions'. The General Board was now forced to abandon the line it had taken in Scotland in the weeks since it was appointed in September. During the cholera epidemic the measures generally adopted in Scotland were those that had been drawn up by Alison in 1832 and developed and supervised in 1848 by a Committee of the College of Physicians, the College of Surgeons and representatives of the Parochial Boards chaired by Alison;[14] in theory at least, the General Board of Health continued to have the power to require Parochial Boards in Scotland to implement these measures and to provide the necessary medicines and medical care.

In 1849, as Lord Campbell had indicated in the House of Lords (above), the government introduced a Public Health (Scotland) Bill but it was rejected by the House of Commons. It was not until 1867 that a Public Health Act was passed for Scotland. Until then, all new Public Health legislation for the removal of nuisances and prevention of disease in Britain was directed in Scotland by the Board of Supervision for the Relief of the Poor and administered by the Commissioners of Police in the towns and by the Inspectors of the Poor in parishes elsewhere.

14. Ibid.

ALISON AND THE COLLEGE DEFEATED
The Registration Act[1]

Almost from its foundation, the College had been made aware of the deficiencies in the system for the notification of deaths and the causes of deaths in Scotland. It was a system that had been in place since the sixteenth century. At the Reformation, each Kirk Session had assumed responsibility for the care of the poor, for the education of the children and for the maintenance of discipline and order in its own parish. In support of these duties, it was expected that each Kirk Session would keep a register of all the baptisms, burials and proclamations of marriage that had been conducted by the parish church. In the first half of the seventeenth century, in the midst of a devastating series of epidemics of the plague, it had become expected that each Kirk Session would also produce Bills of Mortality giving the cause of every death in the parish; the Bills were intended either to give warning of the approach of a new epidemic or, alternatively, to reassure the local community that every death had been examined and that none of the deaths had been caused by plague.

The practice of keeping Parish Registers was only adopted slowly and fitfully across Scotland. The first Parish Registers were kept regularly in parishes in Perthshire from the middle of the sixteenth century; but Edinburgh did not have a register until 1658 and Glasgow not until 1670.[2] By the end of the eighteenth century only 99 of Scotland's 850 parishes had properly maintained registers; the others had either no register or a register that was only kept intermittently or incompetently.[3] Even at best, the Parish Registers were inevitably incomplete; the fee payable to the Parish Clerk deterred poor families from having an entry made in the Register; and families who belonged to denominations other than the Church of Scotland often refused on principle to have entries made in the Parish Register.[4] Bills of Mortality were equally deficient. They only recorded what was known about the deaths of those buried in the Kirk burial grounds and in parishes where there was no Parish Register there could be no Bills of Mortality. Even where Bills of Mortality were drawn up, the few pieces of information they contained were often wildly inaccurate. In a book published by William Creech, it was claimed that in Edinburgh the Bills:

> have been kept in such a manner as to render them the infallible sources of
> error. The register of burial is kept by people whose faculties are impaired by

1. The material and references in this chapter are substantially taken from published work and forthcoming work by Anne Cameron as part of the Scottish Way of Birth and Death project of Glasgow University.
2. Ibid.
3. A. Cameron, Medicine, Meteorology and Vital Statistics: the Influence of the Royal College of Physicians of Edinburgh upon Scottish Birth and Death registration, *Journal of the Royal College of Physicians of Edinburgh*, 2007 (in press).
4. Ibid.

drinking, who forget today what was done yesterday. They enter not into the list of burials any who have died without receiving baptism nor those whose relations are so poor as not to be able to pay for the use of the mort-cloth.[5]

The inadequacy of the Parish Registers was documented in the first volume of Sir John Sinclair's *Statistical Account of Scotland* published in 1791. In his introduction Sinclair explained that his purpose (like Robert Sibbald's in publishing his *Nuncius*[6] a century before) was to assess the human and material resources of Scotland and to determine 'the means of its future improvement'. Between 1791 and 1799, he produced 21 volumes compiled from the replies to a list of 160 questions sent to the Church of Scotland minister in every parish in Scotland. The quality and scope of the replies to his questionnaires varied greatly according to the interests and priorities of the individual ministers and the research they were willing to do in preparing their replies. But it might have been expected that the Parish Register, with its associated Bills of Mortality, would have been a source of factual information immediately available to every minister. However, in the first volume of the *Statistical Account of Scotland* which contained the accounts of the City of Edinburgh and seven adjacent parishes, information on births, marriages and deaths was sparse. Colinton was the only parish for which exact numbers were provided. As was explained in the text, Colinton was quite exceptional; the register of baptisms and marriages 'has been continued with uncommon accuracy from the year 1655 to the present time' and 'the register of burials has been very carefully kept since 1728'. Already in 1791, Sir John Sinclair concluded that 'the parish registers in Scotland have seldom been kept for any length of time with sufficient accuracy'. Bills of Mortality had also been unhelpful; Sinclair noted that while there was clearly documented evidence that some years were 'most remarkable for their mortality', it was impossible to discover the cause of that high mortality.

The College took the public interest roused by Sir John Sinclair as an opportunity to bring about some improvement. At a meeting on 3 May 1791 the President of the College, Andrew Duncan, proposed that it would now be 'proper to set on foot some regulations with respect to the framing and keeping of regular Bills of Mortality'. Charles Stuart, Robert Freer and Thomas Spens were appointed 'to take the matter under consideration and to report their ideas to the College'.

In November 1791, they produced a design for a new form on which all deaths could be clearly recorded and a specific cause assigned to each death; they also presented a set of instructions on how that information should be gathered and distributed. Their 'new mode of keeping Bills of Mortality' was approved by the College and offered for use by the parishes of Edinburgh and its suburbs. In February 1792, the new scheme was recommended to Sir John Sinclair along with a supply of the new forms 'to be sent by means of Sir John to all the different parishes in Scotland with recommendations to the clergy and to the medical practitioners to observe them'.[7] Sir John's work on his *Statistical Account of Scotland* continued until 1799 and during all these years he used his correspondence with clergy and medical

---

5. H. Arnott, *The History of Edinburgh* (Edinburgh, 1779), pp. 322–3.
6. *Nuncius Scoto-Britannicus, sive admonoto deatlante Scotico seu descriptione Scotiae antique et modernae* (Chapter 1).
7. College Minute, 7 February 1792.

practitioners of Scotland to promote the College's new scheme. But while so few parishes in Scotland had properly kept Session Registers there was almost no possibility that the new scheme could succeed.

In 1806, the College acknowledged that the plan that had been drawn up 'many years before for the better regulation of the Bills of Mortality had not been carried into effect'.[8] The College appointed Andrew Duncan, Charles Stuart and James Home to try again. Once again nothing was achieved. The College thanked Sir John Sinclair for his assistance and for a time the matter was allowed to drop. Then, in 1810, Andrew Duncan, Charles Stuart and James Home tried yet again and again with no success. All else having failed, Andrew Duncan now began to prepare for the College his own quarterly reports on 'the number of funerals and the epidemic diseases which in the City of Edinburgh and its liberties;' but after little more than a year Andrew Duncan finally gave up. The movement for reform of the registration of births, marriages and deaths in Scotland continued but the initiative passed from the College into other hands.

The College was not alone in calling for a more efficient system of recording births marriages and deaths in Scotland. Lawyers, for example, found it difficult to prove inheritance claims when their clients possessed no record of their birth or parentage. Many town councils were at a disadvantage in having no certain knowledge of the size and age distribution of the population for which they were responsible. The Church of Scotland accepted that reform had become necessary but was unwilling to pass responsibility to a secular authority.[9] Between 1829 and 1849, no fewer than eight Scottish registration bills were brought into parliament. All were rejected, postponed or withdrawn; on each occasion it proved impossible to resolve what was the same set of difficulties; there were disputes over who should be appointed to keep the new registers; there were claims that a system of civil registration would require the support of a large bureaucracy, would be too expensive and would be unacceptable to the taxpayer; the proposals in four of the bills would make it necessary to amend the laws on marriage. Of these objections the most potent was the last; lawyers, clergymen and the general public were all opposed to any change in the marriage law and on this issue all were united in objecting to the proposed reforms.[10]

A ninth Bill was introduced in 1854. It was drawn up and managed through Parliament by Lord Elcho. It succeed because Elcho sought to keep the costs of administration as low as possible; he placated the Church of Scotland by proposing that the session clerks of the parishes should be appointed as registrars, and he avoided any need to interfere with the marriage laws. The Registration (Scotland) Act took effect on 1 January 1855, establishing a civil system of birth, death, and marriage registration under a General Register Office for Scotland (GROS).

During the 1830s and 1840s the College had taken an active but subsidiary part in the movement for reform. They had appointed committees to report on each new registration Bill

---

8. College Minute, 4 February 1806.
9. A. Cameron, 'The establishment of civil registration in Scotland', *Historical Journal,* 2007, Vol. 50, pp. 1–19.
10. A. Cameron, *Journal of the Royal College of Physicians of Edinburgh.*

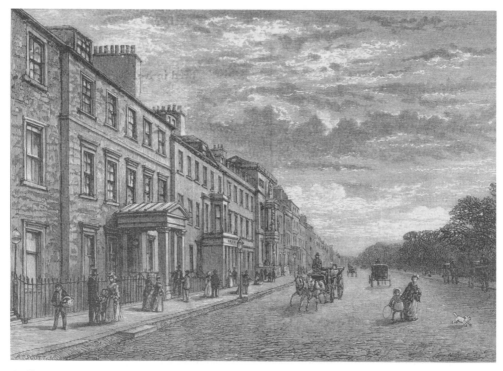

College in Queen Street in the nineteenth century

as it was put forward and submitted suggestions for its improvement; when the campaign seemed to have lapsed and no new Bills were being put forward, the College had agitated for the campaign to be renewed. But during these twenty years the College concerned themselves with two particular issues. When new Bills were under discussion the College tried to ensure that the form on which deaths were to be registered was designed to record the most useful information on each death in the most efficient way. When the Registration Act became law, the College tried to have their preferred medical candidate appointed as Superintendent of Statistics at the new General Register Office in Edinburgh.

THE REGISTERING OF THE CAUSE OF DEATH

In November 1835, a Registration Bill was introduced for England: 'it appearing that the subject had lately been under the consideration of Parliament', Richard Poole reminded the College of 'the steps adopted by Andrew Duncan in 1791 for procuring the establishment of regular Bills of Mortality and stated that so desirable a matter ought not to be lost sight of.[11] A committee under the chairmanship of W. P. Alison was appointed 'to take such measures as to them might seem advisable;' over the next months the committee took note of the provisions of the Act being introduced in England but decided that, since the Act applied only to England, there was no call for the College to comment. The matter was raised again in 1840; from a meeting of the British Association in Glasgow, its Statistical Section sent to the College a copy of its recommendation that a better system of registration of births, marriages and deaths was

11. College Minute, 3 November 1835.

much needed in Scotland. The College replied that they too were aware of the 'essential advantages to be derived to medical science from accurate registration of births, marriages and deaths;' once more a committee was appointed under the chairmanship of W. P. Alison, this time instructed more particularly 'to consider and recommend an effective and uniform system of Registration in Scotland of all Births and Deaths, *specifying in regard to the latter, the supposed cause'.*[12] Alison's report in 1841 set out the arguments that the College was to put forward in objecting to the way in which the Registration Bills of 1847, 1848, 1849 and 1854 all proposed that the cause of death should be recorded.

Alison insisted that the English method of recording the cause of death should not be adopted in Scotland. In the death schedule introduced in England in 1836, there was only a single column in which the cause of death could be recorded. Alison pointed out that in many cases, perhaps even a majority, the deceased would have had no medical attendant during his or her last illness; in such cases the registrar would be offered a cause of death by whoever happened to be reporting the death. Registrars in England were instructed that, whenever possible, a cause of death should be obtained from a medical practitioner who had either been present at the death or had personal knowledge of the deceased's recent state of health; but the single column in the English schedule made no provision for a clear distinction to be made between an informed diagnosis made by doctor and a cause of death offered by a witness with perhaps only the most uncertain knowledge of the deceased. Alison argued that to have a useful record, open to meaningful interpretation and capable of statistical analysis, it was essential that the observations provided by doctors should be clearly separated from the speculations of unreliably informed witnesses;[13] he proposed that the schedule introduced for use in Scotland should have two columns: one for what might be described as the 'ascertained' cause of death, and the another for the 'conjectured' cause. He also proposed that in listing the cause of death the shorter, simpler and more practical nosology used in Scotland should be preferred to the more prolix classification of diseases used in England.[14]

When the first in a series of Registration Bills for Scotland was published early in 1847 it was discussed at a special meeting of the College on 23 March. Alison explained his objections to a number of sections in the Bill and the meeting unanimously agreed:

- That it is the opinion of this College that any register of diseases drawn up according to the forms now in use under the authority of the Registrar General in England necessarily be fallacious.

- That by an alteration of the schedule employed for the purpose and by the use of a shorter and simpler nomenclature of diseases, Registers of Mortality might easily be framed in Scotland admitting of easy comparison with those in England but greatly surpassing them in precision and scientific value.

12. College Minute, 3 November 1840.
13. S. M.K. Martin, William Pulteney Alison: Activist, Philanthropist and Pioneer of Social Medicine, unpublished PhD thesis, St Andrews, 1997, p. 309.
14. For a detailed discussion of the RCPE's views and its ensuing dispute with William Farr of the General Register Office for England, see ibid, pp. 304–15.

- That this resolution, with the general approbation of the College, should be communicated to the Lord Advocate.

James Stark (see below) informed the College that he too had been studying the whole problem of registration and that it did not appear to him that the College would have much difficulty in making its point. However, he did second a proposal that Alison and the president, Robert Christison, should call on the Lord Advocate to present the College's objections to the Bill in person.

In May, the President reported to the College that he and Alison had had a very satisfactory interview with the Lord Advocate. The clauses to which College objected had been modified and he was confident that the Bill 'would be brought forward in a shape which would meet the views of the College'.[15] However, when the Bill was brought forward it failed to find sufficient support in Parliament. In 1848, a new Bill was drawn up; the College agreed that provided it did not 'deviate in any essential particular'[16] from the form that had been agreed with the Lord Advocate in 1847, the College would petition Parliament in its support. However this second Registration (Scotland) Bill also failed and in 1849 a third Bill was submitted; the new Bill was discussed by the College; exactly the same conclusions were reached as in 1848; and, like its predecessors, this Bill also failed in Parliament.

Between 1847 and 1849, three Bills had been withdrawn or had been rejected by Parliament because of the unresolved conflicts between the interests of the Church of Scotland, the secular authorities and the taxpayers. The schedule for the registration of deaths proposed by the College and accepted by the Lord Advocate had not been an issue. In 1854 a new Bill was devised by Lord Elcho, the Member of Parliament for East Lothian and now a Lord of the Treasury. On 9 May, at a meeting of the College called to discuss the provisions of the new Bill it was observed that:

> Its clauses are most carefully formed so as to avoid collision with existing interests and to carry out an efficient system of registration with the aid, so far as it can be rendered available, of the existing [Church of Scotland] machinery.[17]

It was probably as part of his plan to avoid every conceivable cause of contention that Elcho omitted from his Bill the description of the schedule to be used in recording deaths and their causes. This omission caused little comment at the meeting of the College on 9 May when every clause of his Bill was discussed in great detail; since Alison's proposals had already been accepted and included in the three earlier Bills, the College was confident that, in due course, they would be accepted again. At the conclusion of its lengthy examination, College found that:

> Lord Elcho's Bill is calculated to advance the interests of the public and to supply an acknowledged deficiency in the social statistics of Scotland and therefore [the College] recommend the measure as worth of support.

15. College Minute, 4 May 1847.
16. College Minute, 1 May 1848.
17. College Minute, 9 May 1854.

However, the College added:

> In the event of this Bill becoming law it would be important to secure that the entire system of nosology and other details necessary to be considered in registering deaths shall be submitted to the Scottish Medical Corporations and in particular to this College whose anxious interest on the subject by elaborate suggestions for the improvement of the English method in the anticipation of its application under a former Bill … On this occasion, the progress of the Bill should be carefully watched and means should be taken to impress the Home Secretary [Lord Palmerston] and the framer of the Bill [Lord Elcho] with the expediency and propriety of giving effect to the views of the College in the practical working of the measure.[18]

The College agreed that Alison should write to the Home Secretary and to Lord Elcho to remind them of the College's views and recommendations. Elcho's reply was encouraging:

> I am about to submit the Registration Bill to a Select Committee of Scottish Members whose consideration I shall not fail to bring to the points to which reference is made. My only object is to make this Bill as complete and perfect as possible and I shall therefore be most ready to adopt whatever mode may appear the most desirable for registering deaths.[19]

On 15 May, the College presented a petition to Parliament expressing their wish that Lord Elcho's Bill should pass into law. The petition also commented:

> Your petitioners have stated on other occasions their conviction that the system of registering causes of death now adopted in England is essentially faulty and ought not to be extended to Scotland without considerable modifications.
>
> That your petitioners are farther of the opinion that under any Registration Bill the system of Registering Deaths ought to be submitted to the Medical Incorporations of Scotland before being brought into operation. In as much as the statement of cause of death involves questions bearing on the cultivation of medical science of which the medical profession alone can judge.

On 26 May, on the understanding that the form of the schedule for the recording the causes of death was still to be formally decided, perhaps even after the Bill had become law, the College wrote to every Scottish Member of Parliament enclosing a copy of Alison's report of 1841. However, on 18 July, Lord Elcho informed the College that his Bill had been read for the third time and had been passed by the House of Commons. The College later discovered that almost at the last minute the Bill had been amended to stipulate that the English schedule for recording deaths and their causes would be used in Scotland.

On 1 August 1854, the College published what was, in effect, a letter of protest in all the Edinburgh newspapers:

18. Ibid.
19. College Minute, 28 May.

It is quite evident that the value of any System of Registration, must depend on the accuracy with which the returns are made, and the manner in which they are classified; and from want of attention it has happened that the elaborate English reports are useless, or in some respects worse than useless if trusted to as the basis of any calculations, the forms now in use in England rendering them naturally fallacious. A Committee of this College have shown, in a Report which can be seen by application at the College, that by an alteration of the Schedule employed, and by the adoption of a simpler and shorter nomenclature of diseases, Registers of Mortality might easily be found in Scotland, admitting of easy comparison with those of England, but greatly surpassing them in precision, and scientific value. It is thus for the interest of Scotland, to see that her system is not in this respect assimilated to that of England, but reaps the advantage of all those improvements which are the result of the attention which has been paid to the subject by the medical men of the country.

The protest achieved nothing and the English system was adopted in Scotland. The College's defeat was later compounded following the appointment of William Pitt Dundas as the new Registrar General for Scotland. In November 1854, in a letter to George Graham, his counterpart in England, Dundas promised that the nosology used in Scotland would be the same as that used in England, 'even tho' the doctors should make out that a more perfect one could be framed'.[20]

THE APPOINTMENT OF A SUPERINTENDENT OF STATISTICS

Alison's efforts over fifteen years had failed. In the system for the registration of births, marriages and deaths to be introduced in Scotland on 1 January 1855, the causes of death were to be recorded in schedules that did not permit a clear distinction to be made between a considered diagnosis supplied by a medical practitioner and the ill-informed supposition of a relative or friend of the deceased. Even a diagnosis offered by a medical practitioner was likely to be imprecise since practitioners were to be encouraged to use the English nosology, a classification of diseases that was itself confused and uncertain. It seemed evident to Alison that if the information on the causes of death collected by the new system of registration was to be used to provide meaningful statistics, the statistician must be someone with extensive medical knowledge and experience.

In 1837, soon after the new system of registration of births, deaths, and marriages was introduced in England, William Farr had been given a temporary appointment to help organize the quantities of data that were being collected. His chapter in McCulloch's *A Statistical Account of the British Empire* in 1837 had already confirmed his reputation as a statistician; but Farr had also studied medicine in Paris and he was a licentiate of the Society of Apothecaries. The importance of his contribution to the setting up of the new system was quickly recognised and

20. W.P. Dundas to Major Graham, Registrar General [England], 3 Nov 1854. National Archives of Scotland [NAS], GRO1/465: General Register Office Letterbook (outletters) 1854, p. 28.

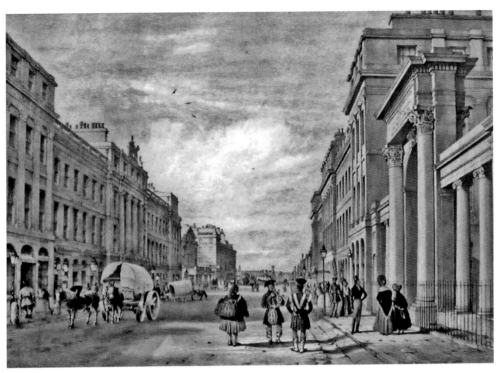

Princes Street from the East, 1840 (New Club)

in July 1839 he was made a permanent member of the staff; by the 1850s it was generally acknowledged that his expertise in both medicine and statistics was essential to the efficient working and reputation of England's General Registry Office.

In 1854, in his report on Lord Elcho's Bill, Alison had recommended 'the institution of some recognised office or offices to be filed exclusively by medical men with a view to the proper superintendence of the registration of the causes of death according to the scientific requirements of the medical profession'. However, the *Act to Provide for the Better Registration of Births, Deaths, and Marriages in Scotland* that became law in July 1854 made specific provision only for the appointment of a Secretary to be nominated by the Registrar General.[21] Alison and the College were concerned that the statistical analysis of the reports on the deaths and the causes of deaths might be delegated to a secretary. In their letter published in Edinburgh on 1 August that year (above) they stressed that 'to carry out with real accuracy a scientific system no mere clerk will suffice. A medical man who understands the nomenclature of diseases and can, from his own knowledge, check inaccuracies should be conjoined with the Registrar; one of business habits and who could dedicate his whole time to the work might easily render these returns valuable public documents'.

21. Elcho may have made no provision for the appointment of a statistician as part of his plan to reduce the cost of the new system down to the minimum possible, Cameron, Medicine.

Alison made the same points privately to the Registrar General, William Pitt Dundas:

> We consider the drawing up of these Reports a matter of real importance for the elucidation of various points in medical science and consider it extremely desirable, that this duty should be assigned in Scotland, as it is in England, to a medical man ... We have paid a good deal of attention to the subject and are confident that we could give such advice to a medical man, employed in drawing up these Reports, as would enable him to make very considerable improvements on the plan adopted in England and thereby lay a foundation for various conclusions, particularly as to the external causes of diseases on which no such satisfactory statistical evidence is to be obtained anywhere else.[22]

Dundas was persuaded. He conceded that only a qualified medical practitioner could present the statistics accurately and he accepted that the medical profession in Scotland would never be satisfied until the General Registry Office in Scotland had its own 'William Farr'.[23] Having first discovered Farr's terms of employment from the Registrar General in England, Dundas applied successfully to the Treasury for permission and to appoint a Superintendent of Statistics for Scotland.

Several medical practitioners put themselves forward for this position. Alison's preferred candidate was George W. Bell. Bell was known to have an interest in vital statistics and he had been an early and active contributor to the movement to have a national registration system established in Scotland. Alison thought him a man of amiable character, well fitted for the post both from 'his intelligence as a medical man and his habits of business.' He was well known in Edinburgh; both his father and his uncle had successful medical practices in the town and he was the Rev. Thomas Guthrie's chief assistant at Edinburgh's Ragged School. He was also the brother-in-law of the Lord Advocate. Alison was confident that his appointment would be widely welcomed.

However, the Registrar General had his own candidate, James Stark. Stark was a member of the Statistical Society of London, Convener of the General Assembly of the Church of Scotland's committee on registration, and the author of several articles on the subject of vital registration.[24] He was a Fellow of the College and he did taken an active part in all the College's discussions on registration. His wife was the eldest daughter of Adam Black, a former Lord Provost of Edinburgh, and it was probably through this connection that, in 1846, he had been commissioned by the Town Council to compile monthly mortality tables for Edinburgh and Leith. For almost a decade he had been investigating the possible influence of weather conditions on mortality rates; his mortality tables included not only the cause of each death

22. Alison requested a mutual friend at General Register House to relay his comments to Pitt Dundas. NAS, SRO8/78, Item 42: W. P. Alison to Alexander Pringle, 11 July 1854 (enclosed with item 43, Alexander Pringle to Pitt Dundas, 14 July 1854). Quoted in A. Cameron, Medicine.
23. W. P. Dundas to Major Graham, Registrar General [England], 23 Oct. 1854. NAS, GRO1/465, pp.14–15. Quoted in Cameron, Medicine.
24. NAS, AD56/225, copy letter James Stark to Thomas Headlam, 12 Mar. 1855 (enclosed with a letter from Stark to the Lord Advocate, 12 March 1855). For an example of his publications, see J. Stark, 'Contribution to the vital statistics of Scotland', *Journal of the Statistical Society of London* 14 (1851), pp. 48–87. Quoted in A. Cameron, Medicine.

but also 'the state of the barometer, thermometer, and rain-gauge' at the time. James Stark's credentials as a statistician were more impressive than those of George Bell. He was also a practising physician; when offered the post of Superintendent of Statistics on 11 July 1855, he accepted on the understanding that the duties of the office would not interfere with his private practice.

Stark and the clerks assigned to assist him were soon issuing weekly, monthly, quarterly, and in due course, annual reports. But Stark began to suffer recurring attacks of 'nervous' illness that confined him to bed for weeks at a time. In 1857, having accumulated substantial fines for absenteeism, he asked that his name be removed from the College's attendance roll. He explained that his delicate state of health would not permit him to attend 'exciting meetings such as those of the College'.[25] Stark's repeated and lengthy absences from the General Registry Office disrupted the production of routine reports of statistics and even delayed the completion of the 1871 Census Report. Eventually in 1874 the Registrar General felt compelled to force Stark's resignation. Another medical man, Dr Robertson, replaced him as Superintendent of Statistics. Stark subsequently retired to the village of Bridge of Allan, and died in 1890.

Of all W.P. Alison's campaigns in the field of public health his effort to secure for Scotland the best possible system for the notification of the causes of deaths was the most disappointing. He had hoped to build on the experience and evident shortcomings of the system introduced in England in 1837. In his system the cause of death would have been given according to a classification of disease that was at the same time more precise and more easy to use than that in use in England. He also promoted the use of a schedule that would have presented the cause of every death in Scotland in a way that was more carefully adapted for statistical analysis than the schedule used in England. However, even with the support of the College, Alison's was only one voice. There were other influential bodies pursuing their own quite different objectives in securing a Registration Act for Scotland. Their differences had caused eight Bills to fail. In securing the passage of a ninth Bill last minute compromises were made, other interests prevailed and Alison's plans were over ridden. In 1835 Alison had been confident that he could secure for Scotland a system of Registration much in advance of that being proposed for England. In the event a workable system was not introduced in Scotland until long after Alison's death; even then it did not include the improvements on the English system that Alison had proposed.

25. College Archive: copy letter Douglas (RCPE Clerk) to James Stark and his answer, 10 December 1857.

13

THE STRUGGLE FOR EQUAL RECOGNITION
Medical Reform

In the 1860s, Britain was at the beginning of a period of peace and prosperity, confidence and reform. The country was at last able to throw off the relics of the eighteenth century. In the first years of the nineteenth century, the country had still been embroiled in the wars that had followed from the revolution in France; the end of those long and expensive wars had brought economic recession, unemployment and hunger. In the 1840s, civil unrest had revived fears of revolution and provoked a return to reactionary and repressive government. In the 1850s there had been the 'sufferings and disgraces of the Crimea'.[1] But thereafter there had been peace; there were no more major foreign wars until the end of the century. In the 1860s, Britain was at the centre of the greatest empire since Roman times and had become the most successful trading nation in the world. No longer dependent only on the empire, Britain had found new and profitable markets in Europe and in the Americas. Agriculture was still the country's largest employer of labour and it too prospered as never before.

Britain, now 'a colossus astride the world',[2] owed its rise to pre-eminence to the phenomenal success of its industry, no longer the separate industries of England, Scotland and Wales but a complex of British industry. Since 1830, seven thousand miles of railway track had been laid forming a network in which each of the great regional centres of industry was rarely more than fifty miles apart from its nearest neighbour and no centre was more that a day's journey from any other.[3] The achievements of British industry generated new wealth that was enjoyed most conspicuously by the entrepreneurs whose vision, courage and endeavours had created it; but there were rewards too for those whose services were essential for industry's success – the professional men, the managers, the merchants and, at a time when industries were still without sophisticated machine tools, the skilled artisans. With the exception of the unskilled, the socially handicapped and the unemployable for whom the issue was not progress but survival, the people of Victorian Britain could look forward to some improvement, not only in their incomes and their standard of living, but also in their freedom to influence the society in which they lived. The proper exercise of that new influence required reform.

REFORM
In 1832, the Reform Act had extended the franchise to include numbers of the new prospering middle class and had given at least some of the new industrial towns the right to send MPs to

---

1. W. S. Churchill, *A History of the English Speaking People* (London, 1958), Vol. IV, p. 227.
2. L. James, *The Rise and Fall of the British Empire* (London, 1998), p. 117.
3. N. Davies, *The Isles: A History* (London, 2000), p. 639.

Parliament. However, these changes had not been enough to deprive the aristocracy and the old landed interest of their dominance in the House of Commons and their control of the government of the country. Now, in the 1860s, a second Reform Act extended the franchise to include virtually the whole of the (male) middle class and the great majority of the skilled (male) working class. The House of Commons was at last made somewhat more representative of the new urbanising industrial Britain. The result was 'a long delayed avalanche of reforms'.[4] The chief reforms were in the public services. In the Civil Service, appointments were no longer to be made by patronage; a new administrative class was created and entry was by competetive examination. In the Army, the Commander-in-Chief was made subordinate to the Secretary of State, the purchase of commissions was prohibited and flogging was abolished. The higher levels of the judiciary were reformed, and there were important reforms in education. And some order was brought to the practice of medicine. In the new prospering Britain, there were many more people who could afford to pay for medical care and, in a country that was being rapidly and heedlesly and unhygenically urbanised, there were many more occasions for that aid being sought. But for prospective patients there was little to guarantee the professional competence of those who offered their services. By the 1860s the profession had been reformed not, as had been in the case of the other reforms of in public service, by government but by the profession itself.

MEDICAL REFORM

In the first half of the nineteenth century, a great many of those offering medical and surgical services were unlicensed charlatans. There could be no doubt that everywhere in Great Britain and Ireland:

> many and great inconveniences have arisen, to the detriment of the king's subjects from the ignorance of persons who have assumed these callings without authority derived from regular education or other legitimate and proper sources.[5]

But even among those medical practitioners who had obtained a licence to practise from a 'legitimate and proper source' there were many who were poorly educated, inadequately trained and professionally incompetent. There were no fewer than twenty authorities in Great Britain and Ireland (Table 13.1) with the power to license medical practitionners. Each one set its own standards for its licentiates, standards that in some cases were so low as to defeat the purpose of the licensing system. Confidence in the integrity and competence of the whole medical profession was inevitably undermined since 'in every one of its ranks, medical, surgical or obstetrical, numerous and melancholy examples of utter incompetence of licensed charlatans present themselves daily'.[6] Reform of the licensing of medical practitioners in Great Britain and Ireland was therefore unquestionably in the interest of the general public.

4. Churchill, *A History*, p. 225.
5. Preamble to Latham's Outline of a Plan for an Intended Bill for the Better Regulation of Medical Practitioners, Chemists, Druggists and Vendors of Medicine, in 1804, quoted in Sir George Clark, *A History of the Royal College of Physicians of London* (Oxford, 1966), p. 625.
6. Ibid, p. 339 quoting Professor George Watt of Glasgow

TABLE 13.1 Licensing authorities for Great Britain and Ireland

The Royal College of Physicians
The Royal College of Surgeons of England
The Apothecaries Society of London
The University of Oxford
The University of Cambridge
The University of Durham
The University of London
The Royal College of Physicians of Edinburgh
The Royal College of Surgeons of Edinburgh
The Faculty of Physicians and Surgeons of Glasgow
The University of St Andrews
The University of Glasgow
The University of Aberdeen
The University of Edinburgh
The King and Queen's College of Physicians in Ireland
The Royal College of Surgeons in Ireland
The Apothecaries Hall of Ireland
The University of Dublin
The Queen's University of Belfast.
The Archbishop of Canterbury.[7]

THE COLLEGE AND REFORM

Not all the licensing bodies in Britain and Ireland welcomed the prospect of reform. For several, reform could only mean loss of ancient privileges and had to be resisted. For the College of Physicians in Edinburgh, however, reform promised an end to problems that had remained unresovled since the eighteenth century. In 1774, William Cullen, then President of the College, had written in a memorandum:

> The Universities of St Andrews and Aberdeen have frequently given degrees in absence upon a certificate of two physicians, very often obscure persons, and it is commonly believed that little else than the payment of the usual fee is necessary to obtain a degree. As to the Unversity of Glasgow, though they do not commonly give degrees in absence yet they often give degrees without requiring any certificated of the candidates' previous study.
>
> The abuses complained of are particularly a hardship on the Royal College of Physicians of Edinburgh who are obliged by their charter to grant licences without examination to any person who has obtained a degree from any of the universities of Scotland.[8]

7. An authority vested in the Archbishop of Canterbury in 1533 and never repealed.
8. College Archive.

Cullen's memorandum was addressed to the Duke of Buccleuch, the government's chief minister in Scotland. He was appealing for legislation to be introduced that would impose on the other Scottish universities the rigorous standards that had recently been introduced for the awarding of medical degrees at Edinburgh. Cullen wrote to his friend, Adam Smith, seeking his support; Adam Smith's answer was interesting but, for Cullen, unhelpful:

> You propose, I observe, that no person should be admitted to examination for his degree unless he brought a certificate of his having studied at least two years in some University. Would not such a regulation be oppressive upon all private teachers such as the Hunters, Hewson,[9] Fordyce?[10] The scholars of such teachers surely merit whatever honour or advantage a degree can offer, much more than the greater part of those who have spent many years in some Universities, where the branches of medical knowledge are not taught at all or are taught so superficially they had as well not been taught at all. When a man has learned his lesson very well it surely can be of little importance where or from whom he has learnt it.
>
> The monopoly of medical education which this regulation would establish in favour of Universities would, I apprehend, be hurtful to the lasting prosperity of such bodies-corporate. Monopolies very seldom make good work, and a lecture which a certain number of students must attend, whether they profit by it or no, is certainly not very likely to be a good one.[11]

Cullen's appeal for reform failed in 1774. Over the next few years, practices at Glasgow University were brought into line with those at Edinburgh. At St Andrews and Aberdeen, however, the abuses continued well into the nineteenth century with unfortunate consequences for the reputation of all Scottish medical degrees. The Royal College of Physicians in London was particularly scornful. As early as 1754, William Hunter, writing from London to William Cullen in Edinburgh, had commented on 'how contemptuously the College of Physicians here have treated all Scotch degrees indiscriminately'.[12] That indescriminate contempt continued into the next century, creating problems for a great many of those graduating with valid medical degrees from Edinburgh and Glasgow.

In the first half of the nineteenth century, the universities of Edinburgh and Glasgow both produced more than 150 Doctors of Medicine (and an equal number of Masters of Surgery) each year. The great majority were Irish or English and almost all in that majority intended to practise in England. Although only a minority were Scots, they were nevertheless too many to find congenial employment north of the border; many of the Scots also looked to practise in England.

9. William Hewson (1739–1774), partner in William Hunters's anatomy school in Windmill Street London. He later established his own very successful school in Craven Street where he taught anatomy and physiology.
10. George Fordyce (1736–1802). One of Cullen's early and favourite students; graduated MD at Edinburgh in 1754. He moved to London where he became a successful teacher of chemistry, materia medica and the practice of physic.
11. College Archive.
12. College Archive.

For centuries the legally recognised licence to practise medicine in England was a medical degree awarded by Oxford or Cambridge; since the foundation of the universities their medical degrees had been accepted as licences to practise medicine 'per universum Angliae regnum;' in the nineteenth century they were still the only university degrees that were accepted as licences to practise in the three kingdoms of England, Scotland and Ireland.[13] In the first half of the nineteenth century, each of the ancient English universities produced, at most, fifteen medical graduates each year. Since neither Oxford nor Cambridge had ever attempted to enforce its monopoly in England, the great majority of medical graduates practising in Great Britain in the early nineteenth century were graduates of Scottish universities. But, in England, they practised not by right but 'on sufferance'.

To practise medicine legally in England, a Scottish graduate could offer himself for examination and become a licentiate of the Royal College of Physicians of London.[14] Since the Apothecaries Act of 1815 he could be licensed to practise both medicine and surgery by the Society of Apothecaries but that required the completion of a five year apprenticeship. If he wished to practise surgery he might become a member of the Royal College of Surgeons of England by examination. However, beyond the major towns there was little attempt to police the exclusive privileges of the College of Physicians, the Society of Apothecaries and or the College of Surgeons and in the middle years of the nineteenth century many Scottish graduates practised medicine and surgery without a licence but undisturbed.

The disabilities suffered by Scottish graduates were at their most severe when they looked for employment in state services. Then they suffered from the prejudices the Royal College of Physicians of London. For many years Edinburgh and Glasgow had been among the leading medical schools in Europe yet to Fellows of the London College their degrees were disparaged and considered 'as common as blackberries;' it was said that degrees 'from many of the Scotch universities may be sent for by stage coach on paying eleven pounds'.[15]

The London College was not only the most venerable medical corporation and the most powerful licensing body in Britain, it was also physically and administratively close to the seat of government. By its ready access to government departments and by its personal contacts with ministers, it was able to promote its own objectives and ensure that it was consulted on medical issues, if need be, to the disadvantage of other professional bodies. In 1796, the president of the Royal College of Physicians of London was able to direct that graduates of Scottish universities or diplomats of the Scottish Medical Corporation would be debarred from promotion in the Army Medical Department.[16] In 1842, the Poor Law Commissioners were persuaded to order that Scottish graduates were to be excluded from appointments in the new Poor Law medical service; according to the relevant Order 'an English licence to practise to be a necessary qualification of a Medical Officer';[17] it was later even more specifically stated

13. Following the Medical Act of 1854, graduates of London University were given the same extensive privileges of Oxford and Cambridge except the right to practise in London.
14. Initially the jurisdiction of the Royal College of Physicians had extended only within seven miles of London but it had latter been extended to include the whole of England.
15. Sir N. Cantlie, *A History of the Army Medical Department* (London, 1874), p. 181.
16. Ibid.
17. Cantlie, *A History*.

that 'a degree or diploma of a Scotch university or other body having power to confer authority to practise in Scotland' was not an acceptable qualification.

The Edinburgh College of Physicians looked principally to the proposed new Medical Act to remove the disadvantages suffered by graduates of Edinburgh and Glasgow by enforcing common criteria for the awarding of medical degrees at all universities in Great Britain and Ireland, and at St Andrews and Aberdeen.

The College also hoped that the proposed Medical Act would extend the privileges of its licentiates. It looked for the removal of the uncoordinated historical geographic and professional limits that still defined the privileges granted to the licentiates of all the medical corporations in Britain. In the middle of the nineteenth century, the Faculty of Physicians and Surgeons of Glasgow[18] still licensed both physicians and surgeons to practise but only in the counties of the old Roman Catholic diocese of Glasgow. The Royal College of Physicians of Edinburgh had the exclusive right to license physicians to practise in Edinburgh and its suburbs. The Royal College of Surgeons of Edinburgh had the authority to license surgeons to practise in Edinburgh, the Lothians, Fife, Peebles Selkirk, Roxburgh and Berwick. In England, the area of jurisdiction of the Royal College of Physicians, which originally included only London and the seven miles round London, had later been extended to the whole of England and Wales. When the London Company of Surgeons became the Royal College of Surgeons in 1797 it was re-created on a somewhat different model from the older Royal Colleges; those who passed its entry examination became, not licentiates, but members of the College with a right to practise anywhere in England and Wales. An Act of 1533 had given the Archbishop of Canterbury the authority to grant licences to practise medicine in England; although seldom used, that authority still existed into the nineteenth century.

There can be little doubt that the Edinburgh College also hoped that the proposed Medical Act would put some limit on what was felt as the overriding power and influence of the Royal College of Physicians of London. In brief, the College hoped for uniformity in the regulation of medical and surgical practice throughout Great Britain and Ireland.

THE EARLY MOVES FOR REFORM

On 25 June 1804, a London physician, Dr Latham submitted to the Royal College of Physicians of London the draft of a *Plan for A Bill for the Better Regulation of Medical Practitioners, Chemists, Druggists and Vendors of Medicines Resident in the Country Districts of the United Kingdom*. A copy of the draft was sent to the College of Physicians in Edinburgh and the other Royal Colleges in the United Kingdom to 'be carefully perused and such alteration made as may be thought necessary'. In a long and detailed document Latham proposed that England, Scotland and Ireland should each be divided into a number of districts. In each district 'the Senior Physician of the respective Royal College of Physicians' in each of the three countries was to be appointed as Resident District Physician with powers to draw up and maintain a register of all the properly qualified practitioners (physicians, surgeons, apothecaries and druggists)

---

18. Not yet a Royal Faculty or a Royal College.

licensed to practise in that district. The Plan included the provision that 'no physician who is not a regular graduate of the Universities of England, of Ireland or of Scotland shall be permitted to practise in the United Kingdom'. It was also required that physicians should be more than 36 years of age, have been a Fellow of one of the Royal Colleges of Physicians for more than ten years and that 'no surgeon who shall not have served a regular apprenticeship of five years and afterwards attended two years in a provincial hospital or at least one year in any of the hospitals of London, Dublin or Edinburgh shall be permitted to practise in the United Kingdom;' and 'each person shall pay for his annual licence two pounds two shilling and one shilling to the Clerk of the Peace for registering and inserting a notification of the same in a list to be published after the summer Assizes in the country newspaper'. There were similarly restrictive criteria for the registration of apothecaries and druggists.

The Edinburgh College of Physicians appointed a Medical Reform Committee to formulate its response. The committee decided that the *Plan* was 'attended with so many difficulties that in its present state' it must be rejected. For the College, the chief objection was that the conditions for inclusion in the proposed register were too demanding both in the duration of training and in the expense of registration and would exclude many well trained, competent and experienced practitioners. On the other hand, the Committee strongly objected to the graduates of the universities of St Andrews and Aberdeen 'which grant degrees without residence or examination' being 'put on the same footing as the other universities of the United Kingdom'.

On 14 August 1805, the College was sent an amended version of Latham's *Plan* but when it arrived it was accompanied by a letter in which the London College of Physicians announcing that Latham's *Plan* had been 'for the present suspended'.[19]

In August 1806, an alternative *Plan for a Bill* was submitted to the Lords of the Treasury (the Prime Minister and members of his Cabinet) by Dr Edward Harrison, a physician practising in Lincolnshire. An investigation in Lincolnshire had shown that there nine out of ten of those practising as physicians were not licensed, had no formal training and were 'empirical pretenders'. Dr Harrison's plan was for one central register to which all properly trained physicians, surgeons, men-midwives, women-midwives and apothecaries in the United Kingdom would be admitted without further examination. Physicians were required to be over 24 years of age, graduates of any university in the United Kingdom who had completed five years of study, two of these years at the university from which they had taken their degrees. Surgeons were to be over 23 years of age, have completed five years of apprenticeship with one year of study at a medical school and hold a licence from one of the corporations of the United Kingdom. Men-midwives were to have attended a course of lectures and had one year of practical training; women-midwives need only have a certificate from a reputable practitioner. Apothecaries were to have served five years as an apprentice. The fee for registration and all other financial considerations were to be settled later.

The Lords of the Treasury referred Harrison's Plan to the medical corporations for their

19. College Minute, 5 November 1805.

views. On this occasion the Edinburgh College's Medical Reform Committee was more forthright in its objections. It considered the proposed Register to be far too exclusive and questioned its true purpose:

> Whatever reform takes place or whatever regulations be enacted they should
> have chiefly in view the benefit of the community at large and not merely the
> emolument and respectability of the medical profession.[20]

The College feared that Harrison's Plan would have the effect of severely limiting the number of medical practitioners in the United Kingdom at a time when the 'health of the nation' required that it should be made easier rather than more difficulty for members of the public 'to obtain proper advice and assistance in sickness or in bodily injuries'. The College recommended that physicians and surgeons should be allowed to enter the profession at twenty-one, the age at which they 'are entitled by law to manage their affairs'. The College also believed shorter periods of training would be perfectly acceptable; for physicians it recommended three years study at a university 'where there was proper instruction in all the branches of medicine and where degrees were awarded only after strict and impartial examination'; for surgeons it recommend an apprenticeship of only three years provided that in that time they had attended for two years at classes given by reputable teachers of anatomy, surgery and medicine; for apothecaries the apprenticeship should also be for three years and, since 'they are generally engaged in medicine', they should attended the same classes in anatomy, surgery and medicine as the surgeons. The College also considered that it would be unfortunate if the expense of registration, 'in addition to the already considerable expense of entering on practice', were to discourage potential recruits from entering the profession. The College also pointed out that there was:

> no doubt that good education both in medicine and surgery may be obtainable
> in universities besides those of the United Kingdom in some of which no, or at
> best very imperfect, medical education is provided.[21] The College cannot
> therefore approve of limiting the practice of physic to the graduates of these
> universities.[22]

Harrison failed to find effective support for his plan in 1806. However he persisted, and, supported by the Lincolnshire Association and a committee of 'discontented and critical licentiates of the London College of Physicians', in 1810 he drew up a *Bill for the Improvement of the Medical and Surgical and Veterinary Sciences and for Regulating the Practices thereof* for submission to Parliament. This was a more radical extension of his *Plan* of 1806 that now included the creation of a Board of Commissioners with powers not only over the maintenance of a Register but also for the establishment of new medical schools and the building of new

---

20. College Minute, 3 February 1807.
21. In 1805, the College had already objected to the graduates of the universities of St Andrews and Aberdeen 'which grant degrees without residence or examination' being 'put on the same footing' as the other universities of the United Kingdom'.
22. Ibid.

hospitals. In July 1810, the Edinburgh College of Physicians was asked by the Lords of the Treasury for its 'sentiments upon the subject of medical reform in general and upon the provisions of the proposed Bill'. The College replied:

A) With regard to the necessity of reform:

1. Abuses do exist in the practice of medicine arising from many persons engaging in it who are not qualified by a previous education; from deceptions daily practised by advertising empirics; and from the incompetence of existing authorities to prevent these abuses.

2. That the legislature is competent to prevent these abuses.

3. That these abuses may in great measure be corrected by Temperate Reform.

B) With respect to the particular provisions of the proposed Bill:

1. The Royal College are of the opinion that the measure of obliging every person who shall hereafter enter upon the practice of any of the branches of the Medical Profession to undergo an examination before obtaining a licence is very proper.

2. They approve of the plan of obliging persons who practise any of the branches of the Medical Profession to register their names and capacities and to take out a certificate of such Registration.

3. They are persuaded that if the above regulations and registrations were duly enforced many of the abuses now existing in the practice of medicine would be prevented.

4. They disapprove of the proposed scheme of creating a Board of Commissioners invested with extensive powers of levying large sums of money from the medical profession, of establishing medical schools, of appointing professors, of building hospitals, of forming botanic gardens etc, etc.

a) Because the appointment of such a Board is not necessary for attaining the essential object of reforming the practice of medicine.

b) Because the existing Medical Institutions are competent to undertake all the necessary duties of the Board.

c) Because it imposes a very heavy pecuniary burden on the profession of Medicine.

d) Because the duties to be conferred on this Board interfere with the rights and privileges of existing Establishments.[23]

Harrison's efforts came to an unsuccessful end in 1811. He failed to win the support of the medical profession and an attempt to rouse public opinion in favour of his Bill was equally

---

23. College Minute 11 February 1811.

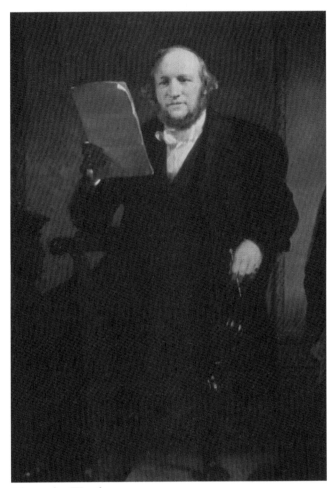

Alexander Wood

unsuccessful.[24] Frustrated by the failure, after many months of negotiations, to find agreement on any of the plans put forward by Latham and Harrison, the London College of Physicians, the most influential of the medical corporations in the United Kingdom, announced that it 'found the task of suggesting remedies for the abuses so arduous that it was discouraged from persevering at least until a more favourable season'.[25]

While the medical profession delayed and prevaricated, the apothecaries and surgeon-apothecaries were more decisive. In 1815, they successfully promoted an Apothecaries Act which gave the Society of Apothecaries the right to examine and license medical men who wished to practise not as either physicians or surgeons but as general practitioners. This was the first time that the designation 'general practitioner' had been used in an official government document; thereafter it came into general use during discussions on the

24. Clarke, *A History*, p. 631.
25. Ibid., p. 632.

organisation of the medical profession in the United Kingdom.

Candidates for the new licence to practise as a general practitioner were required to have served five years as an apprentice with an apothecary or surgeon-apothecary and to present testimonials of 'sufficient education' at a recognised medical school. It had long been the custom for licensed medical men conducting a general practice in England and Wales to describe themselves as surgeons and to be members of the Royal College of Surgeons; now after 1815, most general practitioners wishing to practise in England or Wales felt obliged to take both examinations. As the Act did not apply to Scotland, the Edinburgh College of Physicians had not been asked for its views on the licensing of general practitioners in England but later recorded its regret that a matter as important as the licensing of general practitioners had been 'entrusted to a trading society of Apothecaries'.

UNRESOLVED ANOMALIES

There were now four medical corporations or bodies in England (including the Archbishop of Canterbury), three in Scotland and two in Ireland with the right to grant licences to practise in their own designated area. There were also four universities in Scotland, two in England and one in Ireland awarding degrees in medicine that were widely regarded as licences to practise; however, whether the graduates of these universities practised within the areas of jurisdiction of the medical colleges by legal right or by 'sufferance' or whether their degrees allowed them to practise both medicine and surgery was still all very uncertain. The founding of London University in 1832 added to the anomalies. Initially its medical degrees were accepted as licences to practise anywhere in England and Wales except London where the Royal College of Physician was the existing licensing body. When Durham University, also founded in 1832, began to award degrees to students who had been trained at the medical school at Newcastle, the degrees were accepted as licences to practise in England but again not in London. In 1854 by a special act of Parliament London University and Durham Universities, but not the Scottish Universities, were granted the same privileges as Oxford and Cambridge.[26]

THE HOME SECRETARY'S BILL

Despite this growing multiplicity of licensing bodies there were still great numbers of quacks and unlicensed charlatans practising without hindrance in every part of the United Kingdom. In 1834 Parliament had appointed a select committee to provide the basis of a Bill for the regulation of the medical profession; unfortunately its records were destroyed later that year when the Palace of Westminster was destroyed by fire and that project was abandoned. In 1842, the Home Secretary, Sir James Graham, announced his intention to introduce to Parliament a new Bill *for the better Regulation of Medical Practice throughout the United Kingdom*; the draft of the Bill was eventually published in August 1844. The chief provision of the Bill was the creation of a central council, made up of lay members appointed by the government with a smaller number of representatives of the medical corporations, to supervise the licensing of the

26. College Minute, 20 July 1854.

medical profession in all its branches in the United Kingdom. For physicians the licensing bodies were to be the Royal Colleges of Physicians in England, Scotland and Ireland; the Society of Apothecaries was no longer to license general practitioners in England. The provisions in the charters of the Colleges of Physicians that had limited their areas of jurisdiction in their respective counties were to be abolished. Medical graduates of all universities were to have the right to be examined and become licensed associates of a College of Physicians provided they undertook not to dispense their own medicines. On reviewing the Bill, the College of Physicians of Edinburgh concluded:

- That the two principles of the measure, a uniform standard of education and qualification and the abolition of all local privileges, are those for the recognition of which the College have on various occasions contended and expressed the same opinion in petition to the legislature.

- That the principles now specified, if carried fully into effect, would confer a great benefit on the profession and public and would remove the evils and abuses now existing and for which for a long time past there has been too good reason to complain.

- That in thus providing the public with a supply of fully qualified general practitioners, the College are of the opinion that Government is undertaking all that can be properly attempted by legislative interference.

- That the College have with regret observed that part of the Bill which proposes to abolish the practice of prosecuting unlicensed and unqualified practitioners has given rise to great alarm and a good deal of opposition. The College are inclined to doubt the practicality of restraining unlicensed practice by penal enactments or the expediency of attempting to do so by such means; such powers, although vested in some of the public bodies in Scotland, have for many years been allowed to lie dormant. But rather than endanger the success of a measure otherwise so beneficial the College are disposed not to urge strongly their own opinion on this head.

- That while the College approve most cordially of the general spirit and principles of the Bill, they allow that in various details it may be desirable to introduce certain changes and modifications not affecting its principles or leading to details and far from impairing the efficiency of the measure would tend materially to facilitate its practical application.

Alone among the medical bodies responding to Sir James Graham's Bill the Edinburgh College of Physicians insisted that the regulation of medical practice must not have the effect of unduly restricting the number of medical practitioners allowed to offer their services to the public. At the same time, the College was no less intent than the other medical bodies that those licensed to practise should be both properly educated and of a high standard of professional competence. The College therefore agreed with Sir James Graham that the examining bodies should be the medical corporations and not the universities; the College took the view that the universities should examine their students on the subjects taught in university lecture rooms but fitness to practise should be tested by practical men who were themselves practising clinicians.

The College was content to support Sir James Graham's Bill although it was hoped that a few small but desirable amendments would be incorporated before the Bill was presented to Parliament. However, the Bill was fiercely resisted by the other medical bodies and especially by the general practitioners and the apothecaries. In 1845, Graham introduced an amended Bill to Parliament; in the hope of overcoming the opposition of the general practitioners and the apothecaries, he included a proposal for the creation of a Royal College of General Practitioners. But after months of further objections and continuing disputes between the various medical bodies, in January 1846, a frustrated Sir James Graham withdrew his Bill informing the House of Commons that he had 'done with medical reform'.[27] Thereafter, successive governments let it be known that they would not initiate any new legislation but would lend support to any private member's Bill that could command the general support of the medical profession and seemed likely to attract a majority in Parliament.

In the years that followed no fewer that eighteen Bills were put forward, each one drawn up and promoted by one or more of the factions within the medical profession. All parties were agreed that there should be uniformity in the licensing of practitioners in the different parts of the United Kingdom, that there should be a register of properly qualified practitioners and that the public should be more effectively protected from the attentions of unlicensed charlatans. However the ancient universities of Scotland, England and Ireland, the Royal Colleges in London, Edinburgh and Dublin, the Faculty of Physicians and Surgeons of Glasgow and the Society of Apothecaries in London all intended that these very necessary reforms should be achieved, as far as possible, with as little disturbance of their existing privileges as was possible. The Provincial Medical and Surgical Association (which became the British Medical Association in 1856) and a more radical group associated with the *Lancet* each took it upon themselves to protect what they saw as the interests of those medical men who were not represented by any of these long established institutions. And the faculty of the new University of London argued that many of the difficulties would be overcome if all the universities in England, Scotland and Ireland were to follow their example by introducing a new Bachelor of Medicine degree which could then serve as the standard qualification for general practitioners in the United Kingdom.

For a decade after the failure of Graham's Bill, the conflicting interests within the medical profession in England proved impossible to reconcile. In 1848, the London Colleges and the other medical bodies in England came together to form one Medical Reform Committee but, by April 1850, all hope that this would 'lead to improvement of the medical polity of Great Britain had been entirely blasted, the Committee having been broken up and all its proceedings rendered null and void'.[28] In 1850, Sir James Y. Simpson became President of the Edinburgh College of Physicians. He was an active advocate of reform and did much to keep

27. P. Bartrip, *Themselves Writ Large: The British Medical Profession 1832–1966* (London, 1996), p. 85.
28. College Minute, 16 April 1850.

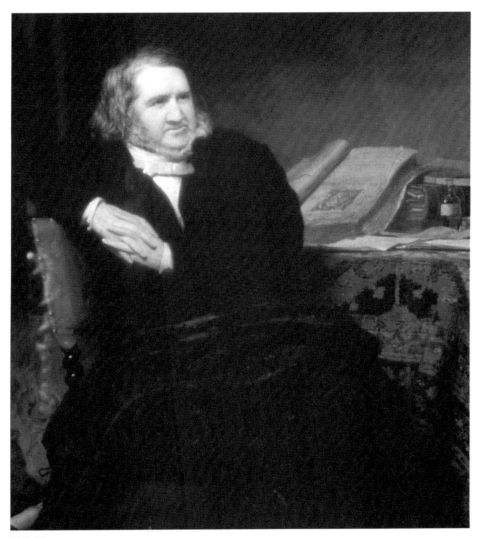

J. Y. Simpson

the issue alive. But until the Medical Act was at last achieved in 1858, the chief negotiator and guardian of Scottish interests was the Secretary of the College, Alexander Wood. In Scotland, positions were much less entrenched: in Scotland the corporations and other medical bodies agreed that they should 'as far as possible, act harmoniously together'. After 1846, when the many and various Medical Reforms Bills were put forward, representatives of the Royal College of Physicians of Edinburgh, the Royal College of Surgeons of Edinburgh and the Faculty of Physicians and Surgeons of Glasgow ('the Scotch Medical Reformers'[29]) joined together to present an agreed response from the profession in Scotland.[30] In Scotland, it

29. College Minute, 21 March 1853.
30. A move to amalgamate the Faculty of Physicians and Surgeon of Glasgow with the Royal Colleges of Edinburgh eventually came to nothing in 1848 but only after prolonged and serious consideration.

continued to be hoped that the reform of medical education and the licensing of medical practitioners would protect or even lead to an increase in the number of doctors practicing in Scotland; the case for such an increase was strengthened in 1852 by the publication of the College's *Statement Regarding the Existing Deficiency of Medical Practitioners in the Highlands and Islands.*[31] In Scotland there was considerable opposition to the idea, championed by the new University of London, that a medical degree from any university in the United Kingdom should be accepted as a licence to practise. However, the 'Scotch Reformers' were willing to set aside this and other considerations in order to secure agreement on a Bill that would achieve what, in Scotland, had come to be seen as the most crucial reform:

> We are quite unanimous in our opinion that former Bills embraced too many objects, and were too complicated, and that a Bill of Medical Reform, in order to be successful, must be directed solely to the determination of the conditions of obtaining the legal status of the general practitioner and to making that status necessary to holding medical appointments and applicable to every part of the United Kingdom.[32]

The medical corporations in Scotland therefore maintained a policy of 'armed neutrality'[33] while the conflicts continued on the medico-political stage in England. In the House of Commons, the Home Secretary, Lord Palmerston, castigated the English medical profession as 'a labyrinth and a chaos'. Shifting divisions, alliances, disputes and temporary agreements within the profession had already delayed reform for the best part of half a century; to many it now seemed that they might look for 'medical reform and the millennium at the same time'.[34]

The seemingly endless self-serving squabbles of the medical profession were brought to an abrupt end by the disasters of the war in the Crimea. *The Times* and other newspapers drew the attention of the British public to the gross deficiencies and mismanagement of the army's medical services and the appalling death rates at the military hospitals at Scutari. The government was shaken by the strength of the public reaction and the stream of protests.[35] A Royal Commission, appointed to inquire into such matters as hospital organisation, food, equipment and supplies focused also on the training of doctors. Medical Reform that before the war had been of interest chiefly, if not entirely, to the medical profession had become a matter of urgent concern for the British public and for the British government.

The war came to an end in April 1856. In August 1856, four months after the end of the war representatives of the Royal College of Surgeons of England, the Royal College of Surgeons of Edinburgh, the Royal College of Surgeons of Ireland and the Faculty of Physicians and Surgeons of Glasgow signed Articles of Agreement to establish a Medical Conference 'of representatives chosen equally by and out of each body that shall consult respecting all matters relating to preliminary and professional education and examination with

31. Royal College of Physicians of Edinburgh, *Statement Regarding the Existing Deficiency of Medical Practitioners in the Highlands and Islands* (Edinburgh, 1852).
32. College Minute, 11 March 1853.
33. College Minute, 1 May 1855.
34. Bartrip, *Themselves*, p. 87.
35. T. Royle, *Crimea* (London, 1999), p. 305.

a view of regulating medical and surgical education and leading to uniformity and reciprocity of privileges of the members of the each division of the profession in the United Kingdom'.[36]

In October, the Medical Conference was expanded to include representatives of the Colleges of Physicians of London, Ireland and Edinburgh and the Company of Apothecaries in London; the elected representatives from each of the centres later made up their own Branch Conferences in London, Dublin and Edinburgh. Later meetings of the Medical Conference were attended by delegates from the universities of Oxford and Trinity College, Dublin.

By the end of October the central Medical Conference had drawn up 'Amended Proposals for a Medical Bill, the heads of which have been settled by the Medical Corporations of England, Scotland and Ireland'. These proposals, drawn up without dissent from the universities of Oxford and Trinity College, Dublin were later 'acceded to' by the universities of Edinburgh, Glasgow and Marischall College, Aberdeen.[37] In May 1857, the Bill was entrusted to F. H. Headlam, MP, to present it to Parliament.

The British Medical Association (formerly the Provincial Medical and Surgical Association) pledged its support for Headlam's Bill. For the BMA the Bill was not perfect but was 'the best that was available and offered the rank and file some representation on the [proposed] governing body'.[38] Headlam had already presented medical reform Bills to the House of Commons on three occasions but each time he had failed to find support. On 1 July 1857, he obtained a majority of 147 for the second reading of this new Bill but was then compelled to withdraw it when it became clear that there was no chance of its completing the committee stage before the end of the parliamentary session. In moving for the withdrawal, Headlam urged the government to bring in a Bill of its own based on the same principles. In December 1857, W. F. Cowper MP, the President of the Board of Health, announced that, on behalf of the government, he would introduce a medical reform Bill in the new year.

In the general election in February 1858, the government was defeated and replaced by a Tory administration. Cowper was now out of office but he introduced his Medical Reform Bill as a private member. His Bill had been drafted by John Simon, the Chief Medical Officer of the Board of Health, and was a skilful compromise of the most generally acceptable of the ideas put forward in the preceding years. There were already two Bills before Parliament, Headlam's Bill submitted for a second time and a Bill put forward by Lord Elcho (the so called 'Edinburgh University Bill' which differed from Headlam's Bill in proposing to allow a university medical degrees as a licence to practise[39]). When Cowper's Bill received its second reading in June 1858, Headlam and Elcho withdrew their Bills and announced that they would support Cowper's Bill. That Bill then passed easily through the necessary stages of consideration and debate in Parliament and on 2 August it received the Royal Assent as *An Act to Regulate the Qualifications of Practitioners in Medicine and Surgery* (its official short title, the *Medical Act*). The chief provisions of the Act were:

---

36. College Minute, 5 August 1856.
37. College Minute, 19 May 1857.
38. Bartrip, *Themselves*, p. 94.
39. When first submitted to Parliament in June 1856 Elcho's Bill had the support of the College but was opposed by the medical corporations of England and Ireland.

- A Council which shall be styled the General Medical Council of Medical Education and Registration of the United Kingdom herein after referred to as the General Council shall be established and Branch Councils for England, Scotland and Ireland respectively.

The General Council shall consist of one person chosen from time to time by each of the following bodies:

The Royal College of Physicians

The Royal College of Surgeons of England

The Apothecaries Society of London

The University of Oxford

The University of Cambridge

The University of Durham

The University of London

The Royal College of Physicians of Edinburgh

The Royal College of Surgeons of Edinburgh

The Faculty of Physicians and Surgeons of Glasgow

The King and Queen's College of Physicians in Ireland

The Royal College of Surgeons in Ireland

The Apothecaries Hall of Ireland

The University of Dublin

The Queen's University of Belfast.

One person chosen from time to time by the University of Edinburgh and the two universities of Aberdeen collectively.

One person chosen from time to time by the University of Glasgow and the University of St Andrews collectively.

and

- Six persons to be nominated by Her Majesty with the advice of the privy Council, four of whom shall be appointed for England, one for Scotland and one for Ireland; and a President to be elected by the General Council.
- The General Council shall appoint a Registrar who shall act as Secretary of the General Council and Act as Registrar for England.
- The Branch General Councils for Scotland and Ireland shall each appoint a Registrar who shall also act as Secretary to the Branch Council.
- Those entitled to be included on the register to include every person possessing any one or more of the qualifications

Fellow or Licentiate of the Royal College of Physicians of London.

Fellow or Licentiate of the Royal College of Physicians of Edinburgh.

Fellow or Licentiate of the Kings and Queens College of Physicians of Ireland.

Fellow or Member or Licentiate in Midwifery of the Royal College of Surgeons of England.

Fellow or Licentiate of the Royal College of Surgeons of Edinburgh.

Fellow or Licentiate of the Royal College of Surgeons of Ireland.

Licentiate of the Society of Apothecaries, London.

Licentiate of the Apothecaries Hall, Dublin.

Doctor, Bachelor or Licentiate of Medicine, or Master in Surgery of any university of the United Kingdom or Doctor of Medicine by doctorate granted prior to the passing of the Act in 1858 by the Archbishop of Canterbury.

Doctor of Medicine of any foreign university practising as a physician in the United Kingdom before 1st October 1858.

- The fee for registration not to exceed £2 in respect of qualifications obtained before January 1859 and not exceeding £5 for qualifications obtained after that date.

THE OUTCOME

When, in May 1857, the draft of the Medical Reform Bill was agreed and ready for presentation to Parliament the College took pride in recording that 'the Royal College of Physicians of Edinburgh have uniformly endeavoured in all their proceeding in regard to Medical Reform to promote the interests of the public and the elevation of the profession rather than to contend for their own advantage'.[40] However, when the Medical Reform Act, as amended during its passage through Parliament, became law in August 1858, it was feared that too much had been conceded and that the future of the College had been put at risk.

In a *Report of the Position of the College under the Medical Act*,[41] the Medical Reform Committee of the College recalled that for many years some 55 per cent of the Fellows admitted to the College lived and practised outside Scotland. Now, Article 49 of the Medical Act made it possible for the Royal College of Physicians of London to become the 'Royal College of Physicians of England' and should it choose to do so 'any Fellow or Licentiate of the Royal College of Physicians of Edinburgh or of the King and Queen's College of Physicians of Ireland who may be in practice *in any part of the United Kingdom* and may be desirous of becoming a member of such a College of Physicians of England shall be at liberty to do so'. The Medical Reform Committee predicted that, should this new college be created, many of the existing Fellows would become Fellows of the English College and the only applications for the Fellowship of the Edinburgh College would come from physicians resident in

40. College Minute 19 May 1857.
41. College Minute, 21 September, 1858.

Edinburgh attracted only by 'the social benefits conferred by the College along with an excellent Library and Reading Room'.

The Reform Committee feared that the future of the College as a licensing body was even less secure. The College was reminded that 'in times past the bye-laws of the College had required that every candidate for the Fellowship should have been at least one year as a Licentiate before being balloted for as a Fellow. The obnoxious Stamp Act had so greatly increased the expense of entrance that the by-law had been abolished in 1829 and since then no licences had been applied for'. It now seemed very uncertain if, after an interval of three decades, the College would now be able to take advantage of the provisions of the Medical Act and once again become an effective licensing body.

Within a few years it became clear that the College's Medical Reform Committee had been unduly pessimistic. In the 10 years before the Medical Act became law, 52 new Fellows were elected; in the 10 years from 1858, there were 56 new Fellows and, as before, the majority lived and practised outside Scotland.

The revival of the College as a licensing body was dramatic. In the first five years under the Medical Act, the College granted no fewer than 974 licences. In the first two of these years, no fewer than 532 licences were granted to doctors practising in England; in the last two of these years the majority were graduates of the new Queen's College of Ireland at Belfast, Cork and Galway. In all five of these years, some 20 licences were granted to doctors practising in Scotland and this number remained constant in the years that followed.[42]

From the early years of the century, the College had contended that the public should be protected from the pretensions of charlatans by the creation of a public register of medical practitioners who had been properly trained and qualified. However, the College had been equally insistent that criteria for inclusion on the register must not be set so high and the register made so exclusive that the number of doctors practising legally in Scotland and in the United Kingdom would be insufficient for the needs of the public.

The Medical Act satisfied both the intentions and the reservations of the College. In 1858 the number of doctors practising in Scotland was 1,552; by 1863 it had risen to 1,674 and by 1868 to 1,725. The College had been particularly concerned that scarcity of doctors practising in the Highlands and Islands should not be made even worse. In the years from 1858 to 1868 the population in the Highlands and Islands continued to fall; during the same years the number of doctors practising there increased from 97 to 136.

A DIFFERENCE IN ETHOS

The Medical Act had been passed to bring harmony and standardisation to the qualifications required of practitioners in medicine in the United Kingdom. But even within the constraints of the Act, the Royal College of Physicians of London, the most influential medical corporation in the United Kingdom, remained determinedly elitist while the Royal College of Edinburgh was more pragmatic in its commitment towards public service. This difference was

---

42. The Stamp Duty was abolished for new licentiates in 1959 but not for Fellows of Colleges.

reflected in the regulations set by the two Colleges for the granting of licences to practise medicine. The London College required that candidates should have reached the age of 25, have completed five years of preliminary medical studies at a university, three years of hospital medical training and have paid a fee of £55. The Edinburgh College proposed that candidates should have reached 21 years of age, have studied medicine for four years, including two years of hospital training, and paid a fee of £10. This caused the London College 'to address a strong and immediate remonstrance' to the Edinburgh College:

> The President and Censors beg to call the serious attention of the Royal College of Physicians of Edinburgh to the injurious effect that their proposed new regulations must have on the character and status of British physicians and especially the character and reputation of the London College of Physicians who, in the event of their obtaining a new charter, would by the recent Medical Act, be compelled to admit into their body any one practising in England who had obtained the licence of the Edinburgh College. Many of those whom the London College would thus be compelled to admit into their number and to the highest rank of medical practitioners in England might be either young men who had just attained their majority or various classes of persons whose qualifications had been insufficiently attested. Such qualifications would not only be in striking contrast with those of the London College but also far below the requirements that must ever be demanded by all who desire to elevate the education and maintain the professional and social status of the English physician.[43]

In reply Sir Robert Christison, the President of the Edinburgh College, gave the assurance that:

> no person will be admitted into its list of licentiates who does not deserve to be enrolled as a Licentiate of a College of Physicians. The only material difference subsisting between the regulation of the College of London and the regulations of that of Edinburgh for the admission of licentiate regards the age of the candidates and the experience presumed to be connected with age … This College is not particularly wedded to the age of 21. It is the age which has been hitherto adopted in Scotland for entering the learned professions for the church, the Bar and medicine. *It is the minimum.* It can be and will be rarely taken advantage of. But in as much as there are medical men, no less than philosophers, politicians, soldiers etc. whose talents and assiduity place them on a level with others at 26 and, more this College cannot see why an arbitrary corporation rule should deprive such men of the advantages with which Providence may have been pleased to bless them … This College deprecates any rigorous rule on that head as being calculated to obstruct the progress of talent

43. College Minute, 26 April 1859.

and to interfere with the public usefulness of a College whose purpose is to foster and not to obstruct talent.[44]

The Royal College of Physicians of London found Scottish university degrees as unacceptable as the licences of the Scottish medical corporations. According to its historian, Sir George Clark, they believed that the Medical Act 'degraded the College's licences by putting Scotch degrees on an equality with them'.[45] The London College felt so strongly that it decided it must 'of necessity abandon all present idea of seeking a new Charter' and of becoming the Royal College of Physicians of England as the Medical Act had proposed. By continuing as the Royal College of Physicians of London, it was relieved of the necessity of admitting persons holding Scottish licences and Scottish degrees. Nevertheless, its 'primacy was decidedly reduced when its representative had to take his seat among the rest' on the General Medical Council. However, according to its historian, 'nothing could deprive the College of Physicians of London of its seniority among the professional bodies nor could any of the others emulate its formal dignity'.[46]

The Royal College of Physicians of Edinburgh took the view that the London College's continuing exclusiveness was not in the interest of the medical profession or the public.

> The great dissatisfaction which has for so many years prevailed throughout the medical profession in Great Britain, originally arose in a great measure from the way and exclusive spirit in which the London College of Physicians and the London Society of Apothecaries guarded the monopolies conferred upon them by their existing charters.[47]

The Edinburgh College saw the Medical Act as 'a great boon conferred on the public of the United Kingdom'. It ensured that the public was provided with a full and reliable list of all properly qualified medical practitioners able to provide medical care in the United Kingdom. At the same time it was of service to the medical profession by removing 'those special disabilities of which complaint has so long justly been made in Scotland'; it ensured that the graduates and licentiates of Scotland, 'possessed of excellent schools of medicine and of the chief requisites for the most complete medical education, were freed from those restrictions which had prevented them from having the whole Empire for their field of Practice'.

44. Ibid.
45. Clark, *A History*, p. 634.
46. Ibid., p. 740.
47. College Minute, 1 May 1848.

14

INCARCERATION OR TREATMENT

The Lunacy Act 1857

At the beginning of the nineteenth century, the laws governing the care and the custody of the insane in Scotland had not changed since the fourteenth century. By a statute of Robert I, the care of those of 'fatuous mind' was the responsibility of family; the care and management of the 'furious' insane was likewise the responsibility of the family but, when the family failed, responsibility devolved on the sheriff of the county, the 'Crown having the sole power of coercing by fetters'.[1] In the first years of the nineteenth century, families who could afford the high fees[2] might devolve the care of their fatuous, deviant or simply inconvenient relatives to a private asylum operating for profit; the great majority of families, however, chose either to care for their fatuous relatives at home or left them free to fend for themselves. Only a few families had the resources to confine their 'furious' relations at home or could find a private asylum willing to accept them; the great majority of the difficult, disorderly or dangerous insane in Scotland were incarcerated in some public institution. In Edinburgh, they were committed to the 'Bedlam'[3] (Charity Workhouse); in Glasgow they were confined in the cells set aside for the purpose in the Town's Hospital; but where there were no public asylums, the 'furious' and the friendless and abandoned 'fatuous' were incarcerated along with the criminals in the country's jails and tollbooths.

The number confined in asylums was small. A survey early in the century found that there were 4,628 insane persons in Scotland.[4] Of these, only 417 were patients in private asylums or public institutions. The conditions in which they were confined were vile and their treatment grossly inhumane and often horrific; having lost their reason, then seen as the defining characteristic of a human being, the insane were treated as if immune to pain or misery.[5] At Inverness in 1815, the mad were confined in a vault between the second and third arches of the old bridge; 'this dark appalling place of durance where the inmates were between the constant hoarse sound of the stream beneath and the occasional tramping of feet and rattling of wheels overhead was not abandoned till the last miserable maniac had been devoured by rats'.[6] In Perth, the tollbooth was a dark and wretched building in the middle of the town. Elizabeth Fry, the prison reformer:

1. Report of the Royal Lunacy Commission for Scotland, 1857 quoted by D.H. Tuke, *The History of the Insane in the British Isles* (London, 1882), p. 322.
2. A week's care in a private asylum cost £5 or more per week, the equivalent of a year's wages for a working man. Even in Scotland's Royal Asylums the standard charge was £1 1s per week or £3 3s for a patient 'with a servant to attend'.
3. Founded early in the eighteenth century in the building that had been the office of the Darien Scheme in 1699.
4. Parliamentary Reports, *Abstract of Returns from Clergy in Scotland Relating to Number of Lunatics in that part of the United Kingdom, 1818.*
5. Tuke, *The History*, p. 148.
6. R. Gardiner Hill, *On Lunacy* (London, 1870), p. 2.

found in it two lunatics in a most melancholy condition; both of them in solitary confinement, their apartments dirty and gloomy; and a small dark closet, connected with each of the rooms, filled with a bed of straw. In these closets, which are far more like the dens of wild animals than habitations of mankind, the poor men were lying with very little clothing upon them. They appeared in a state of fatuity, the almost inevitable consequence of the treatment to which they were exposed. No one resided in the house to superintend these afflicted persons, some man living in the town having been appointed to feed them at certain hours of the day. They were, in fact, treated exactly as if the had been beasts. A few days after our visit, one of these poor creatures was found dead in his bed. I suppose it may have been in consequence of this event that the other, though not recovered from his malady, again walks the streets of Perth without control. It is much to be regretted that no medium can be found between so cruel an incarceration and total want of care.[7]

Gardiner Hill,[8] a Justice of the Peace in Lincolnshire who had visited many asylums in both England and Scotland wrote:

In the early part of this century [the nineteenth] lunatics were kept constantly chained to the wall in dark cells and had nothing to lie upon but straw. Some were chained in dungeons and were gagged, outraged and abused. The keepers visited them, whip in hand, and lashed them into obedience. They were also half drowned in baths of surprise; the bath of surprise was so constructed that the patients in passing over a trap door fell in. Some of the patients were chained in wells and the water made to rise until it reached the patient's chin. One horrible contrivance was a rotary chair in which the patients were made to sit and were revolved at a frightful speed; the chair was in common use. Patients in a state of nudity, women as well as men, were flogged at particular periods, chained, strapped and fastened to iron bars and even confined to iron cages.[9]

The atrocities practised routinely at the York Asylum were even more horrific. 'The cells were in a state dreadful beyond description; some miserable bedding was lying on the straw which was daubed and wet with excrement and urine, the boarded floors saturated with filth; the stench was intolerable'. Patients were emaciated and covered with bruises and marks which 'could be attributed to nothing but the lash of the whip'. One woman, when discharged to her home, was 'dirty, in rags and swarming with vermin; she had 'wounds on her head and her hip was dislocated'. 'There were many instances on record of the female patients being with child by the keepers and male patients'.[10]

Some indication of the horrors practised at York Asylum were revealed during a long and

7. Tuke, *The History*, p. 329.
8. Robert Gardner Hill became the lay Superintendent of Lincoln Asylum in 1835.
9. Hill, *Lunacy*, p. 1.
10. Ibid., p. 4.

very public dispute between its superintendent and the Quaker proprietors of the Retreat in York. In December 1813, the resulting publicity led a private member of Parliament, George Rose, to introduce 'a Madhouse Bill to repeal and render more effective the provisions of the Act of 1774'. In April the Bill was passed by the House of Commons but rejected by the House of Lords. The House of Commons then appointed a Select Committee, chaired by George Rose, to carry out further investigations into the nature and extent of the abuses being practised in the care of the insane and 'to consider of provision being made for the better regulation of mad-houses in England'.

The committee not only confirmed the atrocious conditions and malpractices that prevailed at York Asylum but went on to discover that such abuses were common in England's asylums, even at the Bethlem Royal Hospital (Bedlam) in London then generally 'thought to be equal if not superior to any other asylum in England'.[11] Founded by the Order of St Mary of Bethlem, it had been caring for lunatics since the thirteenth century. In 1815, it was directed by a Fellow of the Royal College of Physicians of London, Thomas Monro, who had been preceded in that office by both his father John Monro and his grandfather James Monro; the resident manager was the apothecary, Mr Haslam. For some years Bethlem had housed, on average, 238 patients of both sexes, many of them kept for long periods under 'restraint'. Those under restraint were manacled and chained by an arm or a leg to the wall. One patient, a Mr Norris who had struck Mr Haslam, had been caged and kept in irons for twelve years:

> A stout iron ring was riveted round his neck, from which a short chain passed to a ring made to slide upwards or downwards on an upright massive iron bar, more than six feet high inserted in the wall. Round his body a strong iron bar about two inches wide, was riveted; on each side of the bar was a circular projection which being fastened to and enclosing each of his arms pinioned them close to his sides. The waste-bar was secured by two similar bars, which, passing over his shoulders were riveted to the waste-bar, both before and behind. The iron ring round his neck was connected to his shoulders by a double link. From each of these bars another chain passed to the ring on the upright iron bar. His right leg was chained to the trough.

At the Bethlem Hospital the Select Committee found abundant proof, not only of cruelty but also of professional incompetence. It was stated 'by Haslam himself that a person whom he asserts to have been generally insane and mostly drunk, and whose condition was such that his hand was not obedient to his will, was nevertheless retained in the office of surgeon'. And in Bethlem, patients were subjected to a regime of medical treatment for their malady. Dr Monro informed the Select Committee that 'the patients are bled about the later end of May according to the weather and after they have been bled they take vomits once a week for a certain number of weeks; after that we purge the patients'. Asked the rationale for such treatment, Dr Monro could only offer that 'that has been the practice invariably for years before my time; it was handed down by my father and I do not know of any other practice'.

11. Tuke, *The History*.

The bleeding and purging practised at the Bethlem Hospital was unusual. In the great majority of asylums in England in 1815 no treatment was offered other than physical restraint. As the Superintendent of one of England's largest asylums explained in the *Lancet*:

> Restraint forms the very basis and principle on which the sound treatment of lunatics is founded. The judicious and appropriate adaptation of the various modifications of this powerful means to the peculiarities of each case of insanity comprises a large portion of the curative regimen of the scientific and rational practitioner. In his hands it is a remedial measure of the first importance and is about as likely to be dispensed with in the care of mental diseases as that the various articles of the Materia Medica will be altogether dispensed with in the cure of the body.

At the Retreat at York the physical restraint of patients had been successfully abandoned in favour of more humane measures. But, in 1815, such a radical departure from established practice was still controversial. When the Select Committee presented its report to Parliament, it did not recommend that physical restraint should be abandoned but it did comment that because asylums were often so overcrowded and inadequately staffed 'there was unavoidably a larger amount of restraint than would otherwise be necessary'. The Report concluded that:

> New provision of law is necessary for ensuring better care is taken of insane persons ... There is not in the country a set of beings more immediately requiring the protection of the legislature than persons in this state a very large proportion of whom are entirely neglected by their relatives and friends. If treatment of those in the middling or in the lower classes of life shut up in hospitals, private madhouses or parish workhouses is looked at a case cannot be found where the necessity for a remedy is more urgent.

In May 1816, Rose introduced a Bill that would have made the inspection of asylums more effective and would have led to the building of new county asylums for pauper lunatics; it was passed by the House of Commons but was rejected by the House of Lords. George Rose died in 1818, but three Bills to the same effect were introduced by other members of Parliament in 1819 but all were defeated in the House of Lords. Until 1844 the legislation on the care of the insane in England remained much as it had been since 1774.[12]

LEGISLATION FOR SCOTLAND

On 18 December 1813, the College met to discuss the Bill for the regulation of Madhouses in England that, George Rose had introduced in Parliament a few days before. Andrew Duncan proposed that the College should recommend to the Lord Advocate that the powers to be granted to the Royal College of Physicians of London for the licensing and regulating of madhouses in England should also be granted to the Edinburgh College for application in

---

12. An Act of 1774 made some provision for the licensing and regulation of madhouses by five Fellows of the Royal College of Physicians of London but was later described by the Commissioners in Lunacy as 'utterly useless'. It did not apply to the lunatic poor and was not operative outside London. Tuke, *The History*, p. 102.

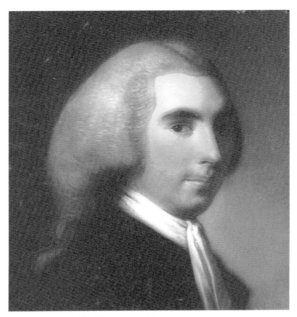

Viscount Melville (New Club)

Scotland. Andrew Duncan's proposal had the support of the Sheriff of Edinburgh who 'considered some such regulations as were proposed in the Bill as highly necessary to be extended to Scotland'.[13] A College Committee was appointed to draft appropriate amendments for the Bill and these were conveyed to Mr Rose in May and July 1814. But, later in 1814, Rose failed to get the necessary support for his Bill in the House of Commons. When he submitted a second version of his Bill in 1815, he did not include the provisions suggested for Scotland. This second Bill was passed in the House of Commons but was rejected by the Lords.

The move for legislation for Scotland was immediately taken up by Viscount Melville (Henry Dundas) and on 7 June 1815 *An Act to Regulate Madhouses in Scotland* was passed by Parliament. The Act provided for the medical inspection of all establishments in Scotland, 'either in the nature of public hospitals or private institutions kept for gain' and for the creation and maintenance of 'an accurate registry of the names, number and description of all lunatics in a state of confinement in houses kept for their reception'. Four inspectors were to be chosen annually by the Royal College of Physicians of Edinburgh and four by the Faculty of Physicians and Surgeons of Glasgow; the Sheriff Depute of each county or his Substitute was to employ one of those chosen to accompany him in inspecting all the houses in the county kept for the reception of lunatics. For the Registration of Lunatics the Sheriff or his Depute or Substitute in each county was to send to the President of the Royal College of Physicians of Edinburgh and to the Clerk of the High Court of Justiciary an annual account of the number of houses that had been licensed during the year for the reception of lunatics; a statement of

13. College Minute, 1 February 1814.

the total number of houses kept in their respective counties for the care of furious or fatuous persons; the names and descriptions of those confined; and a 'report of all that shall have been done by him or under his direction'.

On 3 February 1818, Lord Binning,[14] who had been a members of the Select Committee that Rose had chaired in 1815, introduced to Parliament a Bill for the establishment of district lunatic asylums in Scotland. These asylums were to be state institutions financed by an assessment on the local population. Within days, petitions of protest began to pour in from the cities, towns and counties of Scotland. The nobility, freeholders, heritors, Commissioners of Supply and Justices of the Peace seemed to be united in objecting to this unwarranted intervention by the state. Money was to be raised by compulsory assessment for a purpose that could more fittingly and more effectively be achieved by charity. The objectors could point to the institutions that had already been created by enlightened philanthropy. An asylum had been founded at Montrose by voluntary subscription in 1781 and had later been granted a royal charter. Since then Royal Asylums had been established by the same means at Aberdeen (1800), Edinburgh (1813) and Glasgow (1814). The opponents of the Bill claimed that it could only 'have owed its origin to an unjust and groundless assumption of a want of humanity in the people of Scotland towards objects afflicted with so severe a calamity'.[15] The opposition was so immediate and so overwhelming that Lord Binning's Bill was withdrawn before it reached its second reading.

INTERVENTION BY THE STATE

The College was disappointed at the failure of Lord Binning's Bill but looked to the provisions of Rose's Act of 1815 for some improvement in the care of the insane. The Act gave the sheriffs new powers to license the asylums in their counties, to set the rules for their management, to order the committal of lunatics to an asylum and to order their release. It also fell to the sheriffs to carry out twice-yearly inspections of the asylums and to report on their findings to the Clerk of the High Court of Justiciary. The Act required that, when carrying out his inspections, the sheriff or his deputy should be accompanied on his inspections by a Fellow of the College of Physicians of Edinburgh or of the Faculty of Surgeons and Physician of Glasgow and that a copy of the sheriff's report should be sent to the President of the Royal College of Physicians of Edinburgh. The powers and duties of the inspecting physicians or of the President of the College were not defined in the Act and no provision was made either for the payment of the expenses of medical inspectors travelling beyond their own counties or for medical inspectors to be engaged locally.

> From 1816 a physician nominated by the College[16] accompanied the sheriff or his deputy on a regular six monthly tour of inspection of the establishments for the insane in Midlothian and each May a copy of the sheriff's report was

14. Charles Hamilton, son of the Earl of Haddington.
15. Tuke, *The History*, p. 327.
16. The inspector was invariable a physician of the staff of the Morningside Asylum.

submitted to the President of the College. However, sheriffs elsewhere in Scotland were either reluctant or unable to arrange for the inspection of madhouses in their districts; only the sheriffs of Forfarshire and Aberdeen submitted reports and even theirs were very few. Every June, the Presidents of the College informed the College of the reports that had been received but decreed that as they were not 'proper to be made public' they were to be 'sealed up to be deposited among the papers of the College'.[17]

In 1831, the President informed the Clerk of the High Court of Justiciary that, while the College was still receiving copies of the reports of inspections of asylums carried out by the Sheriff of Midlothian, nothing had been received from sheriffs elsewhere in Scotland for some years; in his reply the Clerk admitted that, since 1816, he had received so few reports from Scotland's sheriffs that he had been unable to maintain the register provided for in the Act. In November 1839, the College at last formally acknowledged that the intentions of the Act of 1815 had been 'altogether frustrated'. A memorial was sent to the Secretary of State for the Home Department expressing the College's 'great regret that owing to causes which lie out of their control, certain clauses of the Act obviously intended for the safety of the public and calculated to yield interesting and important information on the statistics on insanity in this division of the Empire have hitherto been inoperative'.

Statistics on insanity were indeed sadly lacking. The only statistics available in 1839 were those that had been gathered in a survey carried out by Henry Hobhouse, the Permanent Under-Secretary at the Home Department in 1818. The survey found that there were then, in Scotland, 4,628 persons who were recognised as being 'lunatics' or 'idiots'. Of these, 1,357 were cared for at home by the family but the majority, 2,855, had been left to fend for themselves in the community. In England, the proportion 'at large' in the community was even larger; with a population more than six times greater than Scotland's, only 4,782 of the insane in England were confined in asylums. It may be supposed that families were generally reluctant to admit to the stigma of insanity in the family by committing a relative to an asylum but even more reluctant since conditions in the country's asylums were notorious and there was little prospect of an early 'cure'. The revelations of the Select Committee inquiry in 1815 prompted social reformers, notably Lord Ashley (later the Earl of Shaftesbury), to campaign for the massive internment of the insane, for the establishment of district asylums in which to confine them and for improvement in the conditions in which the insane were lodged.

The prospect of state intervention, opening up at a time when the medical profession was expanding more rapidly than the demand for its services, led a number of medical men to opt for 'the mental diseases department of medicine', to devise new regimes of treatment and to create a medical monopoly in the management of the insane. Among the earliest and most prominent of the physicians to adapt his career to the new circumstances was a President of the College, Alexander Morison.

17. College Minute, 1 August 1820.

SIR ALEXANDER MORISON AND THE MEDICAL MANAGEMENT OF THE INSANE

Morison was born in Edinburgh on 1 May 1779. His father, a younger son of a landed family in Aberdeenshire had bought a small estate, Anchorfield, near Leith, and become a successful wine importer, trading with Bordeaux and Portugal.[18] Alexander, his third son, was taught at home until the age of eight when he was enrolled at the High School in Edinburgh. When he was eleven it seemed that he was destined to follow his older brother, Andrew, in making his career at sea[19] but after one voyage to Portugal he wrote to his father 'craving to be restored' to dry land.[20] He was sent off to a tutor in Cumberland, the Rev. Sewel, to be prepared for university. At the age of thirteen, he matriculated at Edinburgh University and, after two years of general studies, he began his medical education. From November 1794, he combined his medical studies at university with a five-year apprenticeship with one of Edinburgh's leading surgeons, Alexander Wood ('Lang Sandy' Wood). He graduated in 1799, his MD thesis, 'De Hydrocephalo Phrenitico', suggesting that he may already have had some interest in neurological and mental disorders.

Within weeks of graduating Morison became a licentiate of both the Royal College of Physicians and the Royal College of Surgeons of Edinburgh and went south for two years to gain further hospital experience in London. At the Westminster Hospital he renewed his friendship with Alexander Crichton. Crichton and Morison's older brother, Francis, had been at Edinburgh University together and both had been apprentices of 'Lang Sandy' Wood. In 1794 Francis Morison had died of typhus while on the staff at Edinburgh Royal Infirmary; his friend Crichton had gone to London to lecture on chemistry, material medica and physic at the Westminster Hospital. When Alexander Morison arrived in London in 1799, Crichton was already established as a physician to the Westminster Hospital and had published his *An Inquiry into the Nature and Origins of Mental Derangement*. His *Inquiry* was much influenced by the philosophy of Thomas Reid;[21] his thesis was that the inappropriate actions of the insane patient were potentially intelligible and that the physician should explore the possibility that the patient's dysfunction might relate to some identifiable disturbance in the modelling of his or her mind during childhood. The patient might then benefit from the exercise of techniques of re-education and re-socialisation. This was a strategy that Morison was to use much later in his private practice.

However, when Morison left London in 1801 he had already abandoned his intention to make a career in medicine. Some months before graduating, he had married his cousin, Mary Anne Cushnie, who was both beautiful and rich, having inherited a major share in a sugar plantation in Jamaica. On his return to Scotland, Morison bought a farm in Galloway and the Bankhead estate in Midlothian. For the next few years he devoted himself to the study of

18. Morison's father was granted arms by the Lord Lyon as Andrew Murison of Anchorfield.
19. His brother had already been drowned at the age of fourteen.
20. Alexander Blackhall-Morison, Biography of Alexander Morison MD, unpublished manuscript, College Archive.
21. A. Scull, C. MacKenzie and N. Hervey, *Masters of Bedlam* (Princeton, 1996), p. 127.

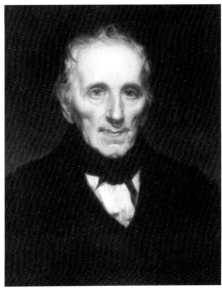

Sir Alexander Morison

agriculture and the management of his estates. In 1804, on his Bankhead estate, he built Larchgrove, the house that he was later to donate to the College.[22]

By 1805 farming was proving to be less rewarding than Morison had hoped and he began to think once again about a career in medicine. He sold off parts of his land to his brother and his brother-in-law and travelled to Russia to visit Crichton, now Sir Alexander Crichton and Physician to Tsar Alexander I, to discuss the possibility of practising at St Petersburg. Nothing came of the visit and he returned to Edinburgh. Then, in 1807 he was invited to become personal 'travelling' physician to Lord Somerville, who was about to travel south to take up residence in London and Surrey. He was in London for only four weeks but in that time he met and was consulted by a number of families of the English aristocracy and several of the French nobility who had fled to England at the outbreak of the Revolution. He decided to practise in London and with that in mind he became a licentiate of the London College of Physicians. He moved to London permanently in February 1808 and with Somerville's support he set up practice at 17 Half Moon Street and in Surrey; in 1809 his practice had not flourished and he accepted an appointment as Visiting Physician to the private lunatic asylums in Surrey.[23] Thereafter he kept on a house and consulting room in London (at 17 Half Moon Street, then 3 St James Square and finally at 26 Cavendish Square) and maintained his connections with Surrey. He established a position on the fringes of court society in London and at Brighton. He accepted warrants as Physician Extra-Ordinary to the Princess of Wales and later as Physician-in-Ordinary to the Household of the Duke of Albany although neither appointment carried a salary or any duties; yet his practice still did not flourish and he remained dependent on the patronage of Lord Somerville.

22. The house was given to the College to endow the Morison Lecture.
23. Blackhall-Morison, Biography.

While Morison struggled to establish himself in private practice in London, his income from the plantation in Jamaica was steadily growing less; at the same time his family continued to grow (his wife had sixteen pregnancies during the marriage). It was now necessary to find another source of income. When, in April 1815, George Rose introduced his Madhouse Bill in Parliament, Morison had hopes of being appointed as one of the Commissioners in Lunacy. Although Rose's Bill failed, Morison had become determined to establish himself as an alienist. Encouraged and probably financed by his brother John, in 1818 he travelled to Paris with letters of introduction to Jean Esquirol at the Salpetriere.

Esquirol had been a favourite student of Philippe Pinel. In 1805 he published *Des Passions considérées comme causes, symptômes et moyens curatifs de l'aliénation mentale* [*The passions considered as causes, symptoms and means of cure in cases of insanity*]. His thesis was that the origin of mental illness lies in the 'passions' rather than in organic diseases of the brain and that madness does necessarily have an irremediably effect on the patient's reason.[24] Esquirol believed that, especially for the insane poor, treatment was best carried out in special institutions. ('A lunatic hospital is an instrument of cure'.) He campaigned to have the ministry of the interior establish twenty public asylums distributed across France. In 1817, he had initiated a course in *maladies mentale* at the Salpêtrière, the first formal teaching of psychiatry in France. When Morison visited Paris in 1818, Esquirol was already attracting large numbers of students from different parts of Europe. Over the next few years Morison made four more visits to Esquirol who became his mentor on the management of the insane.

Back in Britain, in the summer of 1818 Morison visited the Retreat at York, St Luke's in London and the asylums in Wakefield and Glasgow. But he still had no substantial practice either as a physician or as an alienist. He once again became a travelling physician, this time accompanying the Marchioness of Bute on a prolonged tour of Italy. Then in 1822 he became personal physician to Mrs Coutts, the wealthy widow of the banker Thomas Coutts. However he was still determined to 'follow the lunatic department of medicine'.[25] In January 1823 Mrs Coutts decided 'to establish a fund for a professorship to perpetuate the memory of so excellent a man as the late Thomas Coutts'. The offer was rejected by Edinburgh University and by the Edinburgh College of Physicians principally because the terms of the endowment included the provisions that Morison would be a trustee,[26] that he would be the professor and that on his death he would be succeeded by his son.

Morison was undeterred. In Edinburgh he hired a classroom at the university to give a course of lectures on mental diseases. William Cullen and the Professors of Medicine who followed him at Edinburgh had delivered lectures on mental disorders but, in November 1823 Morison became the first man in Edinburgh and in Britain to devote a complete course of lectures on the management of the insane.

On 26 March, he began a similar series of lectures in London at his house at Cavendish

---

24. Strikingly similar to Crichton's earlier *An Inquiry into the Nature and Origins of Mental Derangement*.
25. Morison in a letter to Sir Matthew Tierney on 26 October 1823.
26. The four trustees were to be the Marquis of Bute, the Lord Provost of Edinburgh, the Sheriff of Edinburgh and Alexander Morison.

Square. Thereafter he lectured each autumn in Edinburgh and each spring in London. But without an association with Edinburgh University the project did not have the prestige that Mrs Coutts had envisaged for her memorial to her husband and in 1826 she withdrew her support. Morison found a few new subscribers and managed to continue. In the years that followed, the attendance at his lectures slowly grew, the number of lectures in each series increased from eleven to eighteen and he published the text of his lectures.

In 1827, in a contested election, Morison became President of the College; when he published the third edition of his *Outlines of Mental Diseases For The Use Of Students* in 1829, he was able to identify himself as 'President of the Royal College of Physicians of Edinburgh; Physician to His Royal Highness Prince Leopold; Inspecting Physician of the Surrey Lunatic Houses and Lecturer on Mental Disease, etc'. And in London he was at last becoming established. In 1832, he was appointed Visiting Physician at the Middlesex County Asylum, Hanwell and, in 1835, he was given the privilege of taking his students there to gain practical experience of mental disease under his guidance; in May 1835 he was appointed Physician to Bethlem Hospital with rights to teach there; and he was now Physician to Surrey Asylum, Springfield. His private practice among London's fashionable society was also prospering. Patients who could not be treated at home he admitted to a number of small private asylums to which he had access and others were cared for in private 'lodgings'. In 1838, his long delayed success was recognised when he was knighted.

In his practice and in his teaching Morison continued to follow the precepts of his mentor, Jean Esquirol. In his *Outlines* he discussed the treatment of insanity 'under two heads, Moral Management and Medical Treatment'.

MORAL TREATMENT

Morison advised his students and readers[27] that 'domestic treatment is seldom admissible'. The patient should only be treated at home in his normal environment when the disturbance was 'slight' and when the patient had 'no aversion to the place or the persons about him'. In these circumstances, 'his delusions might be dissipated by judicious intercourse with others'.

However, when insanity was 'completely established' seclusion was 'indispensably necessary'. Seclusion removed the patient from contact with people or situations that had perhaps contributed to his disturbance or might tend to prolong it. Such seclusion was best arranged in a private house where the patient's medical attendant could give him individual attention. The only disadvantage of such an arrangement was that it was inevitably expensive.

For the great majority of cases treatment in a public asylum was strongly recommended; the necessary facilities could be provided at less expense; the patient would be in the care of trained staff capable of carrying out the physician's instructions; and the patient would be open to constant observation. The disadvantages of institutional care were that the idea of having been confined to a mad house was naturally distressing to the patient and his relatives and 'circumstances are said to occur in public asylums that may have an injurious effect on the

27. A. Morison, *Outlines of Mental Diseases* (London, 1829).

insane'. Asylums should be comfortable and as unlike a prison as possible. Males and females should be accommodated separately; the curable kept apart from the incurable; the noisy, mischievous and dirty kept apart from the quiet and clean. There should be a sufficient number of attendants 'in whom mildness and command of temper are indispensable as well as strength and firmness'.

RESTRAINT

Morison was an advocate of the therapeutic use of restraint:

> It has been observed that restraint tends to recall habits of self-control and to check the propensity of acting from the impulses of the moment. The Straight Waistcoat is in general sufficient; the patient ought to be looked after when it is on as it has some disadvantages especially in hot weather. Substitutes for it have been recommended. These are manacles or wrist and ankle cuffs of steel or of leather (what has been termed the muff) and the tranquillizer[28] or armchair. In securing the patient tight ligatures are to be avoided. Blows or ill treatment must not be permitted.

Such restraint was to be maintained until the active stages of the diseases had been subdued. Only then should 'moral treatment' be tried. The objectives of moral treatment were:

> to withdraw the mind from unreasonable ideas and to induce a different train of ideas and feelings ... the advantages of bodily labour are generally admitted, the health is thereby improved and the mind is led to form intellectual combinations ... amusements of various kinds (drawing, music, games etc.) may be useful auxiliaries; even plays have been tried but their utility is very doubtful ... we may endeavour to excite salutary emotions as affection of friends, the hope of liberation, emulation by the example of others and sometimes the feeling of shame ... admitting visits of friends may produce a powerful impression but requires great consideration for when too soon permitted increased excitement may be the consequence.

MEDICAL TREATMENT

Medical treatment was to be mild and simple since 'violent remedies may interrupt the salutary efforts of nature'. And 'a strict watch must be kept on the patient where much irritation or a disposition to suicide exists. The want of decision in taking proper precautions and applying proper restraint may be ascribed the loss of many valuable lives'.

When the patient was in the active state or stage of excitement antichloristic and soothing remedies were indicated. When the patients were 'disposed to be furious:

---

28. The tranquiliser or rotary machine was a chair that could be made to rotate at high speed until the patient was rendered almost unconscious.

benefit is sometimes derived from placing them in darkness … the hair should be cut short or shaved for much hair increases the heat of the head … thirst being often urgent, drink may be given in the night as well as in the day … warm bathing is employed with advantage in many cases but requires caution when feebleness, narrow chest or tendency to apoplexy or haemoptysis exists … costiveness must be prevented and as patients do not give a proper account of their situation in this respect the physician ought to ascertain it himself and feel the course of the colon for its transverse arch has been ruptured from neglect of this … bleeding has been too indiscriminately employed; it is absurd to bleed a madman to calm his fury for he is often rendered more violent after the operation … emetics are not often necessary in mild disease although occasional vomiting is admissible in most cases … heavy columns of cold water poured on the head and sudden immersion in cold water by surprise have been much abused; cooling applications to the head are often useful; a very useful mode of applying this is a handkerchief in the from of a turban applied to the shaved head and kept moist with cold water and alcohol; cold clay and ice applied in the same manner have been recommended … in hysterical insanity the application of cold to the uterine region by means of a sponge soaked in cold water is very beneficial … the rotary machine has a powerful effect in taming the furious maniac but many practitioners consider it hazardous … a course of mercury has been employed empirically.

When Alexander Morison began to lecture on mental diseases, he was a general physician who, according to his grandson, had come to the treatment of the insane 'by accident'. He treated his private mentally disturbed patients at home or in private 'lodgings'. He was also visiting physician to a number of asylums but was content that the administration of these asylums should be in the hands of lay superintendents. In 1823, his views on the management of the insane were those of the leading alienists in Paris and were widely respected in Britain. However, as the internment of the insane in Britain proceeded and new asylums were opened, new ideas emerged on how asylums should be managed and how their patients should be treated. A new generation of alienists challenged Morison's teaching and undermined his public career.

REFORM IN ENGLAND

In the House of Commons in June 1827, Robert Gordon, MP drew attention to frightful conditions in asylums in London. He told of one asylum where he had found a room only sixteen feet long in which sixteen patients were chained in their cribs 'all in a state of great wretchedness'. On Sundays they were left completely unattended and 'wallowing in their filth;' every Monday morning, 'nude and covered with sores and ordure, they were carried into the yard to be suddenly plunged into cold water even when there was ice in the pails'.[29]

29. Tuke, *The History*, p.171.

In February 1828, the House of Commons appointed a Select Committee of Inquiry which found that conditions and abuses in London's asylums were as appalling as Gordon had described. These asylums should, by an Act of 1800, have been visited and reported on every year by Commissioners nominated by the London College of Physicians from among its Fellows. The Select Committee discovered that no such visits had been made for several years; the London College 'had done nothing – literally and strictly nothing'.[30] In June 1828, an Act of Parliament deprived the College of Physicians of its powers to inspect and supervise lunatic asylums and invested them in Commissioners to be appointed by the Home Secretary; these Commissioners were given the authority to revoke the licences of any asylum found 'reprehensible'.

This Act of 1828 also gave the counties of England and Wales new powers to establish public asylums. Over the next fifteen years the number of public and private asylums increased so that at a census on 1 January 1844 there were no fewer than 166 asylums in England and Wales caring for 4,072 private patients and 16,821 pauper patients. This great increase in the institutional care of the insane offered young medical graduates new career opportunities as superintendents of asylums, as visiting physicians at public mental hospitals or as analienist in private practice. In England the most outstanding of this new generation of specialist in the management of the insane was John Connolly.

JOHN CONNOLLY

John Connolly was born at Market Rasen in Lincolnshire in 1794. He studied medicine at Glasgow and, from 1819, at Edinburgh where he was elected a president of the Royal Medical Society. When he graduated in 1821, his MD thesis was 'De statu mentis in insanita et melancholia'. He was briefly in general practice in Lewes and in Chichester before settling in Stratford-on-Avon where he was able to combine general practice with an appointment as Inspecting Physician to the Lunatic Houses for the County of Warwick. In 1828 he applied successfully to be the first Professor of Medicine at the new London University. He may have made it clear to the university authorities, as he did at his inaugural lecture, that it was his intention 'to dwell somewhat more fully on mental disorders, or to speak more correctly, of disorders affecting the manifestations of the mind, than has been usual'.[31] In 1830, he published *An Inquiry Concerning the Indications of Insanity*. In his lectures and in his book he expressed 'his entire disapproval of some part of the usual management of lunatics'. He did not agree that every case of madness must be treated by confinement in an institution. Indeed he held that admission to a madhouse was usually counter-productive; 'the effect of living constantly among mad men and women is a loss of all sensibility and self respect or care … the disease grows inveterate. Paroxysms of violence alternate with fits of sullenness and both are considered further proof of the hopelessness of the case. After many hopeless years [asylum patients] become so accustomed to the routine they are content to remain there, as

30. Ibid., p. 172.
31. Quoted by Scull et al., *Bedlam*, p. 52.

they commonly do, until they die'. His views met a mixed response. The *Lancet* was scornful while the *Medical-Chirurgical Review* was sympathetic. However, within three years Connolly had quarrelled with the authorities at London University over quite separate issues and had resigned his chair.

In 1838, Connolly was appointed superintendent of the Middlesex County Lunatic Asylum at Hanwell, the largest and one of the most prestigious asylums in England. From this eminent position he launched his campaign for reform. He no longer argued against the routine commitment of the insane to institutions. Management there need not be harsh and counter-productive. In particular, he claimed that physical restraint was completely unnecessary.

The abandonment of the routine use of physical restraint had long been advocated by the Tukes at the Retreat at York. In reporting, in 1813, on what could be achieved by a more humane form of treatment, Samuel Tuke had claimed that it had been shown that the use of physical restraint in every case was quite unnecessary but he also wrote that he did not 'anticipate that the most enlightened and ingenious humanity will ever be able to *entirely* supersede the necessity of personal restraint'. Connolly went further. In his hospital reports he claimed, that at Hanwell he had abandoned physical restraint completely and now relied 'wholly upon constant superintendence, constant kindness and firmness when required … Insanity thus treated undergoes great modifications and the wards no longer illustrate the harrowing description of their former state'. His claims at first were met with scepticism by more experienced alienists but by 1840 his policy of non-restraint had been praised by Lord Ashley, the leader of lunacy reform in Parliament, and had won the enthusiastic support of the *Lancet*, the *Times* and the *Illustrated London News*. Connolly had become a national celebrity.

On his appointment as Superintendent at Hanwell, Connolly had at once terminated Morison's association with the asylum. Morison had modified his view and no longer advocated the routine use of restrain in every case of insanity admitted to an asylum. However, he was now yesterday's man and was soon obliged to resign from Bethlem. Nevertheless, he continued to be successful in private practice and he continued to lecture. Morison and many other alienists, including the superintendents of some to England's leading asylums, continued to believe that Connolly's claims were exaggerated and that it was unreasonable to condemn restraint completely simply because it had been abused in the past. They also feared that, if restraint was discontinued, something worse would be substituted in its place.

THE COLLEGE AND PUBLIC ASYLUMS

In Scotland the institutionalisation of the insane ran a different but parallel course. In the early years of the nineteenth century, Scotland was even more poorly equipped with asylums, especially asylums for patients whose relatives could not afford private care. In 1818, fewer than one in eighteen of Scotland's insane were patients in a public asylum. Edinburgh, like London, had its 'Bedlam'. It had been founded in 1740 in Darien House, a once handsome building that had been the headquarters of the disastrous Darien Expedition. In time it had been taken over completely as a public lunatic asylum and had become know locally as 'the

Bedlam'. Edinburgh also had the Royal Asylum at Morningside founded in 1813; at its foundation it had received a grant of £2,000 from the Town Council and many private subscriptions, on the understanding that it would provide accommodation for the pauper insane. The original plan had been for the asylum to have accommodation for three classes of patients: wealthy patients who would be accompanied by a servant; patients paying for their own accommodation; and for pauper patients. However, only the accommodation for the two classes of paying patients had ever been built. The College had played a part in establishing both of Edinburgh's asylums; each year the College nominated two Fellows to serve as managers of the Charity Workhouse and Fellows of the College were both directors and visiting physicians at the Royal Asylum. In November 1834, Richard Poole, a Fellow of the College and one of the managers of the Charity Workhouse, wrote to the President:

> Edinburgh has not one lunatic asylum of size and accommodation sufficient for public demand. It is absolutely surpassed in this respect by some minor towns of Scotland and no less so by others in the sister kingdoms and on the continent. I hold this to be incontestable without deprecating the institution at Morningside which is avowedly imperfect and probably neither will nor ought to be finished according to the design of its founders. However wise and benevolent the intentions of those by whom that establishment was projected and patronised, the metropolis of our country is [still] singularly and deplorably in need of a large asylum for the reception both of insane paupers and of numerous unhappy individuals among the lower and even the middle classes of society.

Poole pointed out that the Charity Workhouse (Edinburgh's Bedlam) admitted pauper lunatics from all the city parishes and patients boarded out from the Canongate and from Leith. It also admitted insane patients who were not paupers, but whose relatives could neither care for them at home nor afford to have them lodged elsewhere. In November 1834, it housed 68 lunatics (42 paupers and 26 paying boarders) and was grossly overcrowded; it was also in need of repair. Since part of the grounds of the Charity Workhouse was then being required for the widening of Teviot Row, Poole suggested that this was an opportune time to build a new Metropolitan or Midlothian Asylum. He proposed that the College should appoint a 'Committee for the purpose of investigating the general condition of lunatics in and around Edinburgh more especially such as are paupers or from the lower ranks of society with a view to an extensive and suitable establishment for their accommodation'.

A College Committee was appointed (Joshua Davidson, John Abercrombie, Thomas Spens, W. P. Alison, Robert Christison, John Smith and Thomas Trail with Robert Poole as its chairman) and on 12 November 1834 it met with the Sheriff, representatives of the Town Council and of the Kirk Sessions who were all 'in favour of the general design'. In a letter to Dr Poole, the Earl of Haddington (the former Lord Binning) offered his support but warned against any attempt to 'extend the plan beyond one county or city':

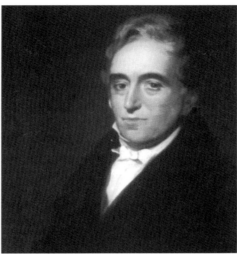

John Abercrombie

I endeavoured to carry a Bill for District Asylums in Scotland generally calling upon a number of counties to contribute to one asylum, more counties being united together in the poorer parts of the country than in the richer and more densely populated. I met with very little support from the Commissioners of Supply who convened in every county to oppose any plan of compulsory assessment and I was obliged to give it up … If the counties were against my proposition fifteen years ago, they are quite as likely to resent any such project in time like the present.[32]

Lord Medwyn, a judge who a few years before had been Sheriff of Fife, also indicated that the Commissioners of Supply, all country gentlemen, were most unlikely to agree to an assessment:

I have a most perfect recollection of Lord Binning's Bill and I well recollect the opposition it met with in Fife. I highly approved of the plan so far as it regarded so large a county as that is; but the plan of assessment which was only to be on the land was so inequitable to the county gentlemen that I used no exertions whatever to carry the measure. When sheriff I was always exceedingly delicate about pursuing any measure the expense of which was to be borne individually by others and not by myself, not being a proprietor in the county. The measure was rejected at the first meeting of the county[33] after it was brought in by Lord Binning and never came before it again.

I have no doubt of the advantage of such a measure but I see no chance of asylums for the poor being built or supported but by assessment. But the assessment should not be confined to the land but should embrace inhabitants

32. The Earl of Haddington to Richard Poole, 29 November 1834, College Archive.
33. The 'county' being the Commissioners of Supply.

of towns and villages according to their 'means and substance' as our Poor Law has it. I am also inclined to think that it should not be restricted to the poor alone but should combine with accommodation for a higher class of the insane. A great establishment of this kind would obtain and admit of the individual attention of a Medical Superintendent as well as probably secure a more kindly treatment from the inferior attendants to pauper lunatics than if they alone were inmates of such an institution.[34]

By January 1835 there seemed to be no prospect of the Commissioners of Supply agreeing to an assessment. Poole next appealed to the church; in May 1835, he sent a circular to the moderators of the Presbyteries and Synods of the Lothians, the Borders and Fife. The few responses that he received 'expressed the opinion that any assessment for a hospital of that kind would be resisted'. In his notes on this correspondence, Poole recalled a statement made only a few years before by the Rev. Thomas Chalmers, the most influential figure in the Church of Scotland:

> Apart from education and institutions for disease, public charity is evil. The blind, the dumb and the deranged may, without mischief, be wholly provided for by philanthropy [which] would reach the limit of that exertion which might be required for the full and permanent relief of all whom nature had so signalised.[35]

Since there seemed no prospect of finding new money either from the Commissioners of Supply or from the Church of Scotland, the College Committee looked to the Directors of the Royal Mental Asylum, Morningside. Poole suggested to its directors that they should now use the £2000 that they had received from the Town Council in 1813 to provide the accommodation for pauper lunatics that they had failed to build. On 23 December 1935, the directors of the Royal Asylum replied that, 'it was impossible, out of the funds at their disposal, to establish an asylum for paupers on the scale required'. Nor could the directors agree to admit even a limited number of paupers to the Royal Asylum since 'that would cause many of the friends of the persons of the wealthier class from sending them to the asylum'. The directors later agreed privately that 'out of proper sense of obligation' they would 'make a contribution out of those funds, whatever the sources of them, had been accumulated'. However, that decision was not communicated to Poole and his committee for over six months. By then the College had come to accept that there was no reasonable expectation that the necessary funds would be found. Meetings of Poole's committee were suspended and the project to build a new large public asylum in Edinburgh was allowed to lapse.

W.A.F. BROWNE

William Alexander Francis Browne was born at Stirling in 1805. As a medical student at Edinburgh University he, like Connolly, was president of the Royal Medical Society. In 1828

34. Lord Medwyn to Richard Poole, 30 November 1834, College Archive.
35. T. Chalmers, *Statement in Regard to the Pauperism in Glasgow* (Glasgow, 1823) pp. 15 and 66.

he qualified, not as a MD of Edinburgh University but as a licentiate of the Royal College of Surgeons of Edinburgh. He was immediately engaged as personal physician to a wealthy lunatic who had been advised to 'seek the benefits of travel and changes of scene'. For two years, as he travelled with his patient in Belgium, France and Italy, he 'attentively examined the arrangements and modes of treatment in some of the most celebrated asylums in the different countries through which [he] passed'.[36] Later, in the summer and autumn of 1832, he returned to Paris for a further period of study with Jean Esquirol at the Salpetriere and in 1834 he was appointed superintendent of the Royal Mental Hospital at Montrose.

At Montrose, Browne created what be believed to be the ideal environment for the moral and physical management of the insane. Chains, manacles, strait-jackets and other means of physical restraint were abandoned. The patients were housed as comfortably as possible; gas lighting was installed everywhere in the asylum, the exercise yards were planted with flowers and shrubs; there was divine service on Sundays. The patients were to be 'treated as much in the manner of a rational being as the state of mind will possibly allow' and measures were introduced that would 'induce them to collaborate in their own recapture by the forces of reason'. Encouraged by the results of his experiment, in May 1837 Browne published his *What Asylums Were, Are and Ought to Be.* His book established his reputation as the leading exponent in the English-speaking world of the new reformed system of managing and treating the insane.

In 1838, Browne was invited to become superintendent of the new Crichton Royal Asylum at Dumfries, the most generously endowed asylum in Britain and one of the best endowed in Europe. His methods began to be adopted in other forward-looking asylums in Scotland. However, in 1838 there were few asylums in Scotland.

THE INTERNMENT OF THE INSANE

Edinburgh's failure to make more provision for the internment of lunatics in 1836 was remarkable; elsewhere in Britain social reformers, led by Lord Ashley were intent on confining the insane in institutions. The primary purpose of the reformers was to rescue the insane from the neglect, hardship and abuse that they suffered in the community. At the same time they had in mind the need to remove the threat that their presence in the community posed to morality and social order:

> It is not calculated to improve morals that half naked maniacs should haunt our paths with tendencies as well as aspects of satyrs. Unchecked, uncontrolled they obey the injunction to multiply their own kind … They are inaccessible to shame, sorrow or punishment, presenting the humiliating spectacle of drunken, ribald rebellious maniacs. Reason or religion cannot reach them and they are abandoned to the dominion of sin.[37]

36. W.A.F. Browne, *Application and Testimonials for the Superintendency of the Montrose Lunatic Asylum* (1834), p. iv, quoted by Scull et.al., *Bedlam*, p. 88.
37. W.A.F. Browne, *Dumfries and Galloway Herald,* 21 December 1843.

In 1818, there were Royal Mental Hospitals at Montrose, Aberdeen, Edinburgh and Glasgow but only a few small public institutions elsewhere in Scotland. New Royal Mental Hospitals were later opened at Dundee (1820), Perth (1826) and Dumfries (1839). Of perhaps even greater significance, an Act of 1841[38] gave sheriffs in Scotland new and very wide powers to commit to an asylum any furious or fatuous person thought to be 'in a state threatening to the lieges'. By 1851, the number of lunatics confined in public asylums had increased to 3,486, some 600 more than the number at large in the community. Unfortunately, however, the reforms that Browne had introduced to Scotland in 1834 had not yet been adopted by all those entrusted with the management of the insane. Outside the asylums the state of the insane continued to be bad and in some of Scotland's asylums it was deplorable.[39]

In 1855, Britain was visited by Dorothea Lynede Dix, a formidable American philanthropist who had devoted herself to the improvement of the care of the insane.[40] In Scotland, her suspicions were first aroused by the great difficulty she had in gaining access to several of the lunatic asylums. When she was eventually allowed entry 'she found the inmates in a most miserable state'.[41] She immediately travelled to London and confronted the Home Secretary. He found her account so startling that, in April 1855, a Royal Commission was appointed 'to inquire into the condition of lunatic asylums in Scotland and the existing state of the Law in that country in reference to lunatics and lunatic asylum'. Following its report an *Act for the Regulation of Care and Treatment of Lunatics and for the provision Maintenance and Regulation of Lunatic Asylums in Scotland* was passed in August 1857. The Act was to bring about 'the massive internment of the insane in what were asserted to be therapeutic institutions.'[42] It also led, in Scotland, to the emergence of psychiatry as a recognised specialism within medicine. The most important and relevant provisions of the Act were:

- A Board of Commissioners in Lunacy for Scotland consisting of three unpaid and two paid Commissioners to be appointed; the Secretary of State to have power to appoint one or two medical practitioners as Deputy Commissioners.

- The Board to have the power of granting (and withdrawing) licences to the proprietors of private asylums; private asylums to be visited and inspected regularly by the sheriff of the county or his deputy; the Board to have the right to visit private asylums as they feel fit.

- Scotland to be divided into districts; each district to have a District Board; District Boards to provide district asylums; the Public Works Loan Commission to lend money for this purpose, the money to be paid back within thirty years. District inspectors to be appointed.

- Public asylums to be visited and inspected regularly by the sheriff of the county or his deputy; the Board to have the right to visit private asylums as they feel fit.

38. *An Act to Alter and Amend Certain Acts Regulating Madhouses in Scotland and to Provide For the Custody of Dangerous Lunatics, 1841.*
39. Tuke, *The History*, p. 339.
40. C.O. Cheney, Dorothea Lynde Dix, *American Journal of Society*
41. *Hansard, cxiv*, HL 28 February 1851, col. 1025.
42. Scull et.al., *Bedlam*, p. 3.

- Patients to be admitted to public and private asylums by order of a sheriff on medical certificates specifying the facts on which the opinion of insanity was founded.

- A medical practitioner to be resident in every asylum licensed for a hundred patients or more; a physician to visit daily those for more than fifty patients; those for fifty or less to be visited twice every week.

The first Report of the Commissioners in Lunacy set out the number and distribution of the insane in Scotland on 1 January 1858. The figures, collected in a very different way, are not strictly comparable with those produced by Henry Hobhouse in 1818; nevertheless, they give a clear indication of the change that had taken place. The proportion of the insane being cared for by family or friends had fallen to from 91 per cent to 31 per cent. The majority were now being managed in public hospitals (42 per cent) poor houses (15 per cent) or private asylums (12 per cent). The internment of the insane in Scotland had been largely accomplished.

The internment of the insane had also been achieved in England;[43] in 1826 the number of insane patients confined in institutions was 4,782 in 1858 that number had increased to 35,347. This great increase in the number of the insane being admitted to asylums in both Scotland and England had a profound effect on the number and standing of alienists in Britain. In the early years of the century a small number of 'mad-doctors' had made an excellent living as proprietors of private asylums. They were not highly regarded by the medical profession. Their success depended on their pretensions to have expertise in the identification and treatment of madness, pretensions which provoked persistent scepticism among more orthodox physicians. Their standing was further damaged by the scandals about treatment in their asylums in the first half of the century.[44] They were also seen to be 'trading in lunacy' and such an association with 'trade' was regarded as an affront to the prestige of a learned profession.

The increase in the number of public asylums, both north and south of the border created many new and more reputable posts for doctors. That all asylums in Britain were now open to the scrutiny and discipline of Boards of Commissioners relieved much of the medical profession's long-standing suspicion and disapproval of the methods employed by asylum doctors; and as salaried officials of the state, mad-doctors, or alienist as many now preferred to be called, no longer had to endure the low status associated with employment in trade.

As the number of asylum doctors increased they came together as a professional organisation; they edited journals and wrote monographs to provide a forum for the transmission of the specialist knowledge and expertise to which they laid. They soon became the public arbiters of mental disorder.[45] The nineteenth-century Lunacy Acts for England and Wales and Lunacy Act for Scotland of 1857 had both interned the insane in asylums and created the medical specialism of psychiatry.

43. By the Lunacy Acts of 1828 and 1845 for England and Wales.
44. Scull et al., *Bedlam,* p. 6.
45. Ibid., p. 7.

15

BRITAIN'S FIRST MEDICAL RESEARCH LABORATORY
The College Laboratory

On 3 August 1886, John Batty Tuke presented to the Council of the College a petition which read:

> We the undersigned are desirous of drawing the attention of the Council of the Royal College of Physicians of Edinburgh to the great need there is for the establishment of a laboratory where scientific investigation could be carried on by those connected with the College. At present there are few facilities in Edinburgh available to those employed in medical practice teaching of hospital work for engaging in such investigation.
>
> The laboratories of the university are primarily for students, are only open to us after they have been accommodated while the professors and assistants in charge have only a very limited time at their disposal for the direction of advanced research. Those of us who are teachers in the Extra Academical School are not as a rule able to keep even a moderately equipped laboratory and are thus to a large extent debarred from carrying on original investigations or the examination of interesting specimens.
>
> Many of us have been taught the new and improved methods of research and feel confident that the establishment of a properly equipped laboratory with a scientific man in charge would enable us to continue our training and investigate some of the many points so urgently requiring solution in the various branches of medical knowledge. These we do not at present state but we are prepared, if the Council wish, to give a list of subjects some of us would investigate in a laboratory such as we earnestly hope the College will see their way to create.

Scientific laboratories had not, at that time, played any great part in the progress of medicine in Britain. Many important advances had been made in medical understanding and practice but these had come chiefly from observations and experience at the bedside and from the verdicts of the post-mortem room. As recently as 1876, the bacteriological studies associated with Lister's work on antiseptic surgery were still being carried on in 'a little passage behind the operating theatre in the old Edinburgh Infirmary' where there was 'no staining of bacteria, no oil-immersion lens, no solid cultivating media, no proper incubators; in fact, everything was in its infancy'.[1] In England, the best and most respected education available for

1. W. Cheyne, *Lister and his Achievements* (London, 1926), p. 76.

medical students was still that offered at the bedside, in the operating theatre and the dissecting room. In London's great teaching hospitals, distinguished clinicians brought up new generations of physicians and surgeons in their own image; that tradition had been continued in the new English provincial medical schools as they were established during the nineteenth century. In the 1880s, Edinburgh University was better provided with laboratory facilities than any other British medical school;[2] the departments of Physiology, Materia Medica and Forensic Medicine all had laboratories but these were used almost exclusively for the instruction of medical students. Edinburgh's continuing reputation as one of the great medical schools of Europe did not rest on the work of laboratory scientists. In medical science Edinburgh could not compete with Germany. From the 1850s Germany had become the major centre for scientific research and education, attracting students from all over the world.

The emergence of this new scientific medicine had begun in Paris in the first years of the nineteenth century. In the aftermath of the Revolution the city's hospitals, which had been founded and presided over by the church, passed into the hands of the state. Salaried physicians and surgeons, given control of public hospitals with a total bed complement of over 20,000, 'turned them into scientific machines for investigating diseases'.[3] Previously the routine examination of the patient had not gone beyond a history of his symptoms, a detailed account of his lifestyle and a limited inspection of his person for external signs of disease; the only common additional investigation was the ritual scrutiny of his urine. In Paris, the physical examination of the patient was extended more deeply with the introduction of Laennec's stethoscope and Auenbrugger's technique of percussion; the urine and other bodily fluids were taken for analysis in a chemical laboratory. Since early in the seventeenth century, post-mortem examination had often provided a clearly visible explanation of the symptoms suffered during life; in eighteenth century Paris, the studies of morbid anatomy were extended to provide evidence that could only be discovered by the examination of body tissues in a histological laboratory.

This new scientific medicine was soon taken up in Germany. In the restructuring of the German states in the years that followed the Napoleonic Wars and the collapse of the Napoleonic empire, the leading universities were transformed from independent corporate bodies to state institutions. State governments gained control over academic appointments and were able to shift the emphasis in academic activities away from the traditional pre-eminence of pedagogy and the acquiring of an encyclopaedic knowledge of existing learning. At first, the shift was simply towards *Wissenschaft*, the pursuit of new knowledge by research. Later, however, state governments encouraged the establishment of research institutes and commissioned research programmes that would yield practical returns; in the 1840s, for example, Baden looked to research in experimental chemistry and Heidelberg for means to improve the quality of the soil, to relieve the prevailing agricultural depression and prevent political unrest among its inhabitants.[4] From the 1850s almost every university in the German

2. J. Burden-Sanderson, *Nature*, 1870, Vol. 3, p. 189.
3. R. Porter, *The Greatest Gift to Mankind* (London, 1997), p. 306.
4. A.M. Tuchman, *Science, Medicine and the State in Germany* (Oxford, 1993), p. 6.

states was being encouraged to found new faculty positions and expensive new institutes for research and education in the natural sciences. This proliferation of scientific activity led to the emergence of the science-based industries that were to transform Germany into one of the leading industrial nations of Europe. The achievements of scientific methods as they were developed in appropriately equipped laboratories were impressive. Applied first in investigations in chemistry and physics they were soon applied to physiology. In Germany, experimental physiology soon replaced clinical trial and pathological anatomy to form the basis of a new scientific and experimental medicine. By the second half of the nineteenth century the great figures in German medicine were the laboratory scientists – Karl von Rokitanscky in Vienna; Rudolf Virchow and Johannes Muller in Berlin; Karl Ludwig and Paul Ehrlich in Leipzig, Herman Helmholtz at Bonn, Jacob Henle at Heidelberg – and physicians and post-graduate students were being attracted from all the most advanced nations to study their methods.

JOHN BATTY TUKE

Batty Tuke was not himself a laboratory scientist. He was of a later generation of the Tuke family who had introduced a new more humane form of treatment of the insane at the Retreat at York in the last years of the eighteenth century. Born in 1842, Batty Tuke was educated at Edinburgh Academy and later studied medicine at Edinburgh University. After graduating in 1856 he became a medical officer in the army, serving in New Zealand during one of the several campaigns of the Maori Wars. On his return to Scotland he became an assistant physician at the Royal Edinburgh Asylum for two years before being appointed as Physician Superintendent of the Fife and Kinross Asylum. It was there that he established his reputation as an alienist with progressive views on the causes and treatment of insanity. He was elected a Fellow of the College in 1871 and, in 1878, he moved to Edinburgh to take charge of Saughton Asylum, then the largest private hospital for the care of the insane in Scotland. He later became President of the Neurological Society of the United Kingdom and a Fellow of the Royal Society of Edinburgh. In 1898 he was elected President of the Royal College of Physicians of Edinburgh and was knighted in 1899.[5]

While at Fife and Kinross in the 1870s, Batty Tuke had made it his practice to conduct post-mortems whenever possible and to make microscopic examinations of the brains and spinal cords of the victims of insanity. His investigations 'started with the proposition that insanity consists in morbid conditions of the brain the result of defective formation or altered nutrition of its substance induced by local or general morbid processes and characterised especially by non-development, obliteration, impairment or perversion of one or more of its psychic functions'. In his Morison Lecture in 1874, he rejected the notion that the 'only entrance to psychiatry was through the dark portals of metaphysics ... the so called mental diseases have never been hitherto in any degree elucidated by metaphysics. It is in the mortuary and the

5. For many years, Batty Tuke represented the College on the General Medical Council. He was made an Honorary DSc by Edinburgh University and an Honorary LLD by Trinity College, Dublin. In 1900 and again in 1906 he was elected Member of Parliament for Edinburgh University.

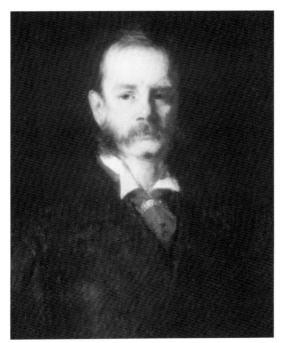

Sir John Batty Tuke

workroom that the arcane of cerebral pathology will be disclosed; the section-knife and the microscope will, at no very distant period, lay open secrets which the iteration of theory of the abstract philosopher can never discover'.[6]

In Edinburgh, but without an appointment at Edinburgh University, Batty Tuke did not have the access to the laboratory space, special equipment and technical assistance that he needed to expand his studies of the pathology of the brain. At a meeting of the College on 4 February 1885 he proposed that 'a committee be appointed to take into consideration the expediency of establishing a laboratory for original research in connection with the Royal College of Physicians'. This he readily withdrew in favour of an amended version that widened the remit of the proposed laboratory:

> That it be remitted to a Committee of the College to consider what means might be devised for encouraging the prosecution of scientific work and proficiency among the Fellows and Members of the College as well as amongst those who are studying with a view to obtaining the Licence of the College.

A committee was appointed and in July it presented a scheme for the establishment of a 'Laboratory for Physiological and Pathological Research'. The projected cost of the scheme for the first year was £857 5s. The Committee admitted that the expenditure was considerable but submitted that 'the state of the College funds fully justifies such an outlay [and] by such an

6. John Batty Tuke, *The Morison Lecture: The Insanity of Over-exertion of the Brain* (Edinburgh, 1874), pp. 71 and 72.

expenditure a great stimulus would be given to research and the College would take an even higher position as a scientific body than it at present holds'. A motion that called for the application of any part of College property to other than normal purposes required the support of 75 per cent of the Fellows present; 20 Fellows voted for the scheme and 15 against and the motion was lost.

A new committee was appointed and in April 1886 it submitted a slightly amended scheme now proposing that the College should 'vote from its capital £1000 for the establishment of the laboratory and, year by year, a sum not exceeding a third of the surplus of annual income over annual expenditure for its maintenance including the payment of salaries'. Again a majority of the Fellows were in favour of the plan but a number were still reluctant to devote such a substantial proportion of the College's funds to the creation of a laboratory that would be of advantage only to 'Edinburgh men' and would leave little to encourage research on clinical medicine and therapeutics, 'surely [according to Thomas Clouston] out-doing the play of Hamlet without the Prince of Denmark'. On this occasion 25 Fellows supported the scheme and 13 voted against; again the motion was lost.

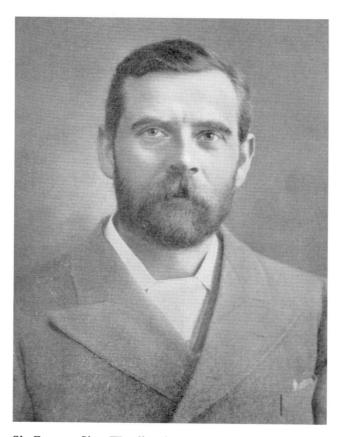

Sir German Sims Woodhead

THE PATHOLOGICAL CLUB

On 22 July, Batty Tuke invited a number of friends to a dinner party at his house, Balgreen, at Murrayfield. They were all young men, professors and lecturers at Edinburgh's extra-mural Medical School, who, for some time, had had it in mind to form a club in which problems of medical science might be discussed informally and where those who had been engaged in research could have their work discussed and criticised before it was submitted for publication. At the dinner were Sims Woodhead, Noel Paton, Barry Hart, Alexander Bruce, Freeland Barbour, George Gibson and Peter McBride and they, with their host, Batty Tuke, now agreed to found a Pathological Club and to invite Byron Bramwell, W.S. Greenfield, John Wyllie, Edward Cathcart, Granger Stewart and William Russell to join them.   The original membership of the club was composed of nine physicians, four surgeons, three psychiatrists, two gynaecologists, one anatomist one physiologist, one ophthalmologist and one laryngologist. The club was to have only one office bearer, the secretary; at each meeting the chair was to be taken by the third person to enter the room. One of the original laws was that 'no communication shall occupy more than half an hour;' the club still exists and that law is still observed.

The Pathological Club had no formal relationship with the College Laboratory but in July 1886 it served to bring together all those still active in the move to found a laboratory even after the move had twice failed. When Batty Tuke submitted his petition to the College in August 1886 (above) members of the Pathology Club were prominent among the signatories.[7]

THE FOUNDATION OF THE LABORATORY

When Batty Tuke submitted his petition in August 1886 it had formidable support. There were eighteen signatories, a majority of the Fellows present at the meeting at which the petition was presented to the College. Of the eighteen, all but five had post-graduate training in the medical science laboratories at Vienna, Berlin, Heidelberg, Frankfurt, Prague or Paris and had published work in prestigious scientific journals; ten were already Fellows of the Royal Society of Edinburgh.   Of the eighteen, only two did not then have teaching posts at Edinburgh Royal Infirmary or at Edinburgh's Extra-Mural Medical School.

When the petition had been read, Batty Tuke once again proposed that 'a Committee be formed to consider the prosecution of original research in connection with the College'. This time his proposal was unopposed. A committee was appointed with Batty Tuke as its convenor. On 23 November 1886, the committee recommended:

1. That the College shall establish and maintain a laboratory to prosecute original research.

2. That the President and Council of the College shall appoint a Curator and Committee whose duty shall be to superintend the establishment and equipment of the laboratory and to supervise and control its expenditure. In the opinion of your committee the

7. D. Guthrie, The Edinburgh Pathological Club, *Medical History,* 1966, Vol. 10, p. 87.

Laboratory Committee should discharge duties analogous to those of the Library Committee, should bear the same relations to the Council and should be appointed annually in the same manner.

3. That the Council of the College shall also be empowered to appoint a scientific man as superintendent of the Laboratory. This officer shall be held responsible for the safe-keeping of all instruments and apparatus. He shall devote such portion of his time as may be determined by the Council to the work of the Laboratory; where under the supervision of the Curator and Committee he shall himself undertake the prosecution of Original Research and be prepared to assist if required to do so in the work of other investigators. Under like supervision he shall also be prepared to furnish Fellows of the College with reports upon such matters as the histology of morbid specimens and of the chemical and microscopic character of urines.

For the first three years after the establishment of the Laboratory the salary of the Superintendent shall be £200 per annum. After the expiry of that period the amount of the salary shall be determined by the Council.
The Superintendent shall be elected annually by the Council at the meeting for the election of Office Bearers.

4. That the laboratory should be open without fee –
(1) To Fellows of the College.
(2) To Members
(3) To any Licentiate who shall obtain the sanction of the Curator and the Committee to use the laboratory for purposes of Scientific Research.
(4) To any Medical Man or Investigator who shall obtain the sanction of the Council of the College, as well as of the Curator and Committee, to use the laboratory for the purposes of Scientific Research.

5. That the College shall vote from its capital funds for the establishment of this Laboratory the principal sum of £1000 and shall empower the Curator and Committee to draw, every year, upon the Treasurer for such sums as may be required for its maintenance and current expenses; it being provided that the whole yearly expenditure including the rent of the premises and the salary of the Superintendent shall not exceed the sum of £650.

6. It is suggested that the fitting up of the Laboratory should be proceeded with cautiously and that apparatus should be procured only as occasion requires. Although £1000 is asked for as probably necessary for the full equipment of the Laboratory it is suggested that only the essentials of a laboratory should at first be procured and that the balance should remain at the disposal of the Laboratory Committee to be employed, if necessary, for its further development.

7. That every year before the Quarterly Meeting of the College in February the Curator shall submit to the Council a written Report regarding the year's work done in the

Laboratory and the expenditures incurred. This Report along with the Report of the Council upon it shall thereafter be submitted to the College at the Quarterly Meeting in February.

8. That the College shall vote a sum of £100 which may be employed by the Council as it deems fit in making grants to investigators, in furthering the publication of Researches made in the Laboratory or elsewhere in offering prizes for original work or for any other allied purpose.

After the Report had been read and approved by the College for a first and second time on 23 November and on 28 December 1886 it was finally adopted by the College on 15 February 1887.

ACCOMMODATION AND FINANCE

The laboratory, commissioned in August 1887, was the first medical research laboratory to be established in Britain. It was housed conveniently close to Edinburgh Royal Infirmary at 7 Lauriston Lane, a building of sixteen rooms on three floors with a large detached hall in the courtyard behind. The hall was equipped for work on experimental physiology; other rooms were for histology, chemistry and bacteriology. There were offices, a workshop, a photographic room and a common room; one large room was furnished for the reception and examination of patients. Number 7 Lauriston Lane was leased by the College from the Directors of the Royal Infirmary for five years at a rental of £80 a year.

By 1891, it had already become clear that larger premises were needed and the College obtained an option to buy 42-44 Lauriston Place.[8] However, the feudal superior, who had strong objections to the building being used for animal experiments, refused to allow the sale. The superior's case was dismissed by the Dean of Guild Court and by the Court of Session but, when it was intimated that the Superior intended to appeal to the House of Lords, the College abandoned the option and renewed the search. Fortunately, the directors of the Royal Infirmary agreed to extend the lease on 7 Lauriston Lane to Whitsun 1896.

In November 1895 the College bought Darien House in Forrest Road, again conveniently near the Royal Infirmary. As we have noted earlier, Darien House had been built as the headquarters of the Company of Scotland Trading with Africa and the Indies (also called the Scottish Darien Company); for many years thereafter it had been the Charity Workhouse (Edinburgh's Bedlam) and more recently it had been the headquarters of the Rifle Volunteer Brigade. Extensive alterations were needed to convert it to a centre for medical research but the first rooms were ready by June 1896. For the College the laboratory was a major investment. The purchase price of the new laboratory was £7,350, almost 12 per cent of the College's total (invested and un-invested) financial resources; the annual running cost of the laboratory during its first years amounted to some 10 per cent of the College's annual income.

In its new and larger premises new skills were developed and made available and demands on the services of the laboratory continued to increase. Within a very few years further

8. Then known as 6 Archibald Place.

expansion was being inhibited by lack of funds. From 1899, the Royal College of Surgeons, a few of whose Fellows made regular use of the laboratory's facilities, made an annual contribution of £200 toward its running costs. The situation was rescued in 1933 when the Carnegie Trustees for the Universities of Scotland bought the Laboratory from the College for £10,000 and assumed responsibility for the whole cost of its maintenance subject to the College making an annual payment of £750 to the Trustees and transferring to them the annual contribution being made by the College of Surgeons. This financial support made it possible for the laboratory to report on 'morbid specimens' (bacteriological or histological) submitted by medical practitioners without charge.[9] This arrangement with the Carnegie Trust continued until 1950.

THE SUPERINTENDENTS (1887–1918)

The first Superintendent of the laboratory was G. Sims Woodhead (later Sir German Sims Woodhead). He was born into a prosperous Yorkshire Quaker family in 1855. He was educated at Huddersfield College and, from 1873, at Edinburgh University, graduating MB CM in 1878. In his final year as a student he had been President of the Royal Medical Society. After terms as House Surgeon and House Physician at Edinburgh Royal Infirmary, he studied bacteriology under Robert Koch in Berlin and with Pasteur in Paris before moving to Vienna for experience in pathology.[10] He returned to Edinburgh in 1881 where he was awarded a Gold Medal for his MD thesis on the pathology of the medulla oblongata;[11] later that year he became senior assistant to William Greenfield, the newly appointed Professor of Pathology at Edinburgh University. While at Edinburgh University he acted as pathologist to the Royal Hospital for Sick Children and Edinburgh Royal Infirmary and in 1883 he published the first of the four editions of his *Practical Pathology: A Manual for Students and Practitioners*, a textbook which remained in print for many years. In 1885 he published (with A.W. Hare) his *Practical Mycology*, the first systematic book on bacteriology in English.

Woodhead had become a Fellow of the College in 1882. In 1887 he was invited to become the Superintendent of the College Laboratory. As Superintendent he gave support and advice in the eleven research projects completed and published from the Laboratory during his short time in office. However, he was able to do very little research of his own since his time was devoted to setting up and organising the new laboratory. When that was successfully accomplished, in 1890 he was invited to set up and become the first Director of the Joint Laboratories of the Royal College of Physicians and the Royal College of Surgeons in London. But within a year the London laboratories were in financial difficulty. In 1891, the Colleges could not afford to install equipment necessary for animal experiments; in 1892, the number of research workers had to be reduced and those who remained were required to provide their own instruments; by 1898, the finances of the London College of Physicians were 'so

9. Fellows of the College were already entitled to receive this service gratis; it was calculated that the fees that could be recovered from all other practitioners would not cover the cost of the clerical work involved.
10. H. Woodhead, *German Sims Woodhead* (Edinburgh, 1923), p. 50.
11. G. S. Woodhead, Some of the Pathological Conditions of the Medulla Oblongata, *Journal of Anatomy and Physiology*, 1882, Vol. 16, pp. 364–90.

lamentable that it was necessary to borrow £1000 for current expenses'[12] and further economies were demanded in the laboratories. In 1899, Sims Woodhead left to become Professor of Pathology at Cambridge. 'By 1901 the laboratories were doomed and the attendants and laboratory assistants were given notice'[13] and in 1902, all research in the London Colleges' laboratories came to an end.

While in London, Woodhead had published his *Bacteria and their Product* in 1891 and had founded the *Journal of Pathology and Bacteriology* in 1893. At Cambridge he continued to work on tuberculosis and was made Assistant Commissioner to the Royal Commission on Tuberculosis. When war broke out in 1914 he was already a Lieutenant-Colonel in the Royal Army Medical Corps (Territorial Force); he served with distinction during the war, was twice mentioned in despatches and was made KBE for his military services in 1919. After the war he continued as Professor of Pathology at Cambridge until his death.

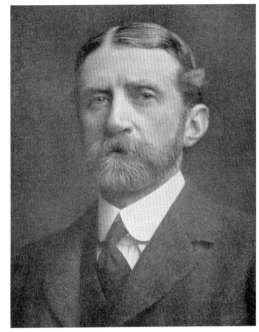

Diarmid Noel Paton

When Woodhead left Edinburgh in 1890 he was succeeded as Superintendent of the Laboratory by Diarmid Noel Paton. Paton was born in 1859, the son of the distinguished painter and academician, Sir Joseph Noel Paton. At Edinburgh Academy he seemed inclined to follow in the footsteps of his father but at the age of thirteen, and probably influenced by his friends and classmates, J. S. Haldane, D'Arcy Thomson and W. Herdman, he became interested in science, natural history and later in medicine. At Edinburgh University he graduated B.Sc. with honours in 1881 and MB CM, again with first-class honours, in 1882. He then spent a year studying in Vienna, Strasburg and Paris. Back in Edinburgh, he was House Physician first at Edinburgh Royal Infirmary and then at the Royal Hospital for Sick Children. In 1884 he was awarded a Fellowship in the physiology department of Edinburgh University; his researches there on bile secretion became the basis of his MD thesis, awarded a gold medal in 1886. He now set up in private practice as a physician with appointments at Edinburgh Royal Infirmary and at the Royal Dispensary. Later that year he was appointed as lecturer in physiology at Surgeons' Hall.

When appointed as Superintendent of the College's Laboratory, Noel Paton gave up medical practice to devote all his time to research and teaching. His chief interest was then in chemical pathology and at the College's Laboratory he became the first physiologist in Britain

12. A.M. Cooke, *The History of the Royal College of Physicians of London* (London, 1972), Vol. 3, p. 924.
13. Ibid.

to devote serious study to the problems of metabolism.[14] His early work was on the physiology and pathology of the parathyroid glands but he later became well known for his important studies on the relationship between poverty, nutrition and growth. In addition to his own researches, he advised, assisted and encouraged the many medical researchers who took advantage of the laboratory's services and facilities while he was its superintendent. After sixteen very productive years at the College Laboratory, he was appointed Regius Professor of Physiology at Glasgow University. There he became most widely known for his contributions to the understanding of rickets, a disease that, at the beginning of the twentieth century, still afflicted very large numbers of children in Britain's industrial towns. But rickets was only one of his important studies; he was elected a Fellow of the Royal Society in 1906.

In Edinburgh, Noel Paton was succeeded by James Ritchie. Ritchie was born in 1864, the son of a Presbyterian minister at Duns in Berwickshire. He was educated at the High School of Edinburgh and at Edinburgh University where he graduated MA in 1884. He then studied medicine, becoming MB CM in 1888 and BSc in public health in 1889. He was House Surgeon to Professor Cheyne and in the same year was President of the Royal Medical Society. He was invited to be an assistant surgeon at the Radcliffe Infirmary in Oxford and there began researches in bacteriology and the actions of antiseptics that led to his MD degree in 1895. When Sir John Burdon Sanderson became Regius Professor of Surgery in 1895, Ritchie was invited to teach bacteriology to his students and in 1901 he helped to plan, and later came to direct, Oxford University's first Institute of Pathology; in 1905 he was made Professor of Pathology.[15] In 1907 he left Oxford to become Superintendent of the College Laboratory; in 1913 he also became Professor of Bacteriology at Edinburgh. He held both appointments until 1920 when A. G. McKendrick became Superintendent of the Laboratory; from 1920 until his death in 1923 he edited the *Journal of Pathology and Bacteriology*.

From 1920 the Laboratory was directed in turn by A. G. McKendrick, W.F. Harvey, R Cranston Low, W.A. Alexander and John Ritchie. All were eminently successful as Superintendents of the Laboratory and all made their own contributions to medical science. But the ethos, the objectives, the practices and the scope of the work of the Laboratory had all already been set by Woodhead, Noel Paton and Ritchie.

RESEARCH

Between 1890 and 1950, the results of the researches carried out in the laboratory were reported in 624 articles published in British and European medical and scientific journals. Over a third of these articles appeared in Journals of particular interest to medical scientists – *Journal of Physiology, Journal of Anatomy and Physiology, Journal of Pathology and Bacteriology, Journal of the Chemical Society, Biochemical Journal, Nature* and others. In these publications the career scientists working in the laboratory made important contributions to comparative anatomy, the physiology of the nervous system, the endocrine glands, metabolism and nutrition. The career scientists who directed these studies made up only a small minority of those working on their

14. E.P. Cathcart, *Proceedings of the Royal Society of Edinburgh*, 1927–8, Vol. 48, p. 221.
15. This was a personal appointment. Oxford did not have a permanent chair of pathology until after Ritchie had left.

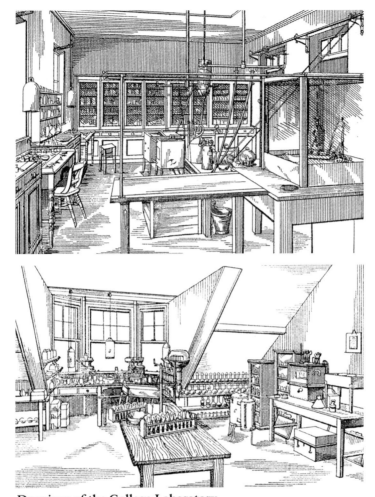

Drawings of the College Laboratory

animal and other experiments; they were often very ably assisted by clinicians devoting part of their time to laboratory research.

However, for the most part, the physicians, surgeons and obstetricians who made up the majority of the laboratory's researchers[16] directed their attention to the pressing medical concerns of the times, the problems that faced them in their everyday practice. They worked on the epidemiology and the bacteriology of the infectious diseases that were the principal causes of death among children at the turn of the century. In 1899, there were 4,469 cases of diphtheria in Scotland with 1,249 deaths, but during epidemics, in which more than 10,000 in Scotland might be infected, the disease 'displayed appalling virulence and killed nearly every child attacked'.[17] In 1899, there were 20,036 cases of scarlet fever; there were only 722 deaths

16. Over the years, a total of 125 full-time and part-time research workers contributed to the work of the laboratory.
17. W. Osler, *The Principles and Practice of Medicine* (New York, 1892), p. 108.

but the late complications of the disease – deafness, arthritis, nephritis, chronic cardiac valvular disease – were common and crippling. Last of these three major diseases was 'enteric fever' (typhoid); in 1898 there were 4,519 cases and of these 601 died.

In the spring of 1894, a trial at the Pasteur Institute in Paris had shown that the administration of the appropriate antitoxin serum was a very effective treatment for diphtheria. In December, the College decided to prepare the antitoxin in the laboratory. The necessary equipment, including two horses, was bought, and after a delay of some months, caused by a fire in the laboratory, a potent antitoxin was produced and used successfully. However, the production of antitoxin proved to be a major undertaking which interfered with the laboratory's research work; when a commercial antitoxin serum became readily available in 1898 the laboratory stopped production.

In the first years of the new century the laboratory published important work on milk-borne bovine tuberculosis in children[18] and on the tuberculosis of bones and joints. There were several investigations into the diseases associated with poverty – malnutrition, anaemia, vitamin deficiencies. There were very relevant studies of the physiology and pathology of pregnancy and parturition; even in 1919 maternal mortality in Edinburgh was still 8.2 per thousand births.

In all, some 400 articles on these contemporary and pressing medical problems were published in variety of prominent medical journals including the *Lancet, Edinburgh Medical Journal, Proceedings of the Royal Society of Medicine* and *Scottish Medical and Surgical Journal.*

Already within thirty years of the foundation of the College Laboratory its medical scientists, working in collaboration with clinicians devoting part of their time to laboratory research, had contributed more to medical science than Scotland's universities and had gained for the Laboratory a reputation as one of the foremost centres of medical research in Britain.[19]

PUBLIC SERVICE

First, as the only medical research laboratory in Britain and later because of its growing reputation, the Laboratory was commissioned to carry out investigations by government and other public bodies. These commissions led to the publication of: *Report on the Air of Coal Mines* (1888) for the Mining Institute of Scotland; *An Investigation into the Life History of the Salmon in Fresh Water* (1898) for the Fisheries Board; *Report on Prison Dietaries* (1899) for the Prison Commission; *A Study of the Diet of the Labouring Classes in Edinburgh* (1900) for Edinburgh Town Council; *Observations on the Movement of Pollution in the Tyne* (1901) for local authorities in Northumberland; *Famine Foods: The Nutritive Value of Some Uncultivated Foods Used during Recent Famines* (1903) for the India Office; *Report on an Outbreak of Scarlet Fever Associated with Milk Supply* (1910) for the Local Government Board of Scotland; *Observations on the Pathology of Trench Foot* (1915) for the War Office.

These commissions formed only a small part of the laboratory's public service. At its

18. G. S. Woodhead's study of one hundred and twenty seven cases was quoted in Osler's *The Principles and Practice of Medicine* (New York, 1892) p. 191.
19. S. Sturdy, Knowing Cases: Biomedicine in Edinburgh, 1887–1920 in *Social Studies of Science*, 2007, Vol. 37, in press.

foundation it was agreed that the 'laboratory should be open without fee to Fellows, Members and Licentiates of the College and to any Medical Man or Investigator who shall obtain the sanction of the Council of the College, as well as of the Curator and Committee to use the laboratory for the purposes of Scientific Research'. It was no doubt also expected that practitioners would use the facilities of the Laboratory to make their own bacteriological, chemical and histological examinations as part of the investigation and management of their own patients. In the event most practitioners chose to submit their patients' specimens for examination by the Superintendent or his resident assistant.[20] In the first year 167 such specimens were examined. By 1898 the number of reports had increases to over a thousand, over 70 per cent being bacteriological examinations carried out for public health authorities. It was arranged that from 1900 the Town Council of Edinburgh would pay for examination of specimens of sputum, urine and milk according to an agreed tariff. Little more than a year later Edinburgh Town Council proposed to accept an offer from the Usher Institute to undertake all bacteriology examinations required by the Medical Officer of Health, the Fever Hospital and general practitioners in Edinburgh. The Town Council's own Public Health Committee objected to this proposal and a large meeting of Edinburgh medical practitioners also voted unanimously against it. Nevertheless the Town Council persisted and, from May 1902, it terminated its contract with the Laboratory. However, Edinburgh's general practitioners opted to continue their arrangement with the College Laboratory as did other local authorities in the south of Scotland.

The number of specimens submitted for examination continued to increase. From 1903, medical officers of Scottish Command, for an annual payment of £20 paid by the War Office, were allocated space in the laboratory for their bacteriological investigations. In 1905, the Local Government Board, then the central health authority in Scotland, arranged that all bacteriological examinations required by their medical officers should be made by the laboratory. By 1907 the annual number of specimens being examined had increased to well over 3,000. The Laboratory Committee decided that there was 'some degree of laboratory abuse:' the laboratory was being asked to carry out examinations that were 'within the competence of any practitioner'. Such requests were 'not consonant with the dignity of the laboratory and the reputation it possesses'. The Laboratory Committee decided that reports would continued to be given free to Fellows and Members of the Royal College of Physicians, Fellows of the Royal College of Surgeons and 'such hospitals and charitable institutions as might from time to time be determined'. But practitioners not connected with the Colleges would be required to pay 2s 6d for an 'ordinary public health report and for other examinations according to a tariff'. Even under this new arrangement the work of the Laboratory continued to increase and in 1909 the Committee found it necessary appointed a full-time bacteriologist.

On the outbreak of the First World War in 1914, eight of the laboratory's researchers and two of its senior technicians left immediately to join the armed forces. The medical officers of Scottish command were withdrawn from the laboratory and their work devolved on the

20. With some occasional assistance from practitioners working in the Laboratory.

laboratory's civilian staff. At the same time the demands on the laboratory increased; pathology services were required by the Royal Navy at the greatly expanded naval base on the Forth; large quantities of anti-tetanus and anti-typhoid serum were produced for the Belgian army. In 1916 new Public Health Regulations were published requiring local authorities to set up schemes for the treatment and control of venereal disease; all blood specimens taken in Edinburgh for Wasserrmann tests were examined in the Laboratory. As the war continued the young laboratory technicians became old enough for army service and were conscripted. Nevertheless, the laboratory was able to fulfil all its very many service commitments

In the years between the wars the routine work increased to new levels as more modern practices in the diagnosis of illness, particularly in Edinburgh Royal Infirmary and Edinburgh's other voluntary hospitals, called for more and more laboratory investigations. When, after the Second World War, the College Laboratory's routine diagnostic services were absorbed by the National Health Service and its buildings and property were handed over to Edinburgh University Laboratory, the number of reports being issued each year had reached 30,909.

LEGACY

For over sixty years the Laboratory had provided the medical community in Scotland with an excellent diagnostic service. It had also made substantial contributions to medical science and in doing so had advanced the careers of a substantial number of its researchers. It was not surprising that some of those who, early in their careers, had helped to establish the Laboratory's reputation as a centre of medical research went on to greater recognition as medical scientists. Twelve were to hold university chairs:

R. J. A. Berry, Professor of Anatomy, University of Melbourne

E. P. Cathcart, Professor of Physiology, University of Glasgow

J. N. Davidson, Professor of Biochemistry, University of Glasgow

W. S. Greenfield, Professor of Pathology, University of Edinburgh.

W. O. Kermack, Professor of Biochemistry, University of Aberdeen

S. McDonald, Professor of Pathology, University of Durham

J. Miller, Professor of Pathology, Queen's University, Ontario

D. Noel Paton, Professor of Physiology, University of Glasgow

J. Ritchie, Professor of Bacteriology, University of Edinburgh

T. Shennan, Professor of Pathology, University of Aberdeen

G. S. Woodhead, Professor of Pathology, University of Cambridge

C. Y. Yang, Professor of Pathology, Hong Kong Medical School.

Others continued full-time in medical research: J.P. McGowan at the Rowett Research Unit, Aberdeen, G.M. Findlay at the laboratories of the Imperial Cancer Research Fund, J.H.H. Pirie, at the South African Institute for Medical Research and J.C. Dunlop as Superintendent of Statistics at the Registrar General's Office in Edinburgh.

It was even more remarkable that a number of those who had early success in laboratory medicine were later appointed to clinical chairs:

F. D. Boyd, Professor of Clinical Medicine, University of Edinburgh

Sir John Fraser, Professor of Clinical Surgery, University of Edinburgh

G. L. Gulland, Professor of Medicine, University of Edinburgh

R. T. Ritchie, Professor of Medicine, University of Edinburgh

R. Stockman Professor of Materia Medica, University of Glasgow

H. A. Thomson, Professor of Surgery, University of Edinburgh.

It was also notable that five Fellows who had first come to notice because of their associations with the laboratory and their work in laboratory medicine – Sir John Batty Tuke, Sir Byrom Branwell, A.H. Freeland Barbour, G. Lovall Gulland, and Alexander Goodall – later became Presidents of the College of Physicians.

In Britain, such merging of the world of the laboratory with the world of consulting room and the close alliance of the medical scientist with the clinician was unique to Scotland. In England, there was physical separation of the leading medical laboratories of Oxford and Cambridge from the great teaching hospitals of London and an equally clear demarcation between the medical scientist and the clinician. In England in 1931, a leading medical scientist at Cambridge wrote:

> There is a certain antagonism between the average clinician and the average laboratory worker. The former resents a certain intellectual conceit on the part of the latter and realises that in his ignorance he ignores the most important side of practice, the art as distinct from the science of medicine. The laboratory man is apt to feel that the clinician is often unprogressive and too content with empiricism and he resents a certain patronage based upon a sense of greater social importance on the part of the doctor.[21]

In Scotland, Noel Paton took a contrasting view:

> The scientific physician is far more likely to make real progress than any of [those] lured into the sheltered groves of laboratory science. They indeed become a real danger to the advance of knowledge. Starting from nowhere and going no-whither, generally ignorant of what has to be done and not seeing what to do, they flicker their lamps in all directions and only obscure the path of reason.[22]

Noel Paton's statement was a vigorous justification of the inclusive and productive relationship between clinician and laboratory worker that had been established in Scotland at the College's Laboratory since 1887.

21. F.G. Hopkins, The Clinician and the Laboratory Worker in J. Needham and E. Baldwin (eds), *Hopkins and Biochemistry* (Cambridge, 1949) p. 207. Quoted in D.F. Smith and M. Nicolson, Chemical Physiology versus Biochemistry, *Proceedings of the Royal College of Physicians of Edinburgh,* 1989, Vol. 8, p. 51.
22. D.N. Paton, The Relationship of Science and Medicine, *Edinburgh Medical Journal* 1928, Vol. 35, p. 10. Quoted, ibid.

NEW QUALIFICATIONS, NEW SCHOOLS OF MEDICINE
Triple Qualification, School of Medicine of the Royal Colleges, Edinburgh School of Medicine for Women

The Medical Act of 1858 established a Medical Register listing all those approved to practise in Great Britain and Ireland. However the Act was an unsatisfactory compromise and left some anomalies and inequalities unresolved. All nineteen[1] of the bodies that had issued licences to practise before 1858 retained that privilege under the Act. But it was generally recognised that there existed a wide variation in the standards that these nineteen different bodies demanded of candidates for their licences; and many of the licentiates who were to be listed in the new Medical Register could only be regarded as 'half-qualified' since they had been examined only on medicine or surgery and not on the full range of medical knowledge and practice.

In drawing up the Medical Bill, John Simon, the Medical Officer to the Privy Council, had intended that, once formed, the new General Medical Council would have powers to exclude from the Register those whose knowledge and skills had not been properly examined. However, the relevant clause was removed from his Bill by the more cautious Home Secretary who believed that such powers should be reserved for the Privy Council.[2] John Simon was not deterred. After the Medical Act was passed, he set out to circumvent the ruling of the Home Secretary and achieve his purpose in a different way. In the following years, he campaigned to have the multiplicity of examining bodies replaced by single conjoint boards of examiners in England, Scotland and Ireland. After twenty-five unsuccessful Bills, two select committees and a Royal Commission, an amending Medical Act was eventually passed in 1886.[3] By then, the College of Physicians and the College of Surgeons in Edinburgh, had already pre-empted the long delayed action by the state.

THE TRIPLE QUALIFICATION
Soon after the Medical Act of 1858 was passed, both colleges realised that their position was under threat. Either the licence to practise medicine granted by the College of Physicians or the licence to practise surgery granted by the College of Surgeons entitled the holder to be included in the Medical Register and to practise anywhere in Great Britain and Ireland. However, three of Britain's principal employers of medical services, the Poor Law Board, the

1. The number was twenty if the Archbishop of Canterbury was included; he still retained the power to license practitioners but it was a power that was no longer used.
2. Under the Medical Act the GMC were given the right appeal to the Privy Council to have holders of substandard qualifications excluded from inclusion on the Medical Register. It was a power that the GMC never used.
3. A. Hull and J. Geyer-Kordesch, *The Shaping of the Medical Profession; The History of the Royal College of Physicians and Surgeons of Glasgow, 1858–1999* (London, 1999), p. 6.

Army Medical Department and the East India Company all insisted that those they recruited as medical officers should have qualifications in medicine, surgery and pharmacy.[4] At the same time the British Medical Association was pressing for it to be made mandatory for all those entering general practice to hold qualifications in medication, surgery and midwifery.[5] It seemed clear that, in the future, those joining the medical profession in Britain would be at an advantage if they obtained their licences to practise from a body that awarded qualifications in all branches of medicine and surgery. It was equally clear that if the Edinburgh Colleges continued to act independently and to offer only single qualifications their financial position would soon be sadly undermined. On 14 June 1859, the two Edinburgh Colleges agreed to hold 'a conference on the subject of granting medical qualifications'.[6] Both Colleges were aware that, By Clause 19 of the Medical Act:

> any two or more of the colleges and bodies mentioned in Schedule (A) [the nineteen licensing bodies] may with the sanction and under the direction of the General Medical Council unite or co-operate in conducting the examinations for qualification to be registered under the Act.

Within ten days, the Colleges had agreed to establish a conjoint examining board. Every candidate for the new double qualification would be examined in both medicine and surgery and 'having passed through the final examination the candidate will receive two separate diplomas, one from each College, so that he will be able to produce them to the Registrar under the Medical Act and register two separate qualifications, L.R.C.P.Ed. and L.R.C.S.Ed'.[7]

On 7 July representatives of the two Edinburgh Colleges met to consider a suggestion by the College of Physicians that they should arrange to meet with members of the Senate of Edinburgh University to discuss the possibility of including the university in the proposed joint examining board. However, it was decided that since representatives of the College of Surgeons had already had an unsuccessful meeting with 'professors of the university' it would be better that the College of Physicians should go to the proposed meeting alone'. On 9 July, Alexander Wood, the President of the College, wrote to the Secretary of the University 'to intimate the willingness of a committee of this College to meet with a committee of the Senatus at such time and place as may be most agreeable to members of the Senatus'.[8] The reply was somewhat discouraging. The Secretary of the University wrote that he had arranged a meeting of the Senate for 12 July but that 'it is not safe to assume that the day will be found a convenient one for the purpose'. No convenient date was found and no meeting with the University was ever held. No reason for the University's reluctance is recorded but, at that time, there was a common perception that the examinations held by the University and by the Colleges were incompatible; College exams were held to be tests of practical skills while University exams were more profound tests of medical knowledge and theory.

4. College Minute, 14 June 1859.
5. P. Bartrip, *Themselves Write Large: The British Medical Association 1832–1966* (London, 1996), p. 98.
6. College Minute, 14 June 1859.
7. College Minute, 24 June 1859.
8. College Minmute, 12 July 1859.

On 23 July, at a meeting of representatives of the College and the Faculty of Physicians and Surgeons of Glasgow, the Faculty was invited to join in an arrangement similar to that already agreed between the College of Physicians and the College of Surgeons in Edinburgh. The Faculty readily agreed and, in August 1859, the GMC gave its approval to both double qualifications (L.R.C.P.Ed., L.R.C.S.Ed. and L.R.C.P. Ed., L.R.C.P.S.G). Over the next quarter of a century, the total number becoming licentiates of the College each year remained almost constant at a little over 200 but the proportion taking the double qualification increased gradually from less than a third to almost half.

In 1881, a new Royal Commission on medical reform was appointed. In 1882 it recommended that holders of only a 'single' qualification should no longer be admitted to the Medical Register. It also recommended that there should be only one conjoint 'divisional' examination board for each 'division' of the country (England, Scotland and Wales) and that these examination boards should provide the only 'portals of entry' to the medical profession. Third, it recommended that the General Medical Council should be reduced in size and be composed of eight members elected by the divisional boards, six appointed by the crown and four directly elected by the profession.

In March 1883, a government Bill based on these recommendations was introduced in the House of Lords. All the Scottish witnesses before the Royal Commissions had been opposed to the creation of conjoint boards. However, there had been no opposition from the profession in England and when, as expected, the Bill before the Lords proposed the creation of conjoint boards for all three 'divisions' (England, Scotland and Ireland) it was assumed that further opposition by the profession in Scotland would be futile.[9] However, all three of Scotland's medical corporations felt that they must make the strongest possible objections to the *composition* of the conjoint board for Scotland as proposed in the Bill. The Scottish board was to be composed of three representatives from Edinburgh University, two from Glasgow University, two from Aberdeen University, one from St Andrews University and one from each of the three Scottish medical corporations. To the Colleges in Edinburgh and the Faculty in Glasgow it was intolerable that eight of the eleven members of Scottish board were to be appointed by University senates on which there were very few members of the medical profession. The proposed composition of the conjoint board was of particular concern to the Glasgow Faculty. The Faculty was already under threat. Evidence presented to the Royal Commission in 1881 had been very damaging to the reputation of the Faculty's examinations;[10] and in 1881, the Medical Reform Committee of the British Medical Association had recommended that, along with the Apothecaries Society of London and the Apothecaries Hall in Dublin, the Faculty of Physicians and Surgeons of Glasgow 'should cease to exist as a medical authority'.[11] The Faculty now feared that if a conjoint examination board were to be appointed with such a small representation of the medical corporations, it was quite possible that the Faculty would not survive.

9. A. Hull and J. Geyer-Kordesch, *The Shaping*, p. 38.
10. Ibid., p. 40.
11. *Glasgow Medical Journal*, 1881, Vol. 16, pp. 360.

In the House of Lords, objections by members defending the interests of the medical profession in Scotland and Ireland delayed the progress of the Bill until eventually it had to be abandoned. The medical corporations in Scotland now hurried to undermine the government's case for compulsory reform by voluntarily reforming themselves. In November 1883, negotiation began on a scheme in which the three corporations would combine to offer examinations that would lead to the granting of 'complete licence' to practise. In October 1884 it was agreed:

- That the three corporations would no longer grant licences to practise separately and independently.[12]

- That the three corporations would co-operate to form an examination board to conduct their examinations in combination.

- That each of the three corporations would elect two members of a Committee of Management

- That there would be three professional examinations.

- That the First Professional Examination would be on:
  Chemistry
  Practical Chemistry
  Elementary Anatomy and Histology

- The Second Professional Examination on:
  Anatomy
  Physiology
  Materia Medica and Pharmacy

- The Third Professional Examination on:
  Principles and Practice of Medicine (including therapeutics, medical anatomy and pathology)
  Clinical medicine
  Principles and Practice of Surgery (including surgical anatomy, operative surgery and pathology)
  Clinical surgery
  Midwifery and Diseases of Women
  Medical Jurisprudence and Hygiene

- That a candidate on passing the third examination would receive the diplomas:
  Licentiate of the Royal College of Physicians of Edinburgh
  Licentiate of the Royal College of Surgeons of Edinburgh
  Licentiate of the Royal Faculty of Physicians and Surgeons of Glasgow.

---

12. Except in cases where the candidate already had a 'single qualification' required a second qualification in order to be included on the Medical Register.

In 1885, the first year in which the new examinations were held, 97 candidates were awarded the triple qualification, L.R.C.P.E, L.R.C.S.E, L.R.F.P.S.G. Ten years later that number had increased to 270. By the ended of the century, 3149 triple diplomas had been awarded and before the outbreak of the World War in 1914 the total had reached 5,069.

THE SCHOOL OF MEDICINE

In May 1895, the College received a proposal that led to the creation of a new School of Medicine of the Royal Colleges, Edinburgh.

At its foundation in 1681, the College had been prevented, by terms of its charter, from competing with the Scottish universities by establishing its own medical school. Edinburgh's surgeons had never suffered such a restriction. In the Seal of Cause by which the Incorporation of Surgeons was founded in 1505, its members undertook to ensure 'that every man that is made freeman or master among us knows the anatomy, the nature and the complexion of every members of the human body ... for every man ought to know the nature and substance of everything that he works'. Towards this end the surgeons asked the Town Council that every year they should be allowed 'one condemned man after he be dead to make anatomy of, whereof we may have experience, each one to instruct the others'.

From the beginning, the Incorporation of Surgeons insisted that their apprentices should be able to read and write. From the beginning the apprentices were given formal instruction on anatomy; from 1656 they were also taught botany and pharmacy and from 1694 they received instruction in chemistry. When the surgeons built their first Hall in 1697 in what became known as Surgeons' Square, it included a meeting hall and museum, an anatomy theatre, a library and a bath house.[13] Into the nineteenth century, this building continued to be the teaching centre of the College of Surgeons.

In the eighteenth and nineteenth centuries there were also private schools conducted by accomplished teachers, most but not all surgeons, in houses in or near Surgeons' Square; John Bell, Charles Bell and later William Cullen[14] at No. 2 Surgeons' Square; John Barclay, Robert Liston and later Robert Knox and William (later Sir William) Fergusson at No. 10; John Gordon and then John Thomson at No. 9; John Lizar at No. 1. As these private schools multiplied in the nineteenth century they spread into Brown Square and Argyle Square and every subject of the medical curriculum was taught at them. Some of Edinburgh's most distinguished medical men launched their teaching careers as lecturers: Andrew Duncan, Sir James Faser, Sir Henry Littlejohn, William Sharpey, Sir James Y Simpson, James Syme, Sir David Wilkie. In all, 62 of those who taught in these extra-mural schools later became university professors in Britain, Canada or Australia. But not all extra-mural lecturers were intent on an academic career. Many were young men supplementing their incomes while they struggled to establish themselves in clinical practice.

In the last years of the nineteenth century there were over 40 lecturers teaching in Edinburgh's extra-mural schools. In July 1892, at a meeting chaired by Henry Littlejohn, they

13. M.H. Kaufman, *Medical Teaching in Edinburgh in the !8th and 19th Centuries* (Edinburgh, 2003), p. 17.
14. The grand nephew of the great William Cullen.

formed themselves into the Association of Extra-Mural Teachers and made tentative plans to apply for a Charter of Incorporation.[15] Two years later, at a meeting in Surgeons' Hall on 9 May 1894, they decided that, rather than forming an Incorporation under the Companies Act, they would prefer to seek 'a closer union of the School with the Royal Colleges of Physicians and Surgeons'.[16] Such a 'connection between School and the Colleges, while not interfering with the great character of the School, its freedom of teaching, and not in any way prejudicing the impartial position of the Colleges towards teaching in the university and other schools preparing students for their diplomas, will be to the mutual advantage of both School and Colleges'.

In a Memorial presented to the Colleges of Physicians and Surgeon in March 1895, they gave as their reason for raising the matter at that time:

> In the first place, the danger which threatens both bodies in the proposed scheme of a teaching University in London in which both the Royal College of Physicians of London and the Royal College of Surgeons of England are represented; and in the second place, the fact that, although since 1697 the School has had a continuous existence, its growth has been so gradual that its constitution has never been clearly defined; and hence it has suffered disadvantages in exercising its legitimate influence on questions of medical education.[17]

The Association proposed the founding of a 'School of Medicine, Edinburgh' (later changed to 'School of Medicine of the Royal Colleges, Edinburgh') and, for this purpose recommended:

> A. That the Royal Colleges recognise lecturers on non-qualifying subjects as well as lecturers on qualifying subjects.
>
> B. That all the lecturers who are thus recognised by the Colleges should form the teaching staff of the School of Medicine, Edinburgh.
>
> C. That the government of the School of Medicine, Edinburgh should be placed in the hands of a Governing Board consisting of five members elected by the Royal College of Physicians, five elected by the Royal College of Surgeons and of five members elected by the lecturers in the School.

The Memorial set out in detail the constitution proposed for the School of Medicine. On 9 July 1895 the proposals set out in the Memorial were accepted by the College of Physicians; it was also readily accepted by the College of Surgeons. The new School of Medicine of the Royal Colleges, Edinburgh proved to be attractive. In the winter session 1897–98, 44 lecturers each taught, on average, a class of 30 students; in the following summer session there were 40

15. D. Guthrie, *Extra-Mural Medical Education in Edinburgh* (Edinburgh, 1965), p. 23.
16. College Minute, 7 May.
17. Ibid.

classes each, on average of 29 students. After this initial peak, the number of students fell slightly; in the winter session of 1899–1900 there were, on average, 26 students in each of 43 classes and in the summer term of 1900, 26 students in 42 classes; thereafter the numbers remained at this high level until the outbreak of the First World War in 1914.[18]

THE EDINBURGH SCHOOL OF MEDICINE FOR WOMEN

The Colleges' School also played an important part in making it possible for women to enter the medical profession in Britain. In 1869, Sophia Jex-Blake had decided to become a doctor. The only woman then practising in Britain was Elizabeth Garret, a licentiate of the Society of Apothecaries and MD of Paris. Sophia Jex-Blake was determined to acquire a British qualification. As she later explained:

> I first applied to the University of London, of whose liberality one heard so much, and was told by the Registrar that the existing Charter had been purposely so worded as to exclude the possibility of examining women for medical degrees. Knowing that at Oxford and Cambridge the whole question was complicated with regulations respecting residence while, indeed, neither of these universities furnished a complete medical education, my thoughts turned to Scotland, to which so much credit is always given for its enlightened views respecting education and where the universities boast of their freedom from ecclesiastical and other trammels. I therefore made my first application to the University of Edinburgh.[19]

At Edinburgh, her application to attend classes on medicine at the university was accepted by the Medical Faculty and by the Senate but these decisions were overturned by the University Court. The Court did not rule on the question of whether women should or should not be taught in the medical classes of the university but it refused to make some temporary arrangement for only one woman. Jex-Blake now recruited five other women, and together they applied this time, not for permission to attend lectures, but for the right to matriculate and attend all

Sophia Jex-Blake (Edinburgh University Library)

18. The number are calculated from the Reports of School of Medicine of the Royal Colleges, Edinburgh published in the College minutes.
19. S. Jex-Blake, *Medical Women* (London, 1886), p. 70.

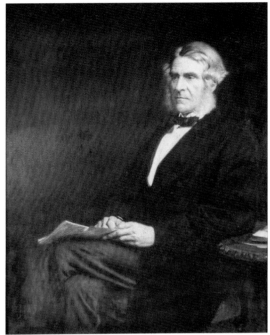

Sir Robert Christison

the classes and examinations required for a degree in medicine. In July 1869, the Medical Faculty, the Senate and the University Court all agreed to their application. However, by the terms of the agreement, university lecturers were permitted to admit women to their classes but not obliged to admit them. Some lecturers were in favour of admitting women to lectures, others strongly opposed, but the majority of the student body were strongly opposed. Less than half of the students who began to study medicine at Edinburgh University ever succeeded in graduating; those who did entered an overcrowded profession and most faced years of struggle and hardship. They were not at all eager to welcome competition from women and they had purchasing power. Lecturers received their fees, not from the university but directly from the students. Lecturers who made themselves unpopular with the student body were therefore likely to suffer a loss in income; many found it politic to refuse to teach women.

When Jex-Blake and her colleagues found it difficult to persuade university lecturers to teach them in the classroom, they were able to enrol in the equivalent class at the Colleges' School. However they were unable to overcome a campaign to exclude them from clinical teaching at the Royal Infirmary and from taking the examinations necessary for graduation. On a number of issues their battles were fought out in the law courts. The publicity brought them the support of the public in Edinburgh and in Britain the lay press[20] was generally sympathetic to their ambitions. Within the university their cause was loyally promoted by David Masson, the Professor of Rhetoric and Sir J. Y. Simpson, the Professor of Midwifery but their advocacy

20. *The Times* and *The Spectator* were particularly supportive.

was overwhelmed by the implacable hostility of Sir Robert Christison, Professor of Materia Medica, President of the Royal Society of Edinburgh, Past President of the Royal College of Physicians of Edinburgh and Physician-in-Ordinary to the Queen. Christison was a member of every committee and every administrative body of importance in Edinburgh medicine and he had the backing of some of Edinburgh's most eminent medical men, including the new Professor of Surgery, Joseph Lister. Unable to overcome the opposition orchestrated by Christison, in March 1874 Sophia Jex-Blake and her colleagues abandoned their attempt to qualify for entry to the medical profession as graduates of Edinburgh University.

Jex-Blake returned to London. There she became active in founding the London School of Medicine for Women in August 1874 and became one of its first students. In January 1877, she graduated MD at Berne and in May she qualified for entry on the Medical Register by passing the examination for the licence of the King and Queen's College of Physicians in Dublin. In June 1878 she returned to Edinburgh and set up practice at 4 Manor Place as Scotland's first woman doctor. In 1881, she suffered a period of depression that lasted for two years. Thereafter she returned to Edinburgh and medical practice, now at Bruntsfield Lodge. At Manor Place she had established a small Dispensary; in 1885 she set up a larger Dispensary with a small five-bed hospital ward.

In 1885 the medical scene was quite changed. Christison had died in 1882 and Lister had left Edinburgh for London. Together the Edinburgh Colleges and the Glasgow Faculty had introduced a Triple Qualification that was open to women. In 1887, Sophia Jex-Blake was able to reassemble several of those who had supported her in her struggles a decade before. They now formed a committee to help her establish a medical school for women. Leith Hospital, which in the 1860s and 1870s had been too small to provide proper clinical experience for students had been enlarged and had been accredited by the Edinburgh Colleges; in the 1889s the staff of the hospital were ready to welcome women students. It was now possible to establish a medical school for women that could offer a complete medical training. The Edinburgh School of Medicine for Women opened at 1 Surgeons' Square in October 1887. In its first years the new school had to overcome some administrative difficulties but it soon became successfully established. Even in its first years there was no shortage of students; in 1900, the number of students who registered to qualify for entry on the Medical Register was 28, more than the number registering at St Andrews and half as many as at Aberdeen University.

THE COLLEGE AT THE END OF THE NINETEENTH CENTURY

These initiatives by Edinburgh's College of Physicians in the last decades of the nineteenth century are best understood in the context of the decline in the fortunes of Edinburgh University's School of Medicine. In the eighteenth century and into the first half the nineteenth, the University's medical school had been the leading medical school in Europe. But, as the nineteenth century continued, Edinburgh was surpassed first by Paris and then by the great city universities and the town medical schools of Germany. At these schools a new more scientific medicine was emerging based on the findings of laboratory studies in

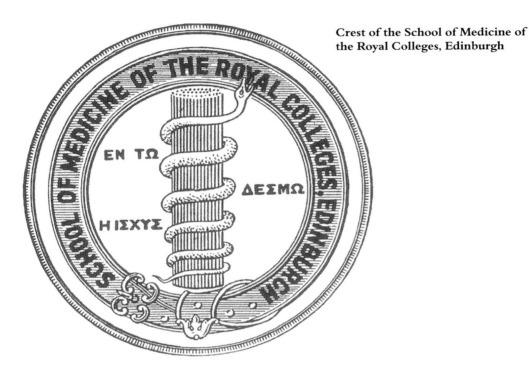

Crest of the School of Medicine of the Royal Colleges, Edinburgh

physiology, biochemistry, histology, cytology, bacteriology and pharmacology. Students who wished to be at the forefront of medicine no longer looked to Edinburgh. They now flocked to Berlin, Heidelberg, Vienna, Leipzig and Munich.

In part, the failure of Edinburgh University to keep pace with the developments in laboratory-based research and practice was due to a lack of the public funding that supported much of the work in Germany. In part, it was due to the widespread opposition to vivisection in Victorian Britain, opposition that led to the Cruelty to Animals Act of 1876.[21] However, an important factor was undoubtedly the innate conservatism of Scotland's universities. In 1870, Professor William Gairdner of Glasgow University wrote that 'the prospects for us are indeed very gloomy unless we can succeed in rousing the public as well as ourselves to the idea that they manage things better in Germany'.[22] In 1887, the College of Physicians did rouse themselves to establish a research laboratory that allowed physicians in Edinburgh to take advantage of the skills they had learned in the laboratories of the leading medical schools in Europe.

The College also roused itself to attract a new flow of medical students to Edinburgh. In the eighteenth century, Benjamin Rush, John Morgan and the other pioneers of American medicine had come to Edinburgh for their education; smaller numbers of medical students had also come to Edinburgh from Russia and other countries of Continental Europe; by the

21. R. Porter, *The Greatest Gift to Mankind* (London, 1999), p. 335.
22. Quoted by D. Hamilton, *The Healers* (Edinburgh, 1987), p. 210.

1850s medical students from these countries had all vanished from Edinburgh. But the introduction of the Triple Qualification by the Colleges brought a new flow of students to Edinburgh from overseas. In the years from 1850 to 1900, 29 per cent of those taking the new Triple Qualification were from India, Australia, Canada, the West Indies or elsewhere in the British Empire.[23] The relationships that the College established with these countries at this time continued long after the Empire had ceased to exist. In 2007, 40 per cent of the Fellows of the College practise in counties that were once part of the British Empire.

The establishment of the School of the Medical Colleges, Edinburgh in 1895 also added to the number of students from distant parts of the empire to study medicine at Edinburgh. Of the students who enrolled for the courses offered by the Colleges' School, a number were matriculated students of the university. The university allowed students preparing for a medical degree to receive their instruction in up to four of the compulsory subjects at the extra-mural school and on some subjects an extra-mural lecturer enjoyed a higher reputation among the student body in Edinburgh than his opposite number at the university. Some students were simply attracted by the lower course fees at the School.[24] Others who had first attended a class at the university and had been disappointed by the quality of the teaching and students who, for any other reason, wished to repeat a course, were all able to enrol at the Colleges' School.

However, each year a substantial proportion of those enrolling at the Colleges' School had come to Edinburgh specifically to study at the Colleges' School and to become candidates for the Colleges' Triple Qualification; in 1900, a typical year, 28 such students registered at the College's School, significantly more than the number of new medical students who registered at the University of St Andrews.[25] These were students who for financial or other reasons had chosen not to enrol for the full number of years study required by a university. At the Colleges' School in a shorter time they were able to complete a sound and comprehensive medical training leading to a respected qualification and inclusion on the Medical Register.

Although not an initiative of the College, the founding of the Edinburgh School of Medicine for Women would not have succeeded without the service of the teaching staff of the Colleges' School of Medicine and its courses would not have led directly to admission to the Medical Register had there been no Triple Qualification.

At the end of the nineteenth century the Royal College of Physicians of Edinburgh was already playing a leading part in preparing for the medicine of the twentieth century.

---

23. 30 per cent were from England and Wales, 24 per cent from Ireland and 17 per cent from Scotland.
24. Fees were 4 guineas for each course at the university and three guineas at the School.
25. Nine registered at St Andrews and 10 at the new University of Dundee.

EPILOGUE

This history ends with the last years of the nineteenth century. At the beginning of that century, the population of Britain stood at little more than ten and a half million, London was the only town with a population over 100,000 and the overwhelming majority of the people made their livings in agriculture or in servicing the agricultural community. By the end of the century, the population of Britain had reached over thirty-five million and well over a third of these millions lived and worked in the seven great industrial conurbations of Clydeside, Tyneside, West Yorkshire, East Lancashire, Merseyside, West Midlands and Greater London; London, Manchester, Glasgow, Liverpool and Birmingham were all among the thirty most populous cities in the world. And outside the great industrial heartlands, new or expanding industries had transformed towns such as Dundee, Cardiff and Bristol. In all, 77 per cent of the people of Britain lived and worked in urban centres of industry.[1] Britain in the 1890s was the most industrialised and, in consequence, the richest nation in the world.

But even by the middle of the century the penalties of such rapid change were already being paid. It had become clear that the nation's industries and industrial towns could not be sustained without a constant transfusion of healthy workers from the countryside. In the centres of industry, great sections of the nation's workforce lived and died in conditions of misery and deprivation. Wages were low; during cyclical periods of unemployment there was no alternative source of financial support; when unemployment was the result of injury or illness there was little skilled medical aid to help the suffering back to work; and chronic poverty inevitably brought the baleful consequences of a poor and insufficient diet. Even for those in regular work, housing was abysmal. There was never enough decent and affordable housing to meet the demands of a constantly increasing population. For decades Britain's industrial towns had grown rapidly and whatever new housing was built was thrown up just as rapidly and after it was occupied it was seldom properly maintained. Worse even than the housing itself was the lack of amenity; there was often no space, no privacy, no clean air, no proper sanitation, no comfort; and misery often led to drunkenness, to violence and to crime.

The ghettos of the industrial poor were places that the great majority of Britain's prospering citizens never visited. But they knew of the 'perishing classes'[2] who lived there and the misery of their existence from the works of Charles Dickens, Mrs Gaskell and Charles Kingsley. What these and other authors presented to the public became the great 'Social Question' of Victorian times. The public response was mixed. For many, the industrial poor

1. K. Robbins, *The Eclipse of a Great Power* (London, 1994), p. 57.
2. D. Fraser, *The Evolution of the Welfare State* (London, 1984), p. 125.

in their ghettos were to be feared as a source of disease and crime; some even feared that the despair of the 'perishing classes' might lead to riots, social disorder and revolution; but for many others the reaction was one of intense humanitarian and religious concern, in some fired by self-conscious guilt about their own prosperity which was so obviously depended on the labour of these same industrial poor.

In the middle years of the century the national importance of Britain's 'Social Question' was well understood. However, there was no expectation that central government would intervene to provide the answer. The political ideology of the time dictated that less government was better government. From the 1840s to the 1870s, in a political climate determined by the ideals of Peel and Gladstone, it was assumed that central government's role should be strictly limited. It was not for the government to determine the structure or working of society. The government's role was to maintain a firmly established and clearly understood framework within which society could be left to run itself. The management of the Social Question was therefore left to existing burgh and county administrations, to established charitable institutions and to new charitable organisations created to meet these specific social problems. Successive governments were confident that without their intervention Britain would continue to prosper.

In the mid-1880s that confidence was first shaken by the 'Great Depression'. Increased competition from Germany and the United Sates and failure to invest in new industries, especially chemistry and electrical engineering, had caused a fall in profits and in interest rates. For the commercial classes there was a significant loss of income; for much of the workforce there was a decade of high unemployment and even greater poverty. In 1885, a Royal Commission was appointed to inquire into the trade depression but it produced no new ideas of any significance. In the 1890s, profits recovered but the confidence of the nation had been badly shaken. And competition from Germany and the United States continued to increase.

The South African War that began in 1899 resulted in an even greater loss of confidence. For three years, British armies of up to 448,435 men struggled to contain Boer commandos that never numbered more than 80,000. The British armies lost 5,774 men killed by enemy action but more than three times that number from sickness and exhaustion. In the end, the war did achieve its declared purpose, but it had been a national humiliation. In Parliament politicians of all parties blamed the quality of the army, not the generals but the men.[3] Over a third of the men who had presented themselves for recruitment in the army – the majority of them volunteering to escape the deprivations and miseries life in the great industrial cities – had been found to be underfed, undersized, unhealthy and generally unfit for service. The conditions in which these men had been born and nurtured was documented in series of sensational reports – William Booth's *In Darkest England* in 1890, Charles Booth's *Life and Labour of the People of London* in 1902, and B. S. Rowantree's *Poverty; A Study of Town Life*, also in 1902. The experience of the South African War and the evidence of these reports convinced the influential sections of British society that Britain's industrial urban population was in a

---

3. *Hansard* cxxxiv, HC 6 July 1903, col. 1324.

process of physical degeneration and that because of the imminent failure in the strength of its workforce and its armed forces, the country was about to lose its empire and its place in the world. Their fears for the future were compounded by the knowledge that the birth rate was falling and the death rate among infants in the first year of life was appallingly high.[4] In a letter to *The Times*, Earl Grey wrote: 'Our successors will be unable to bear the burden of empire as the human reservoirs of the country dry up'.[5]

There was powerful support for a new Eugenics movement in the hope that Britain could breed better people.[6] A campaign for 'National Efficiency', launched by Lord Rosebery, initiated all manner of projects to rescue the nation from decline.[7] But now, at the beginning of the twentieth century, it was at last recognised that the promotion and maintenance of a healthy people could not be safely left to the rudimentary services provided under the Poor Law and the independent efforts of the nation's many charitable institutions, no matter how prestigious. Central government now abandoned its accustomed laissez-faire stance and began to assume direct responsibility for the health of the people. In the first years of the new century, central government formed a series of committees and Royal Commissions to assess the extent of the supposed physical deterioration of the people and to advise on the measures that might improve the physical fitness of the nation's workforce. Following these various investigations,[8] central government reorganised the services provided under the Poor Law, ordered the introduction of physical education in schools, and created a new School Health Service. In 1911, a National Health Insurance Scheme was provided for those in regular employment in industry. In 1913, a free health service was established in the Highlands and Islands. In 1918, a Ministry in England and a Board in Scotland were created to supervise all the health services in Britain. A comprehensive National Health Service followed in 1948.

As the state assumed overall reposibility for health, the orientation of the College changed. For more than two centuries the College had responded directly to what they saw as the changing needs of society. In the twentieth century, the College's scope for independent action became limited. Although still a charitable institution committed by its charter to the service of the public, there was little the College could now achieve in promoting the well-being of society except through the agency of the state.

This social history of the Royal College of Physicians of Edinburgh in the seventeenth, eighteenth and nineteenth centuries is a history of the interaction between *Physicians and Society*. A social history of the College in the twentieth century would be very different. Of necessity it would explore the relationship between *Physicians and the State*.

---

4. The Infant Mortality Rate was 153 per 1000 live births in England and Wales and 128 in Scotland.
5. *The Times*, 26 February 1901.
6. The Earl of Meath, *Hansard* cxxiv, HC 6 July 1903, col. 1324; R. Soloway, *Demography and Degeneration* (North Carolina, 1990), p. 39.
7. M. McCrae, *The National Health Service in Scotland: Origins and Ideals* (Edinburgh, 2003) p. 103.
8. *Report of the Royal Commission on Physical Training*, 1903, Cd. 1507 *Report on the Interdepartmental Committee on Physical Degeneration*, 1904, Cd. 2175 *Report of the Royal Commission on the Poor Laws and Relief of Distress*.

BIBLIOGRAPHY

Alison, W.P., *Observations on the Management of the Poor in Scotland and its Effect on the Health of the Great Towns* (Edinburgh, 1840)

Alison, W.P., *Remarks on the Report of His Majesty's Commissioners on the Poor Law of Scotland* (Edinburgh, 1844)

Alison, W.P., *Observations of the Famine of 1846–47* (Edinburgh, 1857)

Allan, D., *Scotland in the Eighteenth Century* (London, 2002)

Anderson, I.G., *Scotsmen in the Service of the Czars* (Edinburgh, 1990)

Anderson, R.D., Lynch, M. and Phillipson, N., *An Illustrated History of the University of Edinburgh* (Edinburgh, 2003)

Anderson, R.G.W. and Simpson A.D.C., *The Early Years of the Edinburgh Medical School* (Edinburgh, 1976)

Arnot, H., *The History of Edinburgh* (Edinburgh, 1779)

Barfoot, M. (ed.), *To Ask the Suffrage of the Patron: Thomas Laycock and the Edinburgh Chair of Medicine* (London, 1995)

Bartrip, P., *Themselves Writ Large: The British Medical Profession 1832–1966* (London, 1996)

Black, W., *Observations Medical and Political on the Smallpox and the Advantages and Disadvantages of General Inoculation* (London, 1781)

Bower, A., *A History of the University of Edinburgh: Chiefly Compiled from Original Papers and Records Never Before Published* (Edinburgh, 1817)

Brotherston, J.H.F., *Observations on the Early Public Health Movement* (London, 1952)

Brown, C.G., *Religion and Society in Scotland since 1707* (Edinburgh, 1997)

Brown, K.M., *Kingdom or Province* (London, 1993)

Brown, S.J., *Thomas Chalmers and the Godly Commonwealth in Scotland* (Oxford, 1982)

Buchan, J., *Montrose* (Edinburgh, 1928)

Buchan, J., *Oliver Cromwell* (London, 19XX)

Buchanan, George, *History of Scotland* (translated from the Latin by J. Aikman) (Edinburgh, 1827)

Bucholz, R. and Key, N., *Early Modern England, 1485–1714* (Oxford, 2004)

Buckroyd, J., *Church and State in Scotland 1600–1681*(Edinburgh, 1980)

Bynum, W.F. and Porter, R., *William Hunter and the Eighteenth-Century Medical World* (Cambridge, 1985)

Callow, J., *The Making of King James II* (Stroud, 2000)

Callow, J., *King in Exile – James II: Warrior, King and Saint* (Stroud, 2004)

Campbell, R.H. and Skinner, A.S., *The Origins and Nature of the Scottish Enlightenment* (Edinburgh, 1982)

Cameron, J.R.J., *Sir James Young Simpson* (Edinburgh, 1971)

Cantlie, N., *A History of the Army Medical Department* (London, 1874)

Catford, E. F., *Edinburgh: The Story of a City* (London, 1975)

Chalmers, T., *Statement in Regard to the Pauperism in Glasgow* (Glasgow, 1823)

Cheyne, W., *Lister and his Achievements* (London, 1926)

Churchill, W.S., *History of the English Speaking People* (London, 1956)

Churchill, W.S., *Marlborough: His Life and Times* (London, 1966)

Clark, M. and Crawford, C. (eds), *Legal Medicine in History* (Cambridge, 1994)

Clarke, Sir George, *A History of the Royal College of Physicians of London*, Vol. II (London, 1966)

Climenson, E., *Elizabeth Montague: The Queen of the Blue Stockings. Her Correspondence, 1720–1761* (London, 1906)

Cobbett, W. (ed.), *The Parliamentary History of England from the Earliest Period to 1803* (London, 1803)

Cockburn, Lord, *Memorials of His Time* (Edinburgh, 1854)

Coghill, H., *Lost Edinburgh* (Edinburgh, 2005)

Comrie, J.D., *History of Scottish Medicine to 1860* (London, 1927)

Cooke, A.M., *A History of the Royal College of Physicians of London*, Vol. III (London, 1972)

Craig, W.S., *History of the Royal College of Physicians of Edinburgh* (Edinburgh, 1976)

Creech, W. (ed.), *The Works of the Late John Gregory MD* (Edinburgh, 1788)

Creighton, C., *A History of Epidemics in Britain* (Cambridge, 1891)

Crowther, M.A. and White B. M., *On Soul and Conscience; The Medical Aspects of Crime: 150 Years of Forensic Medicine in Glasgow* (Aberdeen, 1988)

Daiches, D., *Robert Fergusson* (Edinburgh, 1982)

Dalzel, A., *History of the University of Edinburgh* (Edinburgh, 1862)

Davies, N., *The Isles: A History* (London, 2000)

Devine, T.D. and Mitchison, R., *People and Society in Scotland*, Vol. I (Edinburgh, 1988)

Devine, T.M., and Young, J.R. (eds), *Eighteenth Century Scotland: New Perspectives* (East Linton, 1999)

Devine, T.M., *The Scottish Nation* (London, 1999)

Devine, T.M., *Scotland's Empire* (London, 2003)

Digby, A., *The Evolution of British General Practice, 1850–1948* (Oxford, 1999)

Dingwall, H.M., *Physicians, Surgeons and Apothecaries: Medicine in Seventeenth Century Edinburgh* (East Linton, 1995)

Dingwall, H.M., *A History of Scottish Medicine* (Edinburgh, 2003)

Dingwall, H.M., *A Famous and Flourishing Society: The History of the Royal College of Surgeons of Edinburgh* (Edinburgh, 2005)

Doig, A., Ferguson, J., Milne, I. and Passmore, R.(eds), *William Cullen and the Eighteenth Century Medical World* (Edinburgh, 1993)

Donaldson, G. (ed.), *Four Centuries: Edinburgh University Life 1583–1983* (Edinburgh, 1983)

Donovan, A.L., *Philosophical Chemistry in the Scottish Enlightenment* (Edinburgh, 1979)

Dormandy, T., *Moments of Truth: Four Creators of Modern Medicine* (Chichester, 2003)

Douglas, A.H., *The Life and Character of Dr. Alison* (Edinburgh, 1866)

Duncan, A., *A Short Account of the Rise, Progress and Present State of the Lunatic Asylum at Edinburgh* (Edinburgh, 1812)

Duns, J., *Memoir of Sir James Y. Simpson, Bart.* (Edinburgh, 1823)

Ferguson, T., *The Dawn of Scottish Social Welfare* (Edinburgh, 1948)

Finer, S.E., *Life and Times of Sir Edwin Chadwick* (London, 1952)

Finn, M.W. (ed.), *Report on the Sanitary Condition of the Labouring Population of Great Britain by Edwin Chadwick* (Edinburgh, 1964)

Fraser, D., *The Evolution of the Welfare State* (London, 1984)

Fraser, W.H. and Morris, R.J., *People and Society in Scotland,* Vol. II (Edinburgh, 1990)

Fry, M., *The Dundas Despotism* (Edinburgh, 2004)

Gairdner, W.T., *The Physician as Naturalist* (Glasgow, 1889)

Gardner, G., *The Scottish Exile Community in the Netherlands, 1660–1690* (East Lothian, 2004)

Geyer-Kordesch, J. and Macdonald, F., *The History of the Royal College of Physicians and Surgeons of Glasgow 1599–1858* (London, 1999)

Graham, H.G., *The Social Life of Scotland in the Eighteenth Century* (London, 1928)

Grainger, J.D., *Cromwell Against the Scots: The Last Anglo-Scottish War, 1650–1652* (East Linton, 1997)

Grant, A., *The Story of the University of Edinburgh* (London, 1884)

Gregory, J., *Lectures on the Duties and Qualification of a Physician* (London, 1772)

Guthrie, D., *Janus in the Doorway* (London, 1963)

Guthrie, D., *Extra-Mural Medical Education in Edinburgh* (Edinburgh, 1965)

Hamilton, D., *The Healers* (Edinburgh, 1981)

Harris, T., *Restoration: Charles II and His Kingdoms* (London, 2006)

Hett, F.G. (ed.), *The Memoirs of Sir Robert Sibbald (1641–1722)* (London, 1932)

Hill, R.G., *On Lunacy* (London, 1870)

Home, F., *Clinical Experiments, Histories and Dissections* (London, 1783)

Houston, R.A.B., *Social Change in the Age of the Enlightenment* (Oxford, 1994)

Houston, R.A.B. *Madness and Society in Eighteenth Century Scotland* (Oxford, 2000)

Houston, R.A.B. and Knox W.W.(eds), *History of Scotland* (London, 2001)

Hutchins, B.L., *The Public Health Agitation, 1833–48* (London, 1909)

Jameson, E., *The Natural History of Quackery* (London, 1961)

James, L., *The Rise and Fall of the British Empire* (London, 1998)

Jex-Blake, S., *Medical Women* (London, 1886)

Jones, K., *Asylums and After: A Revised History of Mental Health Services from the Early Eighteenth Century to the 1990s* (London, 1993)

Lynch, M., *Scotland: A New History* (London, 1999)

Kaufman, M., *Medical Teaching in Edinburgh during the Eighteenth and Nineteenth Centuries* (Edinburgh, 2003)

Lambert, R., *Sir John Simon 1816–1904* (London, 1963)

Lenman, B.P., *Integration and Enlightenment: Scotland 1746–1832* (Edinburgh, 1981)

Levitt, I. and Smout, T.C., *The State of the Working Class in Scotland in 1843* (Edinburgh, 1979)

Levitt, I. (ed.), *Government and Social Conditions in Scotland* (Edinburgh, 1988)

Logue, K.L., *Popular Disturbances in Scotland 1780–1815* (Edinburgh, 1979)

Longford, E., *Wellington: Pillar of State* (London, 1972)

McCrae, M., *The National Health Service in Scotland: Origins and Ideals* (East Lothian, 2003)

McCullough, L.B., *John Gregory and the Invention of Professional Medical Ethics and the Profession of Medicine* (Dordrecht, 1998)

McLachlan, G., *Improving the Common Weal* (Edinburgh, 1987)

Maidment, James, *Analecta Scotia: Collections Illustrative of Civil Ecclesiastical and Literary History of Scotland Chiefly from the Original Manuscripts* (Edinburgh, 1834)

Martin, S.M.K., 'William P. Alison: Active Philanthropist and Pioneer of Social Medicine' (PhD thesis, St Andrews University, 1997)

Miller, G., *The Adoption of Inoculation for Smallpox in England and France* (Pennsylvania, 1957)

Miller, K., *Cockburn's Millennium* (London, 1975)

Mitchison, R., *Lordship to Patronage* (Edinburgh, 1983)

Mitchison, R., *The Old Poor Law in Scotland* (Edinburgh, 2000)

Monro, A., *An Account of the Inoculation of Smallpox in Scotland* (Edinburgh, 1765)

Morison, A., *Outlines of Mental Diseases* (London, 1829)

Morris, R.J., *Cholera 1832: The Social Response to an Epidemic* (London, 1976)

O'Shaughnessy, W.B., *Report on the Chemical Pathology of Malignant Cholera* (London, 1832)

Parish, H.J., *A History of Immunisation* (Edinburgh, 1965)

Passmore, R. (ed.), *Proceedings of the Royal College of Physicians of Edinburgh Tercentenary Congress 1981* (Edinburgh, 1982)

Phillipson, N.T. and Mitchison, R., *Scotland in the Age of Improvement* (Edinburgh, 1996)

Pollock, J., *Shaftesbury: The Poor Man's Earl* (London, 1985)

Porter, R., *The Greatest Benefit to Mankind* (London, 1999)

Porter, R., *Enlightenment* (London, 2000)

Rigley, J., *Lord Palmerston* (London, 1970)

Risse, G.B., *Hospital Life in Enlightenment Scotland* (Cambridge, 1986)

Risse, G.B., *New Medical Challenges during the Scottish Enlightenment* (Amsterdam, 2005)

Ritchie, R.P., *The Early Days of the Royal College of Physicians of Edinburgh* (Edinburgh, 1899)

Robbins, K., *The Eclipse of a Great Power* (London, 1994)

Roberts, S., *Sophia Jex-Blake: A Pioneer in Nineteenth Century Medical Reform* (London, 1973)

Rosner, L.M., *Andrew Duncan MD, FRSE (1744–1828)* (Edinburgh, 1981)

Rosner, L.M., *Medical Education in the Age of Improvement* (Edinburgh, 1981)

Royle, T., *Crimea* (London, 1999)

Royle, T., *Civil War: The Wars of Three Kingdoms* (London, 2006)

Scull, A., MacKenzie, C. and Hervey, N., *Masters of Bedlam* (Princeton, 1996)

Smout, T.C., *A History of the Scottish People* (London, 1969)

Spalding, J., Ellis, R. and Heath, D. (eds) *The Works of Francis Bacon* (New York, 1875)

Stevenson, C., *Medicine and Magnificence* (Yale, 2000)

Thompson, C.Y.S., *The Quacks of Old London* (New York, 1928)

Thompson, F. M. L., *The Cambridge Social History of Britain 1750–1950* (Cambridge 1990)

Thomson, H. W., *The Anecdotes and Egotisms of Henry Mackenzie, 1745–1831* (London, 1927)

Thomson, J., *An Account of the Life, Lectures and Writings of William Cullen, MD* (Edinburgh, 1859)

Todd, M., *The Life of Sophia Jex-Blake* (London, 1918)

Trochler, U., *To Improve the Evidence of Medicine: The 18th Century British Origins of a Critical Approach* (Edinburgh 2000)

Tuchman, A.M., *Science, Medicine and the State in Germany* (Oxford, 1993)

Tuke, D.H., *The History of the Insane in the British Isles* (London, 1882)

Turner, A.L., *Story of A Great Hospital: The Royal Infirmary of Edinburgh, 1729–1929* (Edinburgh, 1937)

Uglow, J., *The Lunar Men* (London, 2002)

Underwood, E.A., *Boerhaave's Men at Leyden and After* (Edinburgh, 1977)

Whatley, C. A., *Scottish Society 1707–1830* (Manchester, 2000)

Williams, H., *A Century of Public Health in Britain* (London, 1932)

Wills, J.E., *1688: A Global History* (London, 2001)

Withers, C.W.J. and Wood, P.B., *Science and Medicine in the Scottish Enlightenment* (East Linton, 2002)

Wohl, A.S., *Endangered Lives* (London, 1983)

Woodhead, W., *German Sims Woodhead* (Edinburgh, 1923)

Zimmer, Carl, *Soul Made Flesh; The Discovery of the Brain* (London, 2004)

INDEX

Page references for portraits and illustrations are given in italics.